Medical Administrator
Cynthia Baron

Ultrafast CT Scan

Healthy Heart Week
Optimal Aging

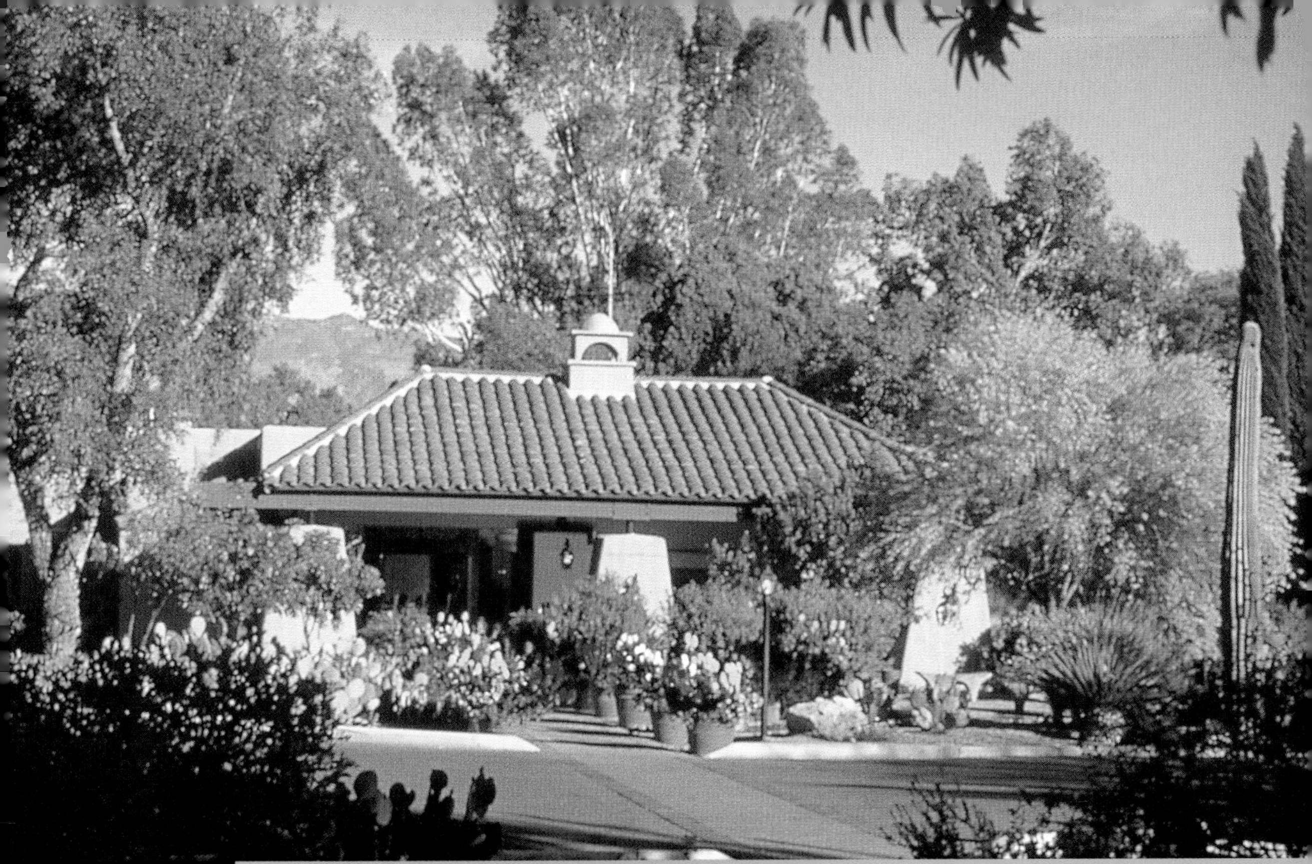

THE Canyon Ranch GUIDE TO Living Younger Longer

A COMPLETE PROGRAM FOR OPTIMAL HEALTH FOR BODY, MIND, AND SPIRIT

THE STAFF OF CANYON RANCH

WITH LEN SHERMAN

INTRODUCTION BY **MEL ZUCKERMAN**

FOREWORD BY Andrew Weil, M.D.

SIMON & SCHUSTER SOURCE

NEW YORK LONDON TORONTO SYDNEY SINGAPORE

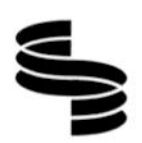

SIMON & SCHUSTER SOURCE
Rockefeller Center
1230 Avenue of the Americas
New York, NY 10020

www.canyonranch.com
Design by Vertigo Design, NYC

Manufactured in the United States of America
10 9 8 7 6 5 4 3 2 1
Library of Congress Cataloging-in-Publication Data
The Canyon Ranch guide to living younger longer: a complete program for optimal health for body, mind, and spirit/the staff of Canyon Ranch with Len Sherman; introduction by Mel Zuckerman; foreword by Andrew Weil.
p. cm.
Includes bibliographical references and index.
1. Health. 2. Exercise. 3. Nutrition. 4. Physical fitness. 5. Spirituality. I. Sherman, Len, 1956–
II. Canyon Ranch.

RA776 .C229 2001
613—dc21

2001031355

ISBN 0-684-87136-X

This book is dedicated, with boundless gratitude,
to the guests and staff of Canyon Ranch.

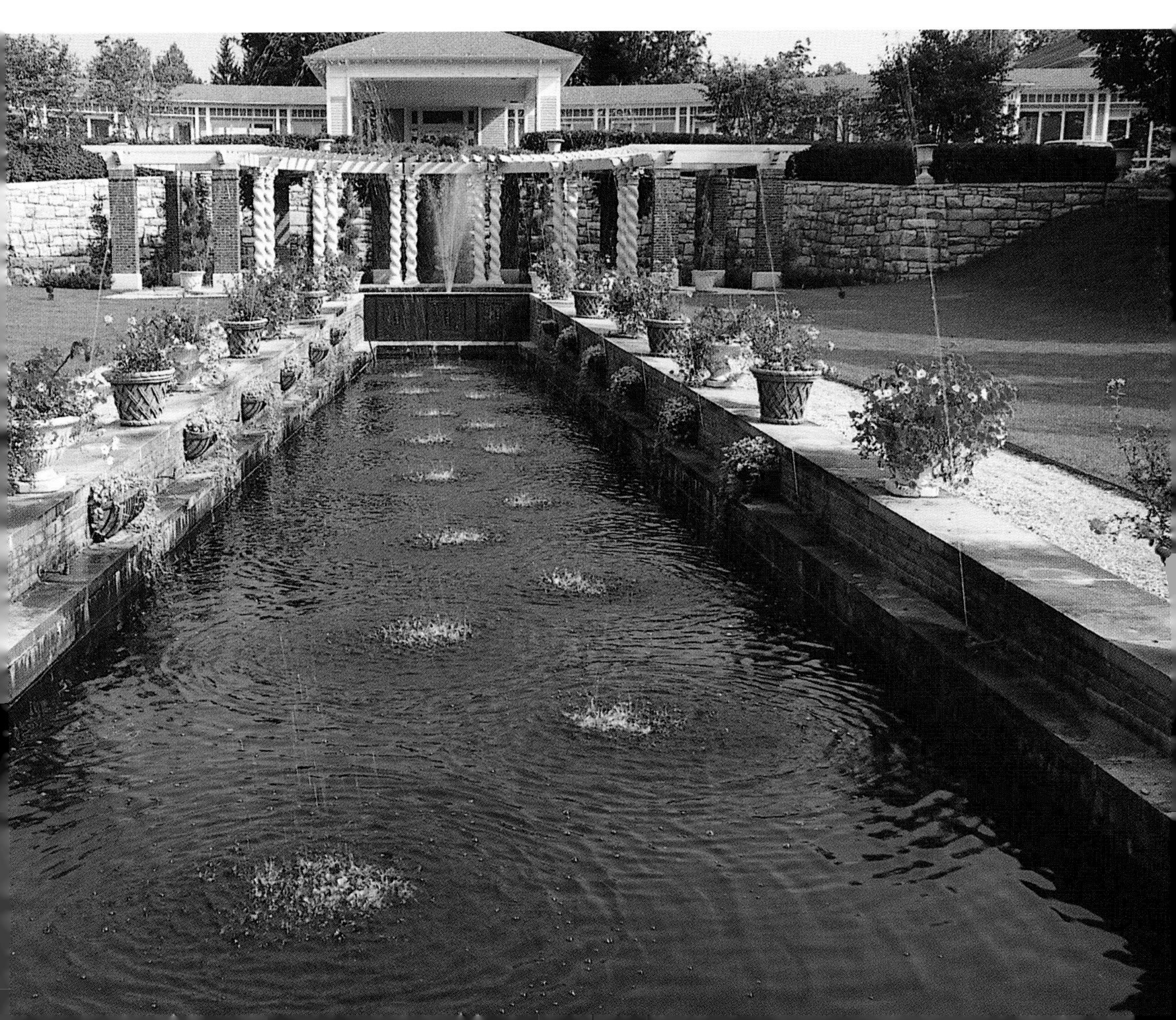

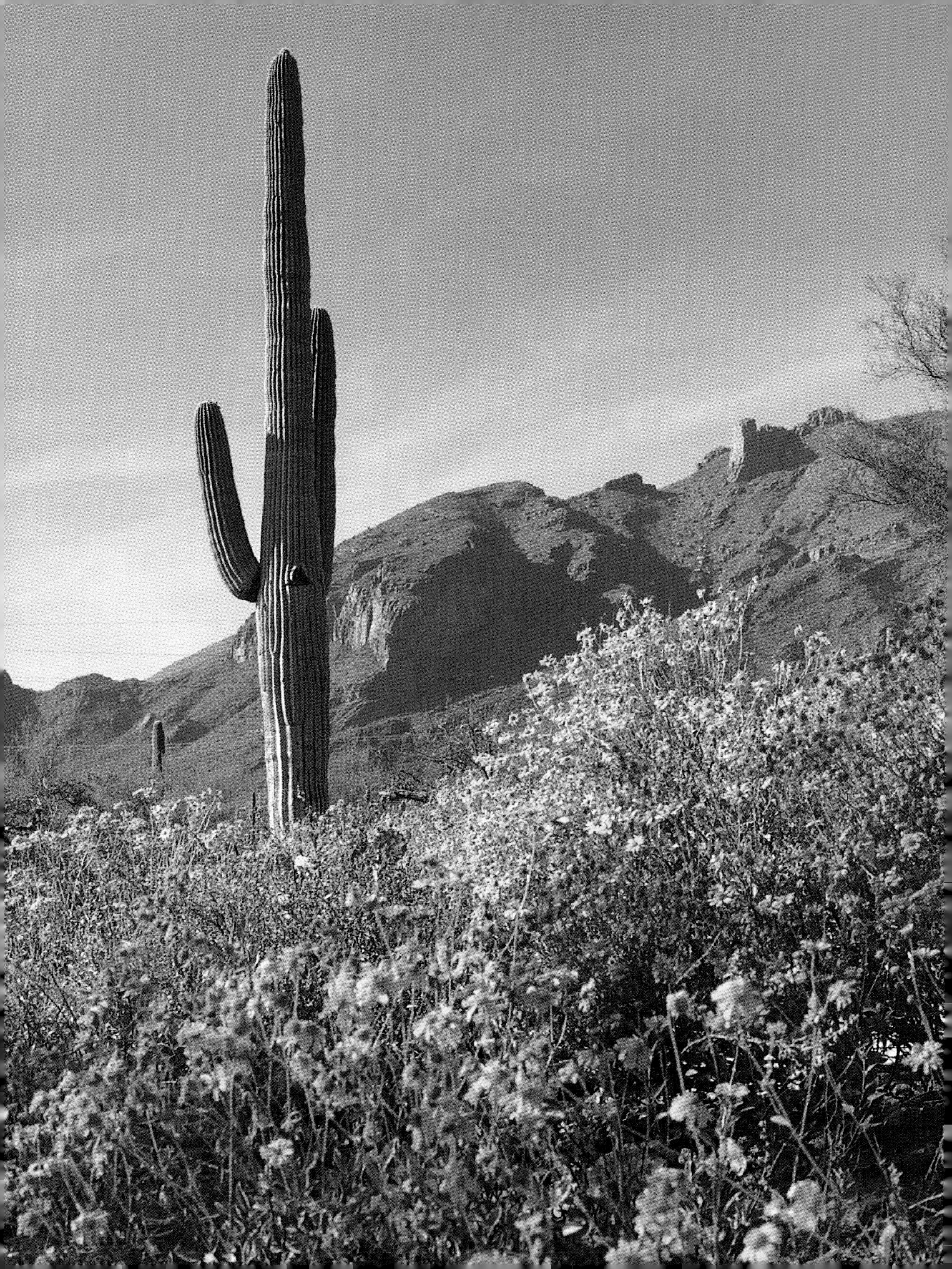

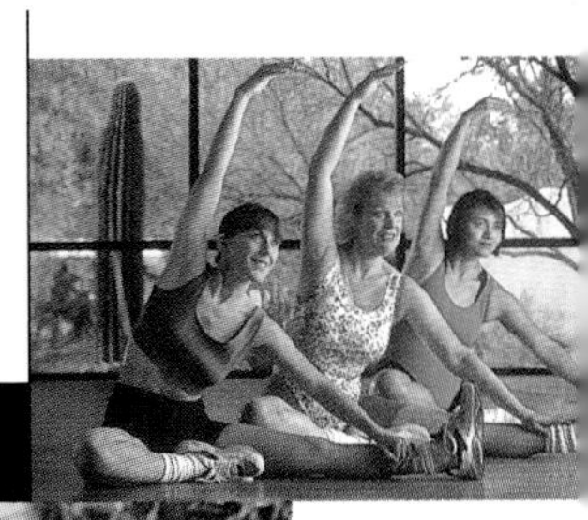

Contents

Foreword

I RETURNED TO TUCSON IN 1975 after several years of traveling through the Americas to study natural and other alternative healing treatments and therapies, while also doing research at the Harvard Botanical Museum on medicinal and psychoactive plants. I was happy to be settled in the desert, living in the Catalina Mountains just beyond the outskirts of the city.

One day a friend of mine, Deborah Morris, stopped by for a visit. She told me about a new venture she was a part of: a spa being built on the site of an old dude ranch just a couple of miles below my house. It seemed that someone named Mel Zuckerman had a vision of opening a different kind of spa, one devoted to fitness and healthy living. About a month before the place opened, Deborah took me on a tour of the facilities.

I had no idea anything so grand was under construction practically in my front yard. I looked around, then gave Deborah my prediction: "This thing will never fly."

For a time it looked as if I might be right. Canyon Ranch had a tough go at first in attracting both guests and the press. But Mel and his wife and associates persevered.

I left Tucson for a year, returning in 1983. When I got back, Canyon Ranch was not only still in business, it was flourishing. Deborah Morris now headed the herbal department, and when I told her I was casting about for something interesting to do, she brought me in to meet Mel. He offered me a job, and I set up a natural healing department at the ranch; I also began to teach medical students at the University of Arizona College of Medicine.

The relationship that I began in 1983 with Canyon Ranch and with Mel continues to this day. It has been a source of personal and professional satisfaction because it gave me the chance to develop the style of practice that evolved into the system I call integrative medicine. I now direct the Program in Integrative Medicine at the University of Arizona, the first program in the world to train physicians of the future to be healers and to combine the best ideas and practices of conventional and alternative medicine. One aspect of the training is to focus attention on lifestyle as a key determinant of health.

Canyon Ranch pioneered the notion that people can take control of lifestyle and of their health and wellness, and it offers many practical techniques for doing so. Unlike any other spa, the ranch has moved beyond concerns with weight loss and explored innovative methods of exercise and nutrition, medicine and psychology, ideas and actions for mind and body. I believe Canyon Ranch is more of a health resort than a spa, perhaps the first health resort in the world.

In building this remarkable place, Mel Zuckerman has been a true visionary. His vision and passion came from his personal experience, as you will soon learn in these pages. Mel is also committed to advancing medical research and treatments. He has been a generous donor to the University of Arizona Health Sciences Center and to the Program in Integrative Medicine.

In my opinion, the model of lifestyle medicine and preventive health care now in place at Canyon Ranch points the way to the future. I hope it will not be too long before most physicians and even insurance companies realize that people of all ages and at all levels of health and fitness need to spend time at institutions like Canyon Ranch to improve their well-being.

If you do not know Canyon Ranch, then this book will introduce you to it, and to many of the ideas and therapies that have made it such a special refuge to so many for so many years. If you are familiar with Canyon Ranch, then perhaps you will gain new insight into its mission. In any case, I am sure you will find here a great deal of information that can affect your life positively and powerfully.

In addition to what *The Canyon Ranch Guide to Living Younger Longer* can do for you as an individual reader, I hope it will stimulate development of the growing movement toward better health and fitness that is visible throughout society.

We will all be better for it.

Andrew Weil, M.D.

Introduction: Living Younger Longer

I GIVE A TALK CALLED "LIVING YOUNGER LONGER" to our guests at Canyon Ranch. I do it at breakfast, at 7:30, to a roomful of people who've mostly been up for an hour or two already, out walking or playing tennis or swimming.

They always want to know what I mean by the title. It's a play on words, based on something I heard the anthropologist Ashley Montague say at a conference on aging. He was explaining that we get the whole concept of fitness from the ancient Greeks, whose ideal, as Montague put it, was "to die young, as late as possible." That's what we all want, I think. (Montague himself died not too long ago, by the way. He was ninety-four.)

Each of us has three clocks running throughout our lives. One is our chronological clock, and we can't do a thing about that. The second is our psychological clock, which measures how old we are mentally and emotionally, how old we think we are. And the third is our biological clock, which is a measure of our physiological and biological age, and which determines how well we function as we age.

Scientists have identified sixteen or eighteen biomarkers, measurements of how old your body really is. They include things like aerobic capacity, how robust your immune system is, how much bone and muscle you have, your sugar tolerance, and so on.

In the last twenty years the medical community has discovered that virtually every biomarker of aging is 70 to 80 percent reversible. While the hands on your chronological clock can't be turned back, your biological clock can be reset. You, however, are the only one who can do it. You must be motivated and even inspired to become responsible for your own health, well-being, and aging process.

In a wonderful book, *Successful Aging*, two physicians named Rowe and Kahn wrote about a ten-year study of several thousand people aged sixty to ninety-five. They found that by the time people reach age sixty-five, 70 to 75 percent of the likelihood of their having good health and functionality is determined by lifestyle. By the time people are eighty to eighty-five years old, how well they're doing is based virtually 100 percent on lifestyle.

Given that information, what will it take for you to decide to become an active, responsible participant in creating a healthy lifestyle? At Canyon Ranch, and in this book, we are very emotional about health, and we want you to become emotional about it too. We want to connect our "intention to health"—our steadfast desire to inspire and motivate people to better health—with your goal of feeling great and living long. We don't just want to give you information; we want to ignite the emotional energy you need for genuine life change. "Getting it" intellectually, in your head, is not enough—you probably already know most of what you need to do to be healthier. You have to "get it" emotionally too. You must desire health and wellness and life.

Health is much more than the absence of disease. One of the pioneers of holistic medicine, Jesse F. Williams, defined that precept in the 1920s and 1930s, yet most of us still tend to think about health simply as not being sick. Consider how little sense that makes. You might as well say that wealth is the absence of poverty, or that knowledge is the absence of ignorance. Here are Williams's own words, the core of the Canyon Ranch philosophy:

> *It's of value to think of health as that condition of the individual that makes possible the highest enjoyment of life. Health, when thought of simply as the absence of disease, is a standard of mediocrity, but when thought of as a quality of life is a standard of inspiration and ever-increasing achievement.*

When do most of us realize that health is a precious and positive thing over which we have some control? For most people, that realization, that critical experience of emotional connection that I like to call the "Aha!" moment, comes too late. Usually it happens in a doctor's office, or in an emergency room or a cardiac care unit. For too many people, the moment when they emotionally "get" the connection between their actions and their state of health is a very painful one.

Let me tell you how I know this, and why Canyon Ranch exists.

I'm seventy-two, and I feel great. I work fifty hours a week, exercise nine days out of ten, and honestly enjoy life. But for the first fifty years of my life I had a health profile I wouldn't wish on anyone.

I have had asthma all my life, and one of my most vivid childhood memories is of getting a shot of adrenaline from our family doctor in New Jersey one morning when I was eight, after an all-night attack. The doctor was telling my mother, "Don't let this boy exercise. He'll get sick if he exercises."

It was 1936, and that was the advice they gave you then if your child wheezed—"Don't let this child breathe too hard." Our doctor was also the school doctor. We'd see him maybe once a year for a ten-minute exam, and I remember him well. He must have weighed four hundred pounds, and he always had a cigarette in his mouth—even when he was examining all these little children—even when he was giving a shot of adrenaline to an asthmatic child. That was how it was then.

High blood pressure ran in my family, and I had it by the time I was twenty. By age twenty-four I suffered from duodenal ulcers, and by my mid-thirties I had diverticulitis and a hiatal hernia. When I was in my forties the doctor told me I had the beginnings of osteoarthritis. And though I had been a very skinny kid, I was overweight for most of my adult life.

I was not happy about any of this, but I didn't know what to do about it. What you were supposed to do in those days—by now it was the late 1960s and I was a home developer in Tucson—was to wait until something went wrong and then go to the doctor.

Just before I turned forty, I decided to see my doctor for a complete physical. He told me about a new battery of tests that compared your results with those of other people of various ages to determine your biological age. These tests were forerunners of the more exact workup available now. This was the first time I'd ever heard of such a thing as biological age.

My doctor told me that it would take a couple of days and that I'd have to go around to various offices to get tests that would measure my physical abilities and my reactions to stress. I would also have to undergo a full medical exam to determine risk factors. I decided to do it. I was curious.

It took about three weeks for the results to come in, and as I waited I became more than curious; I was worried. I'd had health problems my whole life and I was overweight. I started to be nervous that maybe the tests would show that my biological age was four or five years higher than my real age. How would I feel if that was the outcome?

When my doctor called, I was in the basement playing Ping-Pong with my son. I picked up the phone, feeling very tense, and he said, "Well, there's good news and bad news.

"The good news is, we didn't find anything medically wrong that we didn't know about before." And the bad news? "You're in the body of a sixty-five- to seventy-year-old."

I was dumbstruck and didn't say anything for about twenty seconds. I think he could tell I was upset because he said to come in the next day and see him. "There are things we can do about this."

In those days doctors never told you there was something you could do about your health. The doctor was the only one who did things.

I had a bad night. When I went in, he took me into his office and sat down across from me and said something I suppose he thought was really profound. I was certainly hoping it was going to be.

"Mel, the first thing you must do is lose forty pounds."

I saw this doctor often. I was in his office every few months for one problem or another. And this was his big answer?

I said, "Lose forty pounds? Doc, I've lost a thousand pounds in the ten years you've known me."

It was true. I'd go on all these horrible diets—grapefruit diets, protein diets. I'd get desperate and go on one for a few weeks or months until my wife, Enid, was ready to leave me because I was so impossible to live with. Then I'd go off it and put the weight right back on again, because of course all that deprivation hadn't changed the way I lived.

There was, for example, ice cream. I ate ice cream like nobody has ever eaten ice cream. We had a big freezer in the laundry room that I kept full of half-gallon containers of Rocky Road ice cream—that's all that was in there. When I'd come home at night I'd have a big dinner, two helpings of everything and dessert, then sit down to read the paper or do some work. But then, after I'd finished the paper or my work, I'd start feeling bored. That's when I'd think about ice cream.

I'd go to the freezer and get a half gallon of ice cream and bring it into the kitchen, where we had an early microwave oven. I'd put it in there and set the timer. After twenty seconds, I'd give the container a turn, so the whole half gallon would get a little soft, just the way I liked it. Then I'd set it for another twenty seconds. In the meantime, I'd get my spoon—a soupspoon. Never a dish, never an ice-cream scoop, just the spoon. You can see how clearly I remember every little detail; this was an important part of my life.

Then I'd sit down and eat until there were just a couple of spoonfuls left at the bottom of this half-gallon container. That's when the guilt talk would start.

"Zuckerman," I'd think, "surely you are not going to eat a half gallon of ice cream by yourself."

And so, even though I really wanted those last two spoonfuls of ice cream, I'd put the lid back on and put the tub back in the freezer. Less guilt, I guess.

And then I'd go to bed. I never slept through the night back then, although these days I sleep pretty well. I'd wake up after a couple of hours, and what had I always been told you should do when you couldn't sleep? Eat, of course. So it was back to the ice cream freezer, and into the pantry for my favorite cookies and of course the fridge for a container of milk.

You see, I did everything wrong. Continuously!

But let's get back to the doctor's office. "Lose forty pounds" was a very disappointing answer to the fix I was in. I knew I'd gain it back. Then, though, my doctor gave me a piece of news that was important, even profound.

He said, "You're off the charts in your reactions to stress. You're what we call a hot reactor. You must learn to control stress."

I was interested, and I asked him how I could do that.

That's when the profound part stopped. "You just have to learn not to take things so seriously," he told me. That's it?

Today there are maybe fifteen simple techniques you can learn to control stress, and they work. After decades of research, we've learned about ways to reverse biological markers, but in 1968 this was the best advice there was: Go on a diet and learn not to take things too seriously.

I went home, very upset, and said to Enid, "Get me into one of those fat farms. I've got to lose weight."

I went to Rancho La Puerta, in Baja California, and although I really wasn't ready to change, part of me must have been emotionally engaged. Otherwise, my mind never would have let me consider going to a sixties fat farm.

It was very nice, but I was the only man among about eighty women. I remember being in the hall outside one of the exercise rooms, watching these women bend and move. I was just standing there for the longest time, trying to get up my nerve to go in.

When I finally did, it was horrible, even though I tried to hide in the back. There was all this stretching, and the instructor would say, "Now ladies—oh, yes, and you, sir—just grab your ankles and . . ."

And there I was, barely able to get my arms around my knees. It was totally demeaning. And the talk was all about cesareans and teething and clothes—I had nothing to contribute to the conversation. On the third morning I hitchhiked out and flew home.

It had not been the ideal place for me, and, as upset and full of dread as I was, I still wasn't ready. I was still operating from my intellect, not my emotions.

It would be another ten years before my "Aha!" moment came.

My father and mother moved out to Tucson to be close to their grandchildren. My seventy-six-year-old father, who hadn't been to the doctor for years, decided to get a checkup.

I got a call at my office to come with my parents when they went in for the results. The doctor just told me the news was "bad." Enid and I accompanied my parents, and there we sat and listened as the doctor told my father that he had inoperable lung cancer.

My father had smoked all his life. He'd tried to quit a few times, and I have to believe that if he'd known what secondhand smoke does to an asthmatic child, he would have quit for good when I was young.

Now, as we all sat there in a state of shock, I watched him pull out the pack of Camels that had been part of him as long as I can remember. I fully expected to see him tap one out and light up, as I'd watched him do thousands of times before. Instead, he crumpled it between his hands, threw it down on the doctor's desk, and said, "I won't smoke any more! I promise!"

It was his "Aha!" moment—too late.

My father had finally made the emotional connection between his behavior and his health. We buried him six months later.

During those months, I sat and talked with him every day. That's when my father gave Canyon Ranch to the world. Every conversation ended with him sitting with his head in his hands, moaning, "If only I'd quit. If only I hadn't started. If only I'd listened. If only . . ." I can see him now.

That was my "Aha" moment—in time.

When my father died, I was nearing my fiftieth birthday and my weight was out of control. I still have a photo that was taken of me at my parents' fiftieth wedding anniversary, just two months before his death. I'd reached an all-time high on the scales, and I look awful, unrecognizable—bulging cheeks and a forty-one-inch waist.

My biological age at that point must have been eighty-five, or maybe one hundred and five. I didn't know what to do, but I knew I had to do something. So I told Enid, "Get me back into Rancho La Puerta." I was desperate.

But it turned out that Rancho La Puerta had a waiting list, and I could not wait. So I asked her to find me another place.

Enid saw an ad in a magazine for The Oaks at Ojai, in California. Like Rancho La Puerta, it's a very good place, and it's still there. We sent for the brochure, which had an attractive blond in a leotard on the front. Under the photo it said, "Lose a pound a day with Sheila." There was no waiting list.

I thought, "Okay. Maybe I can learn something there."

I drove this time—I wanted to be ready for my getaway. My plan was to stay for ten days. It turned into four weeks.

When I arrived it looked like the same sort of thing as before—all women, plus me. But there was a wonderful person at Ojai, the assistant director, a woman named Karma Kientzler. She noticed me and took me under her wing. (Karma later became executive fitness director at Canyon Ranch, and a vice president.)

I wasn't interested in humiliating myself, so Karma worked with me privately. She took me out walking, away from everyone else, for three miles every day.

Let me make clear that the only exercise I was used to was doubles tennis with friends. And the most strenuous part of that was when we'd wave our rackets for our partners to get the ball. I hadn't walked more than a block in years.

But Karma got me walking, and then walking and jogging. On the tenth day, she had me jog a mile and a half as she timed me. My time was eleven minutes and thirty-eight seconds. Then we walked back to the spa.

When we got there, I found out why she'd timed me. She had a book, by Kenneth Cooper, who'd devised an unscientific rough measure of how fit a person was, based on how fast he or she could traverse a mile and a half. Karma showed me the chart, which plotted ages against times. According to Cooper, if, at age fifty, you could traverse a mile and a half in less than twelve minutes, that put you at the top of your age group.

This gave me the most incredible thrill—I can't even tell you how wonderful it made me feel. And I had done it in ten days. It was a rocket-boosted "Aha!" moment.

Ojai in those days was an old-fashioned fat-farm-type spa—they starved you, worked you out for five hours a day, and then gave you a massage. I'd never felt so good. I wanted to stay, to do more, to feel even better—and never to lose the tremendous feeling I'd discovered.

So that evening I called Enid and told her I wanted to stay, that something very special was happening to me. There was a long silence at the end of the line, and then Enid said, "That special thing that's happening—it better not be Sheila." Funny lady, my wife!

I called again at the end of the third week and begged Enid, "Please come out here. I've found what I want to do with the rest of my life and you have to see. If this can happen to me, we have to teach other people. We have to share this."

In fact, Enid had suggested about five years earlier that maybe we ought to build a fat farm. She'd noticed that there were a lot of places springing up in California and thought Tucson would be a good spot for one. I'd just rolled my eyes and kept on building houses.

By the time we left Ojai, I'd lost twenty-nine pounds, was running three miles a day, and felt better than I had since my early twenties. Twenty months and eight days later, after liquidating all our real estate holdings to finance it, we opened Canyon Ranch. This was our dream—to live healthily ourselves and to educate others who were willing to come to us.

It was a struggle at first. On the day we opened, we had eight guests, only one of whom was full-pay. We never dreamed that we were headed to where we are now—three properties, two thousand employees, and more than seven hundred guests a week at the two destination resorts. Our intention, though, never changed.

Our intention is to help you reach that "Aha!" moment, at which you are emotionally connected to your best intentions for living and aging well. That experience is the difference, literally, between life and premature death, living at home or in a nursing home, enjoying life versus just enduring it.

A good diet, stress control, and exercise—above all, regular exercise and lots of it—are how you create your own opportunities to live well. No one can do it for you, and it's not enough to just know what you should do. You've got to do it.

Seven years ago, when I turned sixty-five, I had a much more sophisticated battery of tests to determine my biological age. This time, according to the tests, I had the body of a forty- to forty-five-year-old man. While my chronological clock had moved forward twenty-five years, I'd turned my biological clock back to where it should have been when I was forty.

There are no guarantees—we all accept that. We don't know how long we'll live. But by creating a healthy life, you create for yourself the possibility of living out your days with vitality, joy, energy, and dignity. And without ever having to look back and say, "If only . . ."

Mel Zuckerman

Mel Zuckerman, founder of Canyon Ranch

How to Use This Book

WHAT YOU HAVE IN YOUR HANDS is Canyon Ranch Health Resort on paper—the closest we could come to it, that is, in fewer pages than the *Oxford English Dictionary*. You're holding ten chapters packed with information and inspiration, as well as detailed, practical advice on issues ranging from turning your bathtub into a spa, to slowing down the aging process, to fixing your aching back. We're confident that 95 percent of what you need to achieve your best possible health is right here between these covers. However, like any visitor to the ranch, you may find the richness of the resources you're tapping into overwhelming unless you have a strategy going in.

Where to begin? Guests at Canyon Ranch start their stay by seeing a program coordinator, who talks with them about their health concerns and goals and then helps them plan their activities. We propose that you, the reader, act as your own program coordinator. You'll get the most out of this book if you decide what, out of all Canyon Ranch has to offer, is important to you right now.

Here's what we suggest. First, think seriously about your health—mental, physical, and spiritual—and particularly about your future well-being. Is there an issue that concerns you, a nagging worry, something you've been telling yourself, perhaps for years, that you need to look into or work on? If several issues spring to mind, focus on the one that seems most pressing.

Next, set a goal. Whether it's losing some weight, improving your cardiovascular health, or getting a handle on the stress that's making you irritable and interfering with your sleep, you'll find practical, state-of-the-art guidance in these pages.

PUTTING TOGETHER YOUR PROGRAM

No matter what your present goal might be, we recommend that you read Chapters 1, 2, and 10. Chapter 1, "Treating Mind, Body, and Spirit: Medicine for Optimal Health," is a primer on the basics of good health and medicine. Chapter 2, "Managing Ourselves: Health, Values, and Human Resiliency," gives our views on how, and why, people save their own lives by changing them. Chapter 10, "Living Younger Longer: Optimal Aging and You," is, quite simply, about where you're headed.

Here are some examples of how you might best use the rest of the book to achieve your main goal.

PROGRAM 1: WEIGHT LOSS

Your ambition is to lose weight and keep it off.

Start by reading Chapter 6, "The Healthy Weight Philosophy: The Dangers of Dieting," for a thorough overview of the issue. The chapter gives you the essence of what our nutritionists, behavioral experts, and medical staff recommend after more than twenty years of helping guests manage their weight.

Your next stop will probably be Chapter 7, "Nutritional Intelligence: The Ten Principles of Healthy Eating," a compendium of advice, tips, solidly supported information, and, of course, healthful recipes from the ranch's famous kitchens.

As you'll find when you read "The Healthy Weight Philosophy," however, exercise is just as important as food to sustained weight loss, so you'll undoubtedly go on to Chapter 3, "Getting Fit, Living Fit: The Basics of Exercise Prescription." There you'll find an overview of fitness, a walking program, simple programs for weight training and stretching, and tips on technique and motivation that have worked for hundreds of our guests.

PROGRAM 2: CARDIOVASCULAR HEALTH

You have the beginnings of heart disease. Your blood pressure is too high, and your last cholesterol test didn't look very good. In addition, your father died too young of a heart attack. Your goal is to improve your cardiovascular health.

You may want to reread "Medicine for Optimal Health," paying special attention to the sections on managing stress, and stress and the heart.

Exercise is your most important weapon in fighting heart disease, so "Getting Fit, Living Fit"—and, in particular, the section on cardiovascular fitness—is for you. If you have injuries that have prevented you from getting the exercise you need, you'll also want to read Chapter 4, "The Strong and Flexible Frame: Musculoskeletal Wellness" for help with musculoskeletal self-healing and injury prevention. "Nutritional Intelligence" will give you the facts you need to develop a heart-healthy eating plan. You may want to pay special attention to the section on phytochemicals and the material on fats: more and more evidence suggests that inflammatory processes are an important factor in cardiovascular disease, and that anti-inflammatory agents in the diet have a real impact.

PROGRAM 3: STRESS MANAGEMENT

Your stress is out of control.

You may wish to reread Chapters 1 and 2 and act on the strategies outlined there for changing both the stressors in your life and your perceptions of them. While you're working on reducing the causes of your stress, you need help in dealing with its symptoms.

Chapter 9, "Emotional and Sexual Intimacy: The Connection Between Happiness and Health" can help you identify and counteract the effects of stress on your personal relationships—and you do want healthy intimacy, since isolation is a major stressor and a predictor of mortality. You may also wish to pursue an exercise program that emphasizes balanced movement and serenity—see Chapter 5, "Balance and Movement: An Essential Component of Fitness" for help. In addition, Chapter 8, "Hands-on Healing:

Bodywork and Massage" is your guide to some of the most effective therapies in the world for integrating and calming mind, body, and spirit. You'll even find instructions there for at-the-office reflexology and preventing headaches.

OTHER GOALS, OTHER PATHS, OTHER PROGRAMS

These programs are just a few examples of the many paths you might take through this book. By presenting them, we simply wish to show that the house of health has many doors. Fitness, nutrition, and mindfulness are not wholly separate entities, and one is certainly not more important than another. Every topic interlocks with the others, and all are part of a healthy, full, and satisfying life.

THE Canyon Ranch GUIDE TO Living Younger Longer

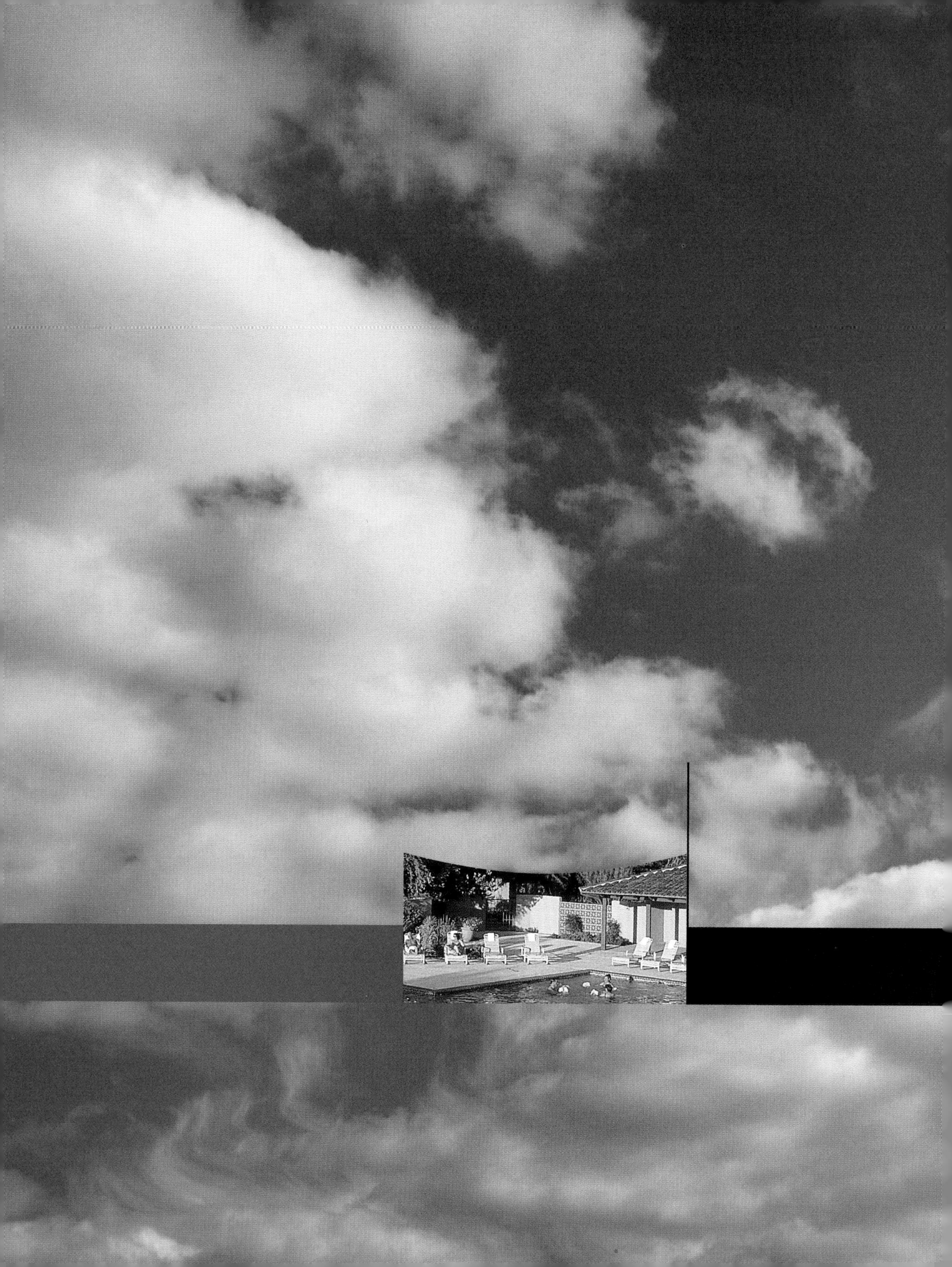

1 TREATING MIND, BODY, AND SPIRIT: *Medicine for Optimal Health*

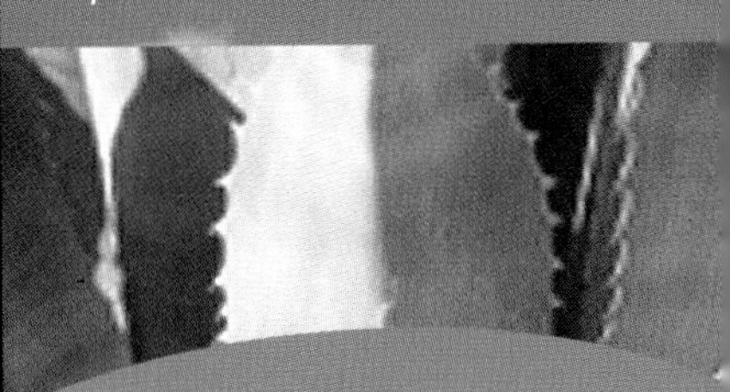

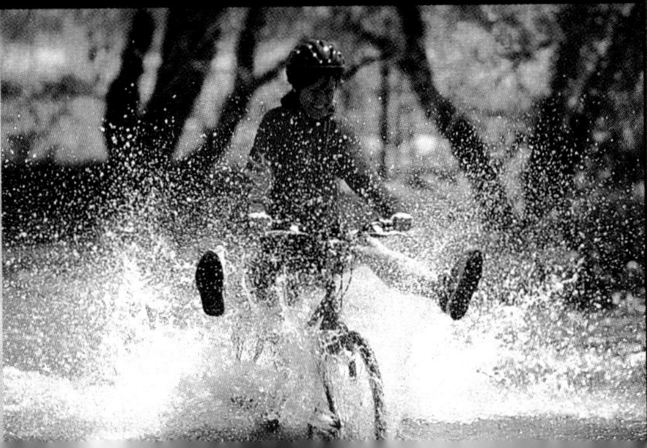

The practice of medicine at Canyon Ranch is holistic, vigorous, proactive, and empowering—and, judging from the events of the past two decades, it's not too much to say that it's the medicine of the future.

Unlike standard Western medical practice, which tends to focus on symptom suppression and the treatment of disease in isolation, the new medicine looks at the whole individual in the context of his genetic inheritance, behavior, health history, and environment. It also tends to view physical, emotional, and spiritual health as equally important aspects of wellness. What unifies the practice of medicine at Canyon Ranch is the concept of *health as a positive and active process of being over which each individual has substantial control.* Canyon Ranch medicine seeks to help each guest take control of his or her well-being to the greatest extent possible.

Medicine at the Millennium

OVER THE LAST HALF CENTURY, a number of factors have contributed to the development of a medical practice that empowers and involves the patient as never before. These factors have come from all over the map, and they're interrelated in complicated ways, but all contribute to a new type of health care that holds tremendous hope for people who are willing and able to take responsibility for their own well-being. The emerging medicine fully recognizes the impact of lifestyle on health, wellness, and aging.

Here are three of the most important developments driving the new medical thought:

1. The most dramatic change in the medical worldview during the last few decades has resulted from the emergence of frightening new infectious diseases and

EXPLORING THE NEW MEDICINE WISELY

THE NEW MEDICINE, accompanied by the rapid diffusion of both empowering information and questionable advice over the Internet, is making self-care more attractive and more confusing every day. Taking control of your health requires attention and plenty of common sense. You must be an informed consumer.

- Check the credentials and training of any practitioner you visit. Is he or she board certified? Did he or she graduate from an institution with a funny-sounding name or one that's well established?
- Watch for individuals who make extravagant claims. If someone promises a quick cure if you change your diet, take a vitamin, and so on, be careful.
- Be sure of the credentials of practitioners who try to sign you up for long and costly treatment packages.
- Do look for a practitioner who keeps you in the driver's seat, whose aim is to help you heal yourself, who

the reappearance of old, "conquered" scourges—including tuberculosis and malaria. This infectious resurgence has helped clarify both the limits of heroic interventions and the vital importance of disease prevention and health promotion. It's become increasingly obvious since the emergence of AIDS, Ebola virus, and the hantaviruses that human beings continue to be part of an evolving, complex biological system, and not the absolute masters of it. As a result, the new medicine tends to treat human health in terms of balance and robustness and functional redundancy, ideas borrowed from ecology and systems analysis.

In an important 1999 article, Lester Breslow of the School of Public Health at UCLA defined two aspects of health: health balance, "the dynamic equilibrium between the human organism and its environment," and health potential, "an individual's capacity to cope with environmental influences that jeopardize health balance." This way of thinking leads to a practice of medicine that is quite different from the standard picture of medicine as a battle—with medical professionals as warriors, drugs as weapons, disease as the enemy, and the body of the passive patient as the battlefield.

Bottom line: there are many, many conditions from which even the highest-tech medicine cannot save us. People who want to increase their chances for long life and good health need to work actively on improving their relation to the world, their internal balance, and their overall wellness.

2. Due in large part to unprecedented prosperity and medical and technological advances, both life expectancy and the incidence of chronic disease related to diet and sedentary lifestyle are increasing in the West. Chronic disease now afflicts many more people in the developed world than the acute illnesses and injuries that, for many good reasons, have been the focus of standard Western medicine. The standard

avoids drugs when possible, and who favors noninvasive treatments over invasive ones. He or she should also be willing to spend the time necessary to get to know you and your medical history and to educate you about your condition and your options for treatment. You have a right to have all your questions answered.

- **Do believe in yourself—in your body's innate capacity to heal itself, and in your ability to choose appropriate ways to enhance that process. Trust in your ability to create your own system of health care.**
- **Do turn to traditional medicine when you feel it is appropriate. The biggest mistake you can make in trying to be your own doctor or in relying purely on "natural" treatments is to miss the diagnosis of a condition that's easily curable by standard medical practice.**

medical model—patient gets sick, patient sees doctor, doctor medicates or operates on patient—simply doesn't work very well for chronic illness or slow debilitation.

The current explosion of research into the biology of disability and chronic disease has begun to yield fascinating insights into the mechanisms of life, and of disease, aging, and death, at the level of the individual cell. As it turns out, our bodies' systems have an order that we are only beginning to grasp, and each of us is biochemically unique, with a one-of-a-kind set of genes. Symptoms and chronic diseases don't appear randomly but develop over long periods of time from imbalances and dysfunctions. These, in turn, are the products of the interaction of genetics, environment, and behavior. We have no control over our genetic inheritance, at present, and little control over our environment. We do, however, have a huge amount of control over how our genetic inheritance expresses itself, once we understand it. We can work with what we inherit by changing our behavior.

Bottom line: the most subtle and important research from the last fifty years strongly supports the significance of cultivating healthful habits and gives us the power to change the way our genes express themselves.

3. Mind and body are no longer treated as separate entities. Drugs that adjust the biochemistry of the brain have revolutionized the treatment of mental illness, while research in new fields like psychoneuroimmunology is revealing the effects of emotion on processes as apparently automatic as immune functioning. Scientists working on stress, for example, have linked chronic anger and fear to physical conditions ranging from hives to obesity to arthritis to heart disease.

Few people probably ever really believed that mind and body functioned independently of one another, but now the relationship has been officially recognized.

Bottom line: all aspects of our lives are interrelated; health is a condition of the whole person.

PATIENT INVOLVEMENT is important in the treatment of all medical conditions: you cannot hand your body over to someone else and expect a good outcome. There are, however, distinct differences in the degree of involvement and personal judgment that various conditions require.

Conditions in which your participation and decision-making power is minimal:

- Treatment of acute illnesses
- Treatment of acute surgical emergencies
- Immunization

Conditions in which your active participation in treatment may help:

- Allergies
- Autoimmune diseases
- Cancer
- Chronic degenerative diseases (like multiple sclerosis)

Taking Control of Your Health

YOU NEED TO take care of yourself—you're convinced. But just how do you do that? Where do you start? And how do you stay motivated?

The most important single principle of health optimization is this: improving your lifestyle doesn't mean you have to be perfect. You don't have to become a vegetarian, marathon-running teetotaler tomorrow, nor should you try. Huge, abrupt lifestyle changes are rarely sustainable and can even cause health problems of their own.

The basic principles of creating a healthy lifestyle are simple, and we'll get to them in just a minute. But as you read through this chapter, and through the rest of the book, don't let yourself become discouraged or overwhelmed. *Of course* you can't do everything right all at once—nobody can. But it is critical that you do *something* and keep after it: remember, *health is a positive and active process of being*, not a thing you can "get" or "lose." Health is in the way you live every day.

Start small, try different things, congratulate yourself for every improvement and healthful choice, and keep at it. Know that you, and only you, can make your life better, more joyful, and, with a little luck, longer. Optimizing your lifestyle can cost almost nothing—the price of some workout clothes and a few dietary supplements. Or it may, eventually, involve hard choices: changes such as creating a balance between work and the rest of life can require financial sacrifice, but bear in mind that we are still just talking about dollars and cents. Length and quality of life, freedom from pain and disability, peace of mind and lightness of spirit belong to a whole different realm of value.

Hundreds of scientific studies show that lifestyle has an enormous impact on health and longevity, but there are, of course, no guarantees, nor any way to predict what the benefits of a healthier way of life will be for *you*. Scientific respectability

- **Genetic predisposition for or diagnosed risk of heart disease and stroke**
- **Hypertension**
- **Viral infections (cold, flu, hepatitis, etc.)**

Conditions in which your active participation in treatment is vital:

- **Arthritis**
- **Asthma**
- **Diabetes**
- **Heart disease**
- **Mental illness**
- **Obesity**

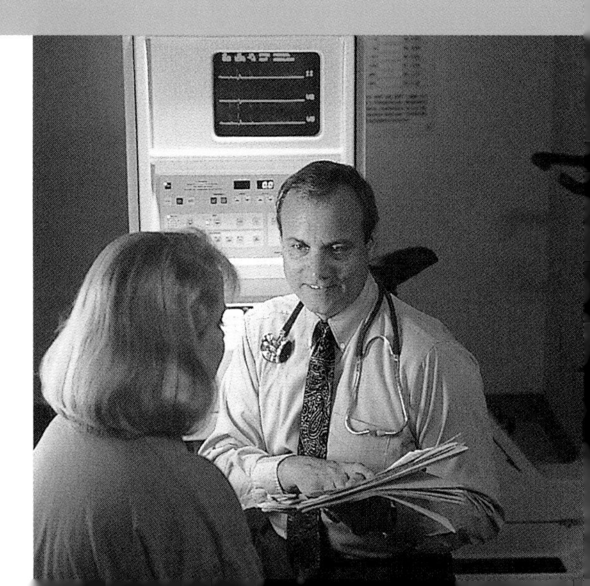

requires controls and statistics, but these only work for populations, not individuals. When you exercise, eat right, and get enough sleep, you simply don't know which bullets you're dodging. It could be the diabetes that runs in the family, the Alzheimer's disease that tragically incapacitated an uncle, or the osteoporosis that crippled your aged neighbor with multiple spinal fractures and made her last months agony. Happily, you'll never know what you missed, but you *will* know that you've done what you could for yourself, and for the people who love you.

Optimizing Your Own Health: The Five Basics of Avoiding Illness and Feeling Great

THE BASICS OF a healthy lifestyle are so simple as to be disappointing, and yet it is impossible to overstate their importance. The finer points are covered in the rest of this book, but the essential actions that will maximize your chances for a long and healthy life are almost embarrassingly obvious. Ironically, your mother's rules for good health cover about 90 percent of what you need to stay alive, happy, useful, and out of the hospital. Research is making the old wisdom look better all the time.

Here is Mom's recipe for health:

I. Go outside and play.

II. Get to bed on time.

III. Eat your vegetables.

IV. Be happy.

V. And if I ever catch you smoking, Mister . . .

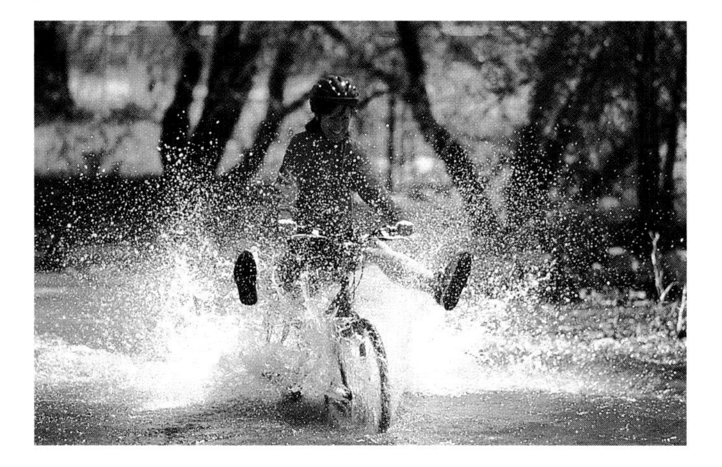

1. "GO OUTSIDE AND PLAY"—EXERCISE REGULARLY

Use it or lose it—the old saw is absolutely correct. Your body was built to move, and nothing good comes of a sedentary way of life.

This book contains everything you need to know to get started on an exercise program. See Chapters 3, 4, and 5—"Getting Fit, Living Fit: The Basics of Exercise Prescription," "The Strong and Flexible Frame: Musculoskeletal Wellness," and "Balance and Movement: An Essential Component of Fitness." All this expert information won't do you a lick of good, however, if you don't put it to use. You must move your body to be healthy.

You know that exercise is good for you, but do you know *how* it benefits you?

1. Exercise prevents or slows heart disease by improving vascular reactivity—the ability of the blood vessels to readily and easily open and close as more or less blood flow is needed.

2. Regular exercise is like taking heavy-duty antioxidants. Our bodies "rust out" over time as tissues are degraded by free radicals. Exercise slows and even reverses the aging process by reducing inflammation and releasing the body's own antioxidants.

3. Exercise lowers the amount of adrenaline circulating in the body, reducing the damaging effects of stress and the propensity of blood vessels to spasm.

4. Exercise increases lean body mass. Greater muscle mass increases metabolism and improves the ratio of "good" to "bad" cholesterol in the blood.

5. Exercise improves vagus nerve tone. This nerve slows the heartbeat, and its tone is so important for heart health that doctors prescribe beta-blockers to improve tone for heart attack patients. Beta-blockers cut the risk of a second heart attack in half; exercise achieves the same result naturally, without side effects, and may well prevent the first heart attack from ever occurring. Good vagus nerve tone is also associated with a low incidence of irregular heartbeat.

6. Exercise relieves stress. Besides lowering adrenaline, the physical release relaxes the whole body and gives the mind a rest.

7. Exercise pumps up immunity, in part by promoting efficient circulation of the lymph, the fluid that clears infection and toxins from the body. The lymphatic system is a huge circulatory network with no pump; it relies instead on voluntary and involuntary muscle movement to circulate the lymph.

8. Exercise promotes good sleep. Regular exercise, by itself, cures many cases of insomnia. Ecclesiastes has it right: "The sleep of the laborer is sweet."

Common Concerns About Exercise

1. *Can I exercise too much?* Use your common sense, follow your doctor's advice, and when you take up a new activity, be moderate. Beyond that, unless you start putting in more than two hours a day, don't worry about exercising too much.

2. *Don't people who exercise get injured more than people who stay safely sitting down?* Sure, but most athletic injuries are minor and limited. A sedentary way of life leads to system-wide degenerative damage that's much more serious and eventually sets the stage for the kind of injury (typically the dreaded broken hip) that puts an end to independent living for so many older people.

3. *Isn't exercise dangerous for older people?* On the contrary—the older you get, the more deadly the *lack* of physical activity becomes. Becoming and staying physically active as we age does, of course, present challenges: we must adjust our exercise regime so that it doesn't injure us. (See "Exercise and Age" in Chapter 3, page 48.) As joints become more susceptible to injury, for example, walking, cycling, and swimming may be better choices than higher-impact activities like jogging. It's also wise—at any age—to ease into a new activity gradually, so that joints and connective tissues have time to adapt to new movements and challenges.

A sedentary lifestyle, however, is *not* a choice if you want to live well and long. Aside from smoking, exercise habits are the best single predictor of longevity and health for people over fifty.

How to Stay Motivated

1. Join a convenient gym. For many people, the desire to get their money's worth out of the membership keeps them moving.

SPECIAL HEALTH CONSIDERATIONS FOR WOMEN

WOMEN ARE MUCH more likely than men to suffer the bone-mineral loss that leads to fragile bones and debilitating fractures in later life. A high-calcium diet; hormone-replacement therapy and/or a diet high in the isoflavones found in soybeans, lentils, and chickpeas; and weight-bearing exercise can prevent, arrest, and, to a degree, reverse bone-mineral loss. Recent research shows that regular weight-bearing exercise is a more important factor than calcium intake in preventing and arresting osteoporosis: bedridden people who take 1,000 mg of calcium a day still lose bone rapidly. The women of China, on the other hand, who consume no dairy and a diet that's relatively low in calcium, but who have few laborsaving devices, have a much lower incidence of bone fracture than their Western counterparts.

Weight training is very beneficial for women of any age. The key is proper form, many repetitions, and consistent effort. Interestingly, older women who regularly do vigorous yard work and gardening seem to get many of the same benefits as their contemporaries

2. Invest in fashionable workout clothes and good shoes, if you enjoy them. Having nice equipment and looking good helps.
3. Look through fitness magazines at the newsstand and consider subscribing to one that appeals to you. The better publications are packed with excellent information, advice, and encouragement. We especially like *Men's Health, Shape, Walking, Self, Yoga Journal,* and *Body & Soul.*
4. Make exercise a priority: don't let it be the activity that goes by the wayside every time your schedule gets tight. Think of it as a serious and necessary investment, one that makes it possible for you to enjoy your financial investments to the utmost. If being physically active seems like a sacrifice, accept it as such and approach it with the same discipline you approach work and financial planning.
5. Start with what you can make yourself do and gradually add more, and if you get bored, try something else that looks appealing. What you do is much less important than the fact that you do *something*: ten minutes a day is a fantastic improvement over no minutes a day and is much, much better than an hour or two of furious exercise once or twice a month. And remember, being physically active becomes easier and more enjoyable the longer you do it. We promise.

II. "GET TO BED ON TIME"—GET AT LEAST EIGHT HOURS OF SLEEP A NIGHT

Length of sleep per night is one of the most powerful predictors of mortality known, but it's the least appreciated of all the major aspects of basic health. Our need for adequate sleep is as nonnegotiable as our need for exercise. Human beings can adjust to many things, but we cannot successfully adapt to lack of either exercise or sleep.

who do formal weight training—and they also enjoy the inestimable benefits of being out in the fresh air doing something they love. It's important to recognize that working out is a substitute for the physical work our bodies need, and a formal exercise regime is not necessarily better than real physical work.

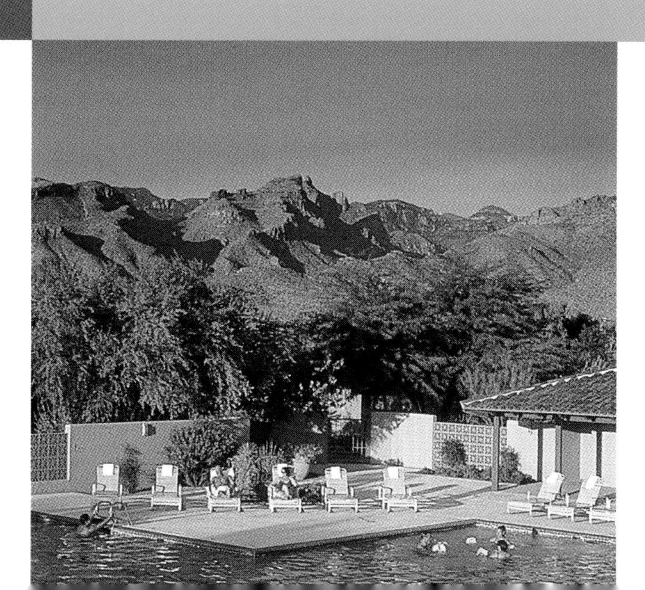

Humans used to go to bed soon after the sun went down and slept until it came up again: Why stay up in the cold and the dark? But with the invention of the electric light, a hundred-watt bulb—the illumination of an unheard-of hundred candles—could be in every room of every house, and at very little expense. Many people decided that, as superior and energetic beings, they needed only four or six hours a night. This is a dangerous self-deception: only rare individuals are truly rested on less than seven hours a night. In addition, it isn't really possible to "catch up" on lost sleep on the weekends—sleeping late a couple of days a week just ensures that your wake-sleep cycle stays out of whack.

While You Were Sleeping . . .

There's still much about sleep that we don't understand, but we do know that it's a furiously active biological state. Sleeping is emphatically not a waste of time. Here's a glimpse into what went on last night:

During the first part of the night, your brain turned into a biochemical factory, churning out antioxidants, growth hormone, antiaging markers such as DHEA and testosterone, and vital immunological factors. Your body's exquisitely complex chemical balances and controls were restored. Later on, you shifted into more vigorous REM, or dream, states while your brain sorted through yesterday's experiences, "tattooing" memories, making connections, and consolidating learning. The last period of sleep, toward morning, was crucial for your creativity and mood—this is the sleep that most people with depression don't get.

When we're sick, we sleep. When we're hurt, we sleep. Babies and teenagers and pregnant women sleep prodigiously. Sleep is our time for healing and growth. Sleep nourishes, renews, and "knits up" body, mind, and spirit. As our ancestors knew—and we forgot—there is no substitute for it. Lack of sleep can produce a variety of serious consequences, including depression, difficulty in weight regulation (due to both depressed mood and increased insulin resistance), and overproduction of stress hormones. In short, lack of sleep tends to make you depressed, fat, and jittery. Get some rest.

There are now more than eighty distinct sleep disorders on the books, and the number continues to grow. The most common and troublesome sleep problems currently recognized are sleep apnea and upper-airway distress syndrome, restless legs syndrome and periodic leg-movement disorder, narcolepsy, sleep phase disorder (sleep cycles out of sync with daily life), REM movement disorder, inadequate sleep disorder (not getting enough sleep by choice), and alcohol- and medication-related disorders. A major cause of poor sleep for many middle-aged women is menopause, due to hot flashes that can cause repeated awakenings during the night. Sleep apnea (short, repeated episodes of not breathing) is by far the most serious and the best understood of all sleep disorders. Apnea is basically a problem with the configuration of the throat that causes frequent collapse of the windpipe. The telltale symptom of sleep apnea, which affects up to 5 percent of the population, is snoring punctuated by periods of silence and sudden snorts. (It's typically a suffering spouse who sends the patient in to be examined.) Apnea not only prevents sound, restful sleep; the repeated short episodes of oxygen deprivation increase risk of

- Sudden death
- Stroke
- Heart attack
- High blood pressure

If either you or your sleeping partner suspects that you have sleep apnea, seek help. Many doctors, whose medical training might have been designed specifically to create sleep disturbances, are still not asking their patients about their sleep, and they often don't know much about sleep deprivation. In general, if you often have trouble getting to sleep, if you wake up during the night, or if you snore heavily, seek evaluation at a sleep center.

Sleep Ecology

If, on the other hand, you're tired all the time just because you go to bed too late, you need to change your habits. Regularity is the key to deep, peaceful sleep. Establish a solid sleeping pattern, beginning with a routine of winding down in the evening. Think of the natural cues that for millions of years told us it was time to rest, and arrange your evening to imitate them.

- Turn the lights lower as the evening goes on, and settle into quiet, restful activities.
- Exercise is enormously helpful for insomnia, but get your workout early in the day: exertion can be stimulating.

HOW SLEEPY ARE *YOU*?

HABITUAL DAYTIME sleepiness is *not* normal.

Do you often

Fall asleep on airplanes?

Need naps to make it through the day?

Get sleepy in afternoon meetings?

Fall asleep in front of the TV?

Need caffeine to drive more than two hours?

If you answered yes to any one of these questions, you're probably sleep deprived.

You're more seriously sleep deprived if you do any of the following:

Fall asleep during church or class

Fall asleep in waiting rooms

Doze off during conversations

Such behavior indicates that your level of sleep deprivation is dangerous. Seek help immediately from a sleep clinic or sleep specialist.

- Cut out caffeine after lunchtime.
- Get out and get some sunlight every day—this reinforces the body's day-night cycle.
- Eat dinner early, so the heavy work of digestion is mostly done by bedtime, and avoid excessive alcohol intake—it has a rebound effect and may cause waking due to dehydration.
- Keep your bedroom slightly cool and dark, and reserve the bed for sleep and sex—don't do anything else there.
- Do not watch the clock—you cannot *make* yourself fall asleep. It's normal to take from 15 to 30 minutes to doze off.
- If you find that you're wakeful, get up and go to another room and do something peaceful. Reading or working on a crossword puzzle are good activities; listening to a book on tape or to someone telling a story is even better—look what bedtime stories do for little children. Listening to music is less effective because music doesn't engage the language centers of the brain. Part of wakefulness is "interior conversation" and a flow of calming words from outside can override the internal chatter. Keep the lights low, have a light snack if you wish, and keep your eyes off the clock.

III. "EAT YOUR VEGETABLES"—EAT WELL

Two chapters of this book are devoted to the finer points of nutrition and healthy weight, and while diet is certainly an important part of good health, our bodies are more forgiving about diet than exercise or sleep.

Recent research indicates, however, that several components of diet unequivocally improve our chances for long, healthy life. This is significant, because in the

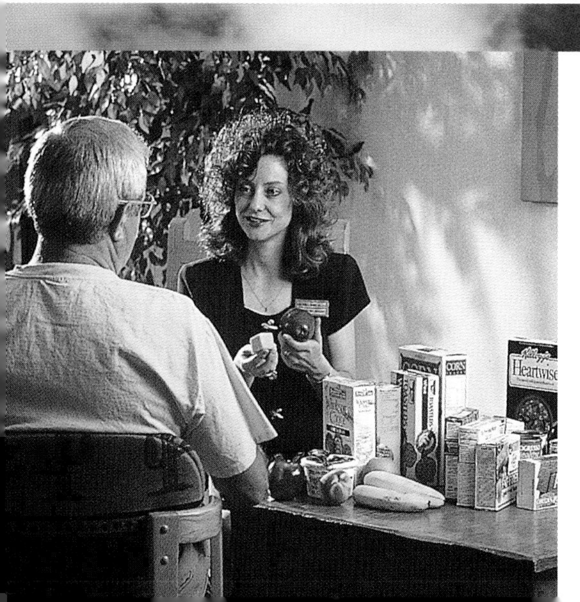

FOR WOMEN: Evidence indicates that a diet high in the isoflavones found in soy, lentils, and chickpeas may help prevent heart disease and reduces the severity of menopausal symptoms. At this time, there's no standard prescription for how much soy you should eat. The usual advice is to work at adding soy-based foods and beverages to your regular diet.

FOR MEN: Current research on lycopene, a phytochemical found in red vegetables and fruits and especially plentiful in tomatoes, indicates that it fights prostate cancer. Some doctors now recommend that men over age forty drink a glass of tomato juice every day and consume one more daily serving of tomatoes, preferably cooked with olive oil.

fast-paced, contentious world of "nutritioneering," disagreement is the norm. *No one* disagrees about these five:

1. Eat eight to ten servings of fruits and vegetables a day: these are the foods with the greatest power to prevent disease. A serving is just one piece of fruit or a half cup of berries, broccoli, or beans—an amount roughly equivalent to a D-size cell battery. If eight to ten servings sounds like too much, consider this breakfast:

- half a grapefruit
- a plain yogurt topped with fresh or frozen berries
- a glass of tomato or orange juice

That's three servings before you walk out the door. (See Chapter 7 for more on portion sizes, a rundown on the wonders of phytochemicals, and the many virtues of fiber.)

2. Eat fish or another source of omega-3 fatty acids several times a week, or take a supplement. These powerful anti-inflammatory agents appear to benefit tissues throughout the body, from the linings of blood vessels to brain cells. (See Chapter 10 for more information.)

3. Avoid animal fats and trans-fats (margarine and shortenings, also known as "hydrogenated" or "partially hydrogenated *anything* oil"). The typical American diet is too high in fats that are solid at room temperature. Reducing consumption of these fats decreases the incidence of heart disease. (Canyon Ranch chefs do not use even a speck of trans-fats.)

   Don't use margarine as a spread, avoid fried foods, and read labels on baked goods and processed foods. (See Chapter 7 for more about fats.)

4. Eat large quantities of dark green leafy vegetables and legumes, or take a vitamin B supplement that includes folic acid once a day. Folic acid clears homocysteine from the blood. High levels of homocysteine, a waste product of metabolism, is a strong risk factor for many age-related diseases.

5. Choose foods rich in dietary fiber (see Chapter 7) and limit intake of refined carbohydrates like added sugar, sweets, and foods made with white flour.

IV. "BE HAPPY"—MANAGE YOUR STRESS

Chronic, unmanaged stress is bad for you—surely you know that already. But did you know that it's so common that the word is currently evolving into an intransitive, active verb? Phrases like "She's totally stressing" express the feel of contemporary life.

Chronic, uncontrolled stress reactions do real physical damage, but that's not the whole story. Life without stress is unimaginable. Without stress we'd never get much done, and we certainly wouldn't have sports to watch on TV. And on those few occasions when a powerful, split-second, all-out physical response is exactly what's called for—your house is on fire and you need to get out—it's that good old fight-or-flight response that gives you a shot at survival.

Stress, like cholesterol, comes in two flavors: "bad" and "good." *Distress* is the official name for what we usually mean when we talk about stress. At the extreme, it's the heart-pounding, stomach-churning, anxiety-ridden state in which we feel driven, agitated, and tormented. At lower levels, however, distress is highly productive—how many completely laid-back people ever accomplished anything?

Eustress is the happy side of stress. It's a positive state of physical readiness and excitement. Children opening birthday presents, a couple flirting at a party, people playing games, an audience watching a thrilling movie—they're all feeling eustress. Life would be pretty dull without it.

There's plenty of evidence, however, that contemporary life keeps many of us continuously running on stress, and that's not good. Physiological stress reactions begin with the release of two chemicals: adrenaline, which is responsible for the "fight or flight" surge in heart rate and blood pressure, and cortisol, which is related to cortisone and prednisone and makes red blood cells sticky (so that blood clots rapidly after injury). Cortisol is implicated in depression and increases appetite. Some people release more adrenaline when stressed: they tend to be anxious and thin. Other people release more cortisol under pressure, and they tend to put on weight and become depressed.

CHANGING THE MIND'S INTERPRETATION OF STRESS, OR BUDDHISM 101

CAREFULLY STUDY THE FOLLOWING ARGUMENT, and set a specified time aside to think about it every day:

- **The world is imperfect.**
- **I suffer because I expect the world to be different.**
- **In order not to suffer, I must change my expectations of the world.**

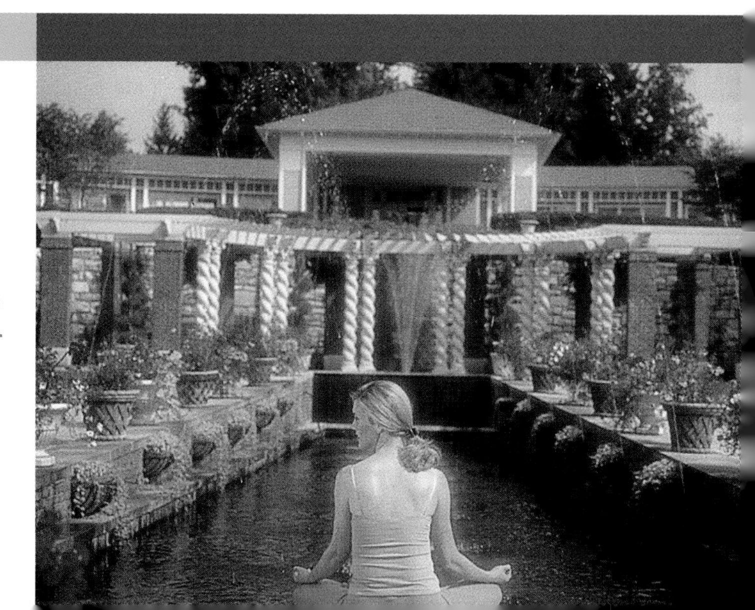

Adenaline and cortisol, though, are only the beginning of a biochemical cascade that, when triggered many times a day over a period of years, can (at the very least) make the following conditions worse:

- headaches
- insomnia
- depression
- anxiety
- skin disorders
- obesity
- musculoskeletal problems
- digestive troubles
- high blood pressure
- cardiovascular disease
- asthma attacks
- ulcers
- diabetes
- arthritis
- alopecia (hair loss)
- poor concentration
- impaired memory and other neurological changes
- panic attacks
- irritable bowel syndrome
- immune deficiency diseases
- infertility and diminished sexual drive

If that list isn't impressive enough, it now appears that there's something even more disastrous for overall health than chronic stress: chronic stress combined with many of the things we do to relieve it—like smoking, drinking alcohol, and overeating.

Stress has three parts:

1. An exterior event or situation—a stressor
2. The mind's interpretation of the stressor as such
3. The body's response to the mind's perception of the stressor

Each of these components of stress is potentially manageable, and if you can master any one of the three, you prevent the damage. You can change your life so as to avoid the event or situation through management of time and tasks; you can modify your mind's interpretation of the event as a stressor; or you can work on modulating your physical response.

Practical Stress Management

Most stress reduction strategies concentrate either on avoiding the stressor (making a habit of leaving early so that being late isn't such a threat, getting enough sleep) or on managing the body's response (taking deep breaths, visualizing a calm and relaxing place, doing relaxation exercises). Both strategies can be very effective.

Damping the second component of the stress response, the mind's interpretation of events, is a much bigger process, requiring both a deepened self-awareness and a more objective view of the world. It takes work to get to the point where you don't *need* to get angry over little things, but the time and effort are worth it, especially if you're a "Type A personality" or a "hot reactor."

The Type A worldview:

- My day is a series of hassles
- I never have enough time
- I need more control
- I'm constantly thwarted in reaching my goals

If this describes *your* world, you're undoubtedly so goal-oriented that you're isolated from other people in the course of the day—a serious health risk by itself—and you are angry a great deal of the time. You also create many of the situations that infuriate you by overscheduling and expecting perfection from yourself and from the world: "This stupid, inept checker needs to work faster because I must get through this supermarket line in two minutes or I won't make it across town in time for my next appointment—which I can just do if I hit all twenty-three lights on the green."

Type A behavior is subtracting years from human lives this minute: anger has been shown to be a bigger risk factor for heart disease than high cholesterol. If you are a cranky, irritable, and demanding person, you can measurably improve your physical health and life expectancy by learning to separate yourself from your anger. The key is to expect less and forgive more—not the easiest advice in the world to follow.

Adjusting the way we see the world is the ultimate in stress relief, and it involves such profound change that it takes us deep into the realm of philosophy and religion, which, by the way, have been shown to have significant health benefits.

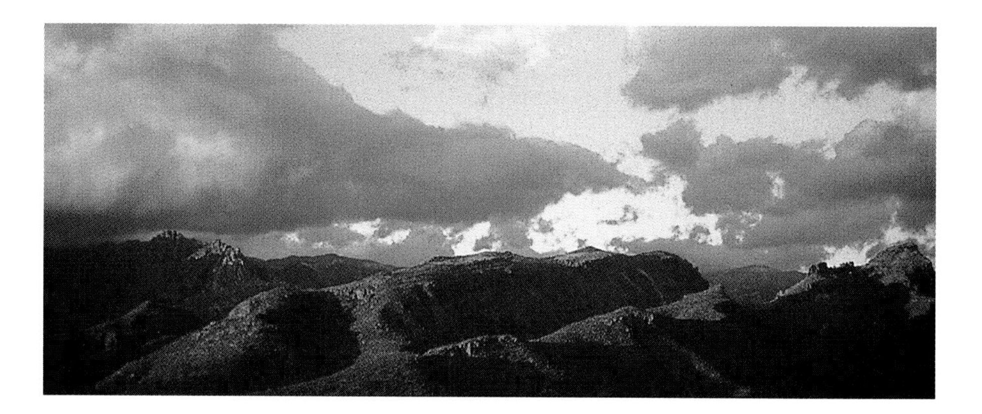

V. "AND IF I EVER CATCH YOU SMOKING, MISTER . . ." —MANAGE YOUR HABITS

Human beings are amazing: we can become addicted to anything. From aerosol propellants to contract bridge, from Cuban cigars to paperwork, there's somebody out there making a habit of it.

Any habit, once it starts to be compelling, reduces our adaptability, flexibility, and, finally, our personal freedom. There's no one less free than a junkie.

Try thinking about it this way: stiffening, or loss of resilience, is the very essence of aging. We're born willing to try anything, but by the time we reach fifty, most of us have worn grooves in our daily lives so deep that change really hurts. Given the fact that time is relentlessly whittling away at our flexibility and function every day, it's just good policy not to help the process along. Studies of centenarians have identified cheerful adaptability and eagerness to try new things as leading characteristics of people who live to be one hundred. Rigidity kills, and addiction is rigidity taken to an extreme.

Some habits are obviously ruinous in and of themselves: smoking, compulsive gambling, and doing drugs are obviously destructive. Any habit, though, however acceptable or virtuous, can limit our freedom.

There's nothing wrong with playing video games, garage-sale hopping, or reading the morning paper, but when any of these activities begins to impinge on our personal choices, it bears looking at. We need to keep an eye on *all* our habitual actions for the sake of continued adaptability. Human beings tend to get into ruts, and that's the way it is. But if we keep surveying ourselves and making adjustments, we'll have no need of professionals to help us extricate ourselves from our own habits.

If, for example, you just don't have time one night for that single beer when you come home, and you find yourself feeling a little cranky about it, then you may want to stop and think about whether you want to go any further down that particular road. The full-blown alcoholic who goes in for treatment has waited until she's heard the snake rattle. It's so much easier to avoid getting anywhere near the danger of addiction in the first place.

Ironically, the more control we humans have over our environment, the wealthier and more personally unencumbered we are, the more likely we are to shape the world to suit us—and to forget how to shape ourselves to fit the world.

The crucial questions to ask yourself about your habits are, "Am I doing this thing I always do because I really like it, or because it's what I always do? Am I becoming overattached to this particular aspect of my day?"

Of course, many habits are useful and even necessary, but even our good habits can use some conscious attention from time to time.

Take brushing your teeth, the very definition of a good habit. Notice how you do it tonight. Maybe you aren't brushing your teeth as well as you might; perhaps

WILLED LOSS OF FREEDOM produces some of the strangest spectacles known: Howard Hughes in his hospital bed, saving his urine in jars and growing his nails long; Elvis Presley gorging himself on prescription drugs, bacon, and peanut butter. Such people not only die before their time; they're functionally near dead long before their hearts stop beating.

you're scrubbing them laterally instead of carefully brushing up and down, the way you're supposed to. It's easy to develop bad habits within our good habits when we don't pay attention.

Other good things we do regularly—religious observances, for example—also benefit from our full attention. Ritual becomes an empty shell when we allow emotion and conscious thought to seep out of it: worship reduced to simple habit offers us no real spiritual help and does no honor to our God.

Another common trap is sticking to the way we've always done things even when circumstances change. Maybe you started jogging twenty years ago, in your mid-twenties, and you've jogged faithfully all these years. Good for you. But now your knees are starting to ache, or maybe they've been aching for years, and there's this thing going on with your Achilles tendons. Still, jogging is what you do for exercise, by heavens, and you're going to keep at it until you need joint replacements.

Well, that's swell news for an orthopedic surgeon somewhere, but there really are other forms of exercise that you might consider trying. If you've become that addicted to jogging, you've given up some of your freedom as a human being. You've let some of your ability to choose slip away, and, with it, part of your connection to the world. What it comes down to is mindfulness.

You can check up on your habits by asking yourself:

- Is this how I did this before? Is this how I always did this?
- Am I doing this because I want to or need to, or out of habit?
- Is that okay?

Pay attention to what you do, think, and feel from one moment to the next, even while doing things you've done hundreds or thousands of times before. We're not only healthier when we don't live by rote—we're more fully alive.

And by the Way, Stay Informed

YOUR MOTHER PROBABLY didn't tell you to keep up with breaking health news, but this is now the Sixth Commandment of basic health. Fascinating and important information from research in exercise physiology, disease prevention, biochemistry, genetics, and a dozen other fields has been pouring forth at an amazing rate in the last few years.

For example, if you look up *homocysteine* in a good home medical reference book published just a few years ago, you won't find any mention of this rogue amino acid. Elevated homocysteine levels, which tend to increase with age, are now considered a major risk factor for heart disease and this significant risk can be controlled simply by getting enough folic acid every day. The strong connection between adequate B-vitamin intake and lowered risk of heart disease is something you need to know about, but the word has only been out for a year or two.

So here's another vital action you can take for optimal health: keep up with the latest news. The best sources we've found for breaking health news are newsletters published by reputable research institutions, and Web sites affiliated with government health agencies, independent research foundations, and universities. We're less enthusiastic about sources sponsored by pharmaceutical companies, hospital chains, and vitamin manufacturers: the blizzard of health news is overwhelming enough without the added confusion of advertising and hidden agendas.

WE PARTICULARLY RECOMMEND

- University of California at Berkeley's "Wellness Letter" (www.berkeleywellness.com)
- Harvard University's "Healthletter," "Heart Letter," "Mental Health Letter," and "Women's Health Watch"
- Harvard School of Public Health's Your Cancer Risk site (www.yourcancerrisk.com.harvard.edu)
- Tufts University's "Health and Nutrition Letter" (www.healthletter.tufts.edu)
- "Nutrition Action Health Letter" from the Center for Science in the Public Interest (www.cspinet.org)

It's Your Life

YOUR MOTHER COULDN'T make you follow the rules, and heaven knows Canyon Ranch can't. It's all up to you. The best general advice the ranch's highly skilled health professionals have to offer is that you take an active role in improving and maintaining your health and function, and that you do it now. Don't let denial or magical thinking get in the way: what you don't know *can* hurt you, and no miraculous new treatment will save you from yourself. Only you have that power.

The way you live can increase both the number and the joy of your days on this earth. Live well.

Chi Gong Relaxation Exercise

Chi (or *qi*) gong, which means "energy refinement" or "vitality cultivation," is one of the four pillars of traditional Chinese medicine. (The others are acupuncture, massage, and herbal therapy.)

This healing and health-maintenance regime is as rich and varied a self-development practice as yoga. Regular chi gong practice, like the regular practice of yoga, is physically beneficial and can be very helpful in regulating emotion and calming the mind.

Simple Chi Gong Relaxation Exercise

Sitting or standing in a relaxed, upright position, close your eyes and take a deep, slow breath. Fill the lungs completely, letting the diaphragm expand. Feel a slight pause in the breath, then exhale completely but without exaggeration. Repeat several times.

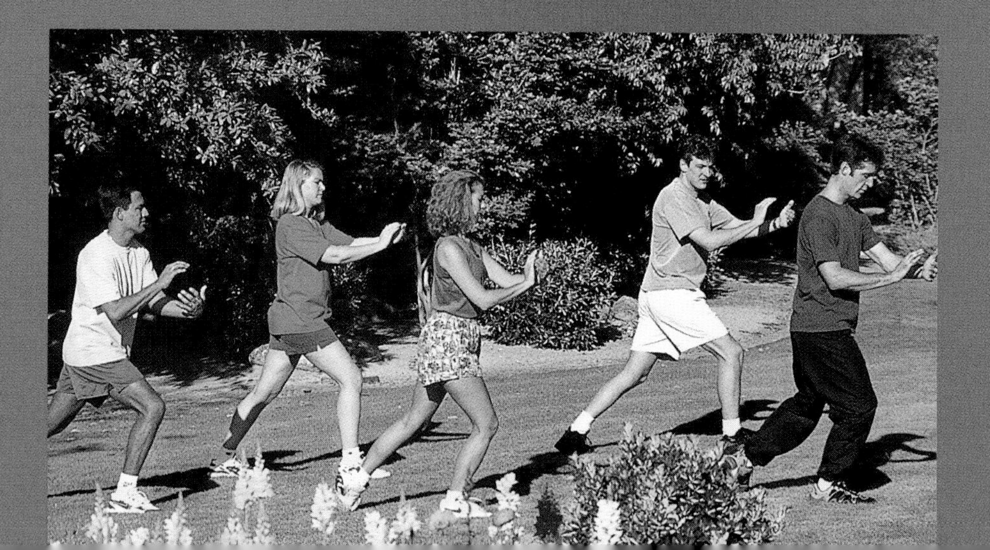

Silently repeat each of the following statements five times while breathing deeply and slowly. Allow yourself to feel what you are describing:

My hands and feet are heavy and warm.

My feet and legs are heavy and warm.

My abdomen is warm and comfortable.

My breathing is deep and even.

My heartbeat is calm and regular.

My forehead is cool.

When I open my eyes, I will remain relaxed and refreshed.

Chi gong teachers recommend doing this exercise several times a day to strengthen and refresh the whole system and to prepare for more advanced meditation.

CANYON
RANCH

2 MANAGING OURSELVES: *Health, Values, and Human Resiliency*

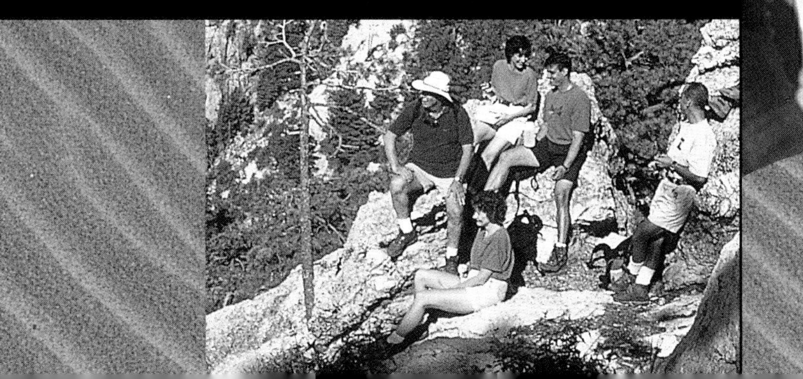

"When you've got your health, you've got everything"—remember the old vitamin commercial? An attractive, well-to-do, fit older couple beam at each other and play with the grandkids while a disembodied voice draws the moral for us. Naturally, the actors on the screen appear to have much more than just their health—they also have money, looks, family, and each other.

It's simply not true that physical health is everything. There's more to life than being healthy in the vitamin-company sense. While no one could ever accuse Canyon Ranch or its founders, Mel and Enid Zuckerman, of undervaluing physical well-being, we also believe that health means more than good lab results and a heart like a bull's. We've seen too many vigorous, attractive, successful, and profoundly miserable people come through the ranch.

We have also seen many folks who have suffered great losses and live with serious physical problems, but who remain healthy in the profoundest way. In spite of great challenges and disappointments, these people enjoy life and contribute to the world. Such people have the emotional and spiritual resources to make the very best of whatever comes along. They are emotionally resilient.

This chapter is about how to cultivate within yourself the emotional and spiritual qualities that contribute to resilience—the capacity to bounce back, and even to learn, when faced with difficulty, loss, disappointment, and tragedy. We need resilience because we cannot, in fact, control anything outside ourselves, and if we're honest, we realize that we can't even completely control ourselves. We cannot, for example, change our basic temperament.

What we can do is take concrete, practical steps toward *managing* our lives and ourselves so that we can find the greatest possible fulfillment in whatever fate hands us. Like physical strength and flexibility, emotional resilience is something we can improve over time by taking positive action.

Managing yourself isn't something you learn to do in a day, or a year: it's a lifelong process. But you can begin working consciously toward greater happiness and freedom right now. It all begins with a willingness to ask questions of yourself and the world. The most important questions center on a single, old-fashioned word: *values.*

Your Foundation

PEOPLE LIKE TO TALK about values, generally without defining them. So what do *we* mean by values? *Values are spiritual and moral qualities that command esteem.* Your most important values are sacred—you would sacrifice for them. (Sacrifice is the heart of the sacred: the connection is right there in the words.) The things you care about most, and are proud to care about, are your values.

Your values are entirely your own, and they're your bedrock. It's crucial that you identify them, because they determine what *you* need to be fulfilled. When our actions are not congruent with our values—when, for example, we behave as if professional success were everything when what we really value most is family, or adventure, or self-expression—we suffer chronic, gnawing distress. The feeling that we're forever pulled in incompatible directions is a sign that our values and actions are out of alignment. Over time, this sort of chronic life stress can be extremely destructive; it depletes the emotional resources we need to handle life's inevitable losses and sets us up for major health risks, personal isolation, and unhappiness.

Values and the Culture

OUR ANCESTORS MANAGED to cope with stress most of us can barely imagine: the possibility of losing those they loved to infection, famine, war, or accident at any time, just for starters. Epidemics, pogroms, and crop failures have been terrifying facts of life for most of human history, and remain so for millions of people in developing countries.

Yet our forebears kept going, and treasured their time on earth, in large part because they lived in a world where spirituality was an essential part of life. When the hard times came, a strong, shared value system, assurances of the future, and the comforts of ritual and community were there for support. Karl Marx never spoke a truer word when he said, "Religion is the opiate of the masses." He meant it, of course, as a condemnation of religion, but if we stop and consider the effects of opiates on the brain, we might want to ask, "And what, exactly, is so bad about *that*?" Suffering is dreadful, and that which relieves pain is a blessing.

Recent research on people who go to church (or synagogue, mosque, or temple) indicates that, on average, believers enjoy

- better health, both physical and mental
- more lasting relationships
- fewer problems with drugs and alcohol
- in general, a stronger sense of well-being

than people with no religious affiliation.

In millennial America, however, even people who have strong beliefs need to sort out their values for themselves: our hypercommunicative, materialist culture leaves nothing unquestioned for long. It's up to us to decide what we value most, and how we want to live.

If we don't, consumer culture will do it for us: our corporate-centered society works overtime to prepackage values and make them ours. In the barrage of commercial messages in which we live, the question of what we value most always has the same answer—we should care about whatever's being advertised at the moment. That's the mantra of Madison Avenue: happiness is the next purchase.

If we aren't in touch with our values, and fully conscious of living in congruence with them, there are any number of people waiting to tell us what should be most important to us, usually something concerned with their financial gain. Since advertisers are very clever, they're able to exploit the emotional power of our bedrock values—our love for our children and desire to protect them, say—and attach it to whatever product they're selling, be it SUVs, bathroom cleaner, life insurance, or Ivy League schools.

If you have children and fall for this particular sell, you're likely to find yourself working seven-day weeks to pay for all the things your kids absolutely must have to be safe and happy, when you know in your heart that what they need more than anything is your time and attention. And will you be chronically, severely stressed? Yes. This is just one of many value-confusion traps that lock even folks who make very substantial livings into a grinding round of overwork and distress, and there are many, many others. The only sure way out is to clarify what *you* really care about, and to work on expressing your values in the way you live.

Stress reduction techniques are extremely useful for treating the symptoms of stress, and they can provide real help in turning off the stress response (see Chapters 3 and 9). Better yet is living meaningfully and with conviction. When our actions arise directly from our values, we leave little space in our days for stress to settle in and set up permanent housekeeping.

THE TRUTH ABOUT TIME

TIME MANAGEMENT is just a surface issue of life management, and time stress is a symptom of underlying life stress. Here's the cold, hard truth about time: there are twenty-four hours in each day—not one second more, and not one second less. You'll never be so smart, so wealthy, so attractive, or so personable that you'll have a fraction of a second more than anyone else. You cannot buy time, nor can you stretch it.

The interesting question is why, with so many laborsaving devices, we run faster than ever. If we're saving so much time, where are we putting it? How is it that we run so hard without ever having the sense of running the good race? It's worth taking time—yes, precious time—to think seriously about how our culture's furious pace shapes our days and nights.

Values can be an inestimable resource for each of us. In times of confusion, we can turn to them for direction; in times of trouble, they give us strength. Our values are our guide to connecting our psychic energy source, our emotions, to our actions. When we do make that connection, we feel inspiration, "the coming-in of spirit." The results can be tremendous.

Sorting Out Your Life, in Six Not-So-Easy Steps

THE FOLLOWING EXERCISE can get you started on learning how to manage yourself by helping you define your values and how your life aligns with them. Find some quiet time and sit down with paper and pencil.

STEP 1

Before we can call on the power of our values, we need to identify those things we hold most dear. Our values evolve throughout our lives—usually while we aren't looking.

Try to answer the following questions, concentrating on those that spark your interest and get your words and thoughts flowing. Don't let the sample answers limit you—they're just there to get you started.

1. What three things do I value most in life? (A few examples: truthfulness, independence, beauty, friendship, tranquillity, being right with my God, nature, courage, responsibility, professional accomplishment, compassion, winning, service to others, close emotional ties, providing for those who depend on me, the respect of the people who know me.) Alternate ways of asking this question: What would I die for? What do I hold sacred? What would I sacrifice for? What do I live for?

2. When do I feel, and have I felt, most alive? What gives life to my life? (List all the times that occur to you, and write a bit about each one.)

3. Whom do I love? What qualities do I love and admire most in them?

4. What words would I like to see chiseled on my tombstone? What would I want people to say about me after I'm gone? What would I want to say on my deathbed?

When you're finished, look back over what you've written. Circle words or phrases that recur, or seem especially significant. Listen to your feelings; you're looking for the core of your life, your heart's blood.

Write down the three words or phrases that strike the strongest chords. You've just identified your three most important values at this moment.

STEP 2

For the purposes of this next exercise, we'll divide life into three domains. The three areas we all need to attend to are:

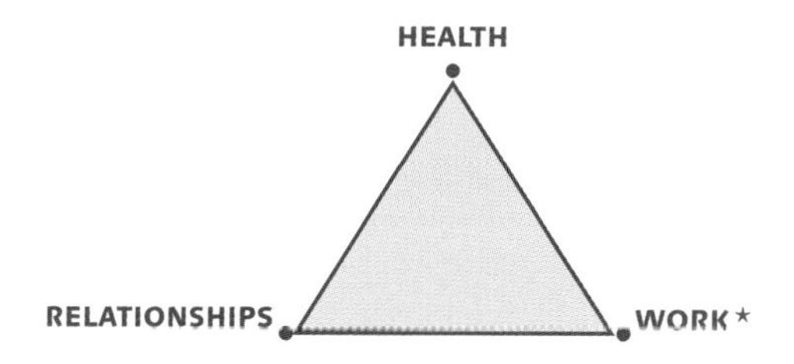

* Not necessarily a job—whatever you do that gives you your sense of purpose.

Of course the domains of life aren't really walled off from each other; they're highly interdependent. You can't have excellent health, for example, if you hate your work and your personal life is a mess. Making these artificial distinctions, however, is useful for now in defining the shape of your life.

Write down under each life domain the top three values you identified in Step 1.

Now for the hard part. Ask yourself, "What behavior would express each of my most strongly held values in each domain?" In other words, what could you *do* in each domain to reflect each of your top three values?

The actions you identify, like your set of values, will be completely individual, but here are some examples that may give you an idea of how the process works.

Say your top value is responsibility. You'll want to write down how you behave, or *could* behave, responsibly in each domain. How could you express the importance being responsible has for you in your work, in your relationships, and with respect to your health?

CANYON RANCH EXISTS only because one man, Mel Zuckerman, consciously threw all the force of his energy, talent, and vision (and every penny he and his wife had) into the full expression of his values. (If you haven't read his introduction yet, you owe it to yourself to go back and do so. His story has probably changed more lives than any other single thing at Canyon Ranch.) The delight and power Mel felt when he found release from chronic sickness and the dread of an early death inspired him to put everything he had into his "crazy dream" of a small health resort near Tucson, Arizona, a resort now famous throughout the world. The passion sparked by the possibilities burned away obstacles, and he ended up creating something that had never existed before. (A student at Harvard Business School who studied the early years of Canyon Ranch for his master's thesis concluded that founding the ranch was "an act of fiscal irresponsibility.") What drove Mel was his

Your first action in each domain might look something like this:

Work: Doing what I'm needed for, and doing it well and on time. I am consistently reliable.

Relationships: Taking good care of my family and being there for them when they need me.

Health: Doing everything I can to take care of myself—exercising, getting enough sleep, eating right, and managing myself in the face of stress.

If your second value were nature, your second set of actions might look something like this:

Work: Doing work that helps the environment, or that gets me outside in a beautiful area, or that somehow connects me to nature.

Relationships: Nurturing my ties to people who also care about nature so that we can share our love of the natural world.

Health: Getting my exercise outside, and doing what I can to stay healthy so I can keep hiking (or climbing, birding, sailing, biking, gardening, etc.).

STEP 3

Look at each of the nine actions you've written down. Ask yourself, "Am I doing this now?"

If the answer's a clear yes, circle it. You've got that taken care of, and you've identified a part of your life that's undoubtedly a source of satisfaction to you. It can also be a source of instruction and inspiration.

When you consider an action and the answer is "Well, sort of" or "No, but I'm getting there," underline it. Try to determine whether there are constraints that you can't do anything about in these areas, or if you could possibly make some changes.

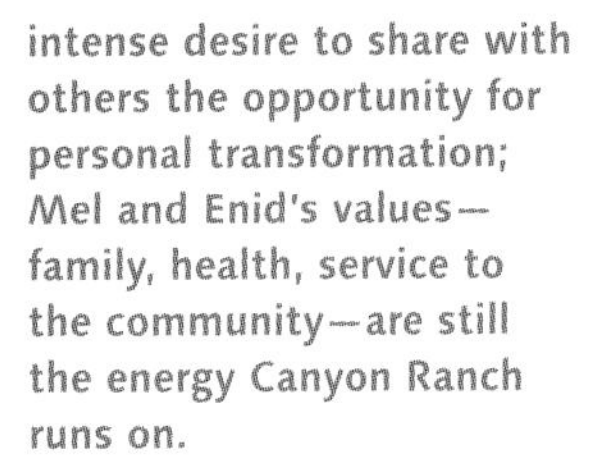

intense desire to share with others the opportunity for personal transformation; Mel and Enid's values—family, health, service to the community—are still the energy Canyon Ranch runs on.

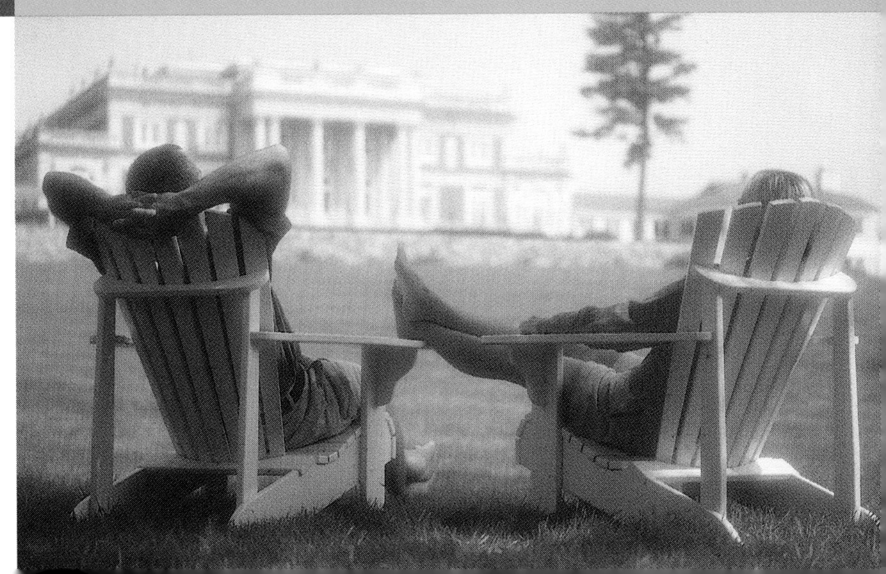

Perhaps you're a little short in some respects because you must to attend to other values or domains of life right now. That's reality.

In the vast majority of cases, we make changes in our lives incrementally, and circumstances often limit what we can do. Say that you've made exercise a priority, but on a particular day you're committed to activities that preclude exercising: you have a big project due at work, and you need to take your daughter to the dentist. You must take care of these things, and that's that. But if you keep your physical activity goal in mind and do what you can, when you can, you'll feel better about the day and yourself. If you park way out in the parking lot, carry your groceries, take the stairs instead of the elevator, and so on, you're trying. Effort always counts.

Now draw a square around actions that you aren't even close to performing. They're aspects of your life that are unsatisfying and very probably sources of distress. Don't start dwelling on these areas right now. You don't want to approach this exercise in a problem-solving mode. The trouble with problem solving is that it takes a lot of energy, energy that you could use to actually live out your goals. No one who's ever accomplished something big started out by anticipating every conceivable problem that might lie ahead. If you try to change your life by problem solving instead of by envisioning possibilities, you probably won't change a thing. When, however, you recognize and experience your real strengths in life, you'll get excited, which generates more energy for change. Finding that energy and setting it loose is the next step.

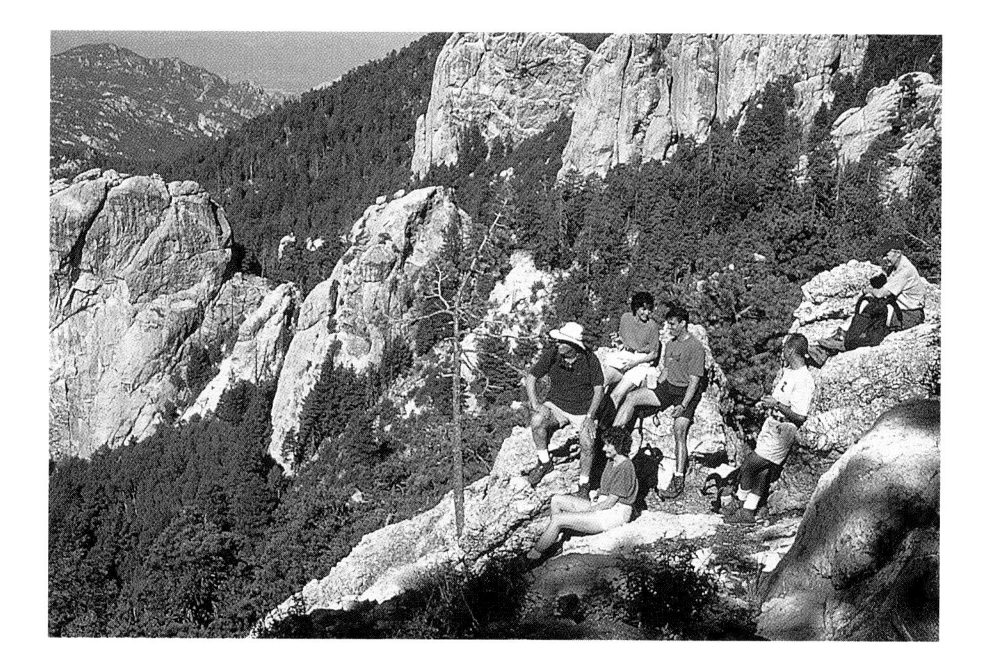

STEP 4

Go back and look at all your circles, the parts of life in which you feel content and in control. Study them carefully. This takes some concentration, because it's natural to focus on what's wrong—and hard to see what's right.

We do hundreds, maybe thousands of things beautifully every day, but we do them intuitively or automatically, without noticing our competence. Since we don't pay attention to much of what we do really well, we often don't have conscious access to the strategies that work best for us.

Look for your patterns of success before you study the areas where you'd like to make changes. It's a basic but little-recognized fact of human nature that we all tend to ignore what's *right*. Evolutionary biology, once again, is at the bottom of our difficulty. The age-old dynamics of survival compel us to be on the lookout for life-threatening emergencies: difficulties of any sort rivet our attention. Most of the problems we face today, however, don't really pose a threat to life or limb, but we continue to use up fantastic amounts of energy keeping watch.

So take time to look at your circled actions—the things you do that satisfy you—and ask yourself, How do I do this? How did I get where I am with this? Did I put a high priority on this? Did I learn and prepare? Did I have the right support systems?

Once we begin to pay attention to what's fine, and how, almost without noticing, we manage to make it that way, we can take the lid off a nearly limitless source of personal energy. *When we recognize our strengths, we can lead from them.*

STEP 5

Once you have a handle on the best parts of your life, try to apply the strategies that work for you to the parts of life you wish to enhance. Write down each boxed action, everything you want to do better or more of, on a separate piece of paper and start brainstorming, taking time to fill each page. Use your life successes as a blueprint, and write down every specific action that pops into your head as you ask yourself, "What can I do that's in line with the congruent behavior I've identified? How could my strengths help me with this? What's possible?"

Try to make all your ideas concrete, because a vague resolution—"Spend more time at home"—is fated to remain a "should do," not a "will do." Your possible courses of action can be huge and improbable dreams: "Bail out of the company and move the family to Fiji." They can be small and immediately doable: "Volunteer to help manage Brett's football team next fall," "Leave the office no later than six on Wednesday," "Set up a regular date night with my mate." But do make them concrete, so you can picture doing each one clearly enough to decide whether or not you want to give it a try.

STEP 6

Underline the actions that you want to take right away, organize them according to priority, and set aside a regular time to plan for the week ahead and review the week that's done. (A half hour on Sunday works for many people.) Write your action commitments for the week in your weekly planner, on your wall calendar, or wherever your keep track of your obligations.

The idea is not to fix everything all at once, but to begin moving in a direction that feels right. If you need more connection to the natural world in your daily life, for example, you might pencil in time on Tuesday to stop by a florist to pick up flowers or dried plants for your office to reflect the current season. If you decide to limit your workload, whether to free up time or to increase your satisfaction in doing a thorough job, you might write in a reminder to resist taking on more than you can handle at the weekly department meeting.

The individual steps you take may be very small, even microscopic, and that's just fine. You didn't get to where you are now in a year, and you won't arrive at where you'd like to be overnight, either. It's very, very important that this "gap analysis" not become just another source of frustration and stress: know and believe that small changes add up. Savor them, and see where they take you. Like every other human being on earth, you are finding your own way, moment by moment.

When you sit down to look back over the past week and plan for the next one, notice what worked and what didn't and think about why. You may very well find that your self-management record starts to outgrow your planner, so pencil in time to find a beautiful blank book to use as a life-management journal.

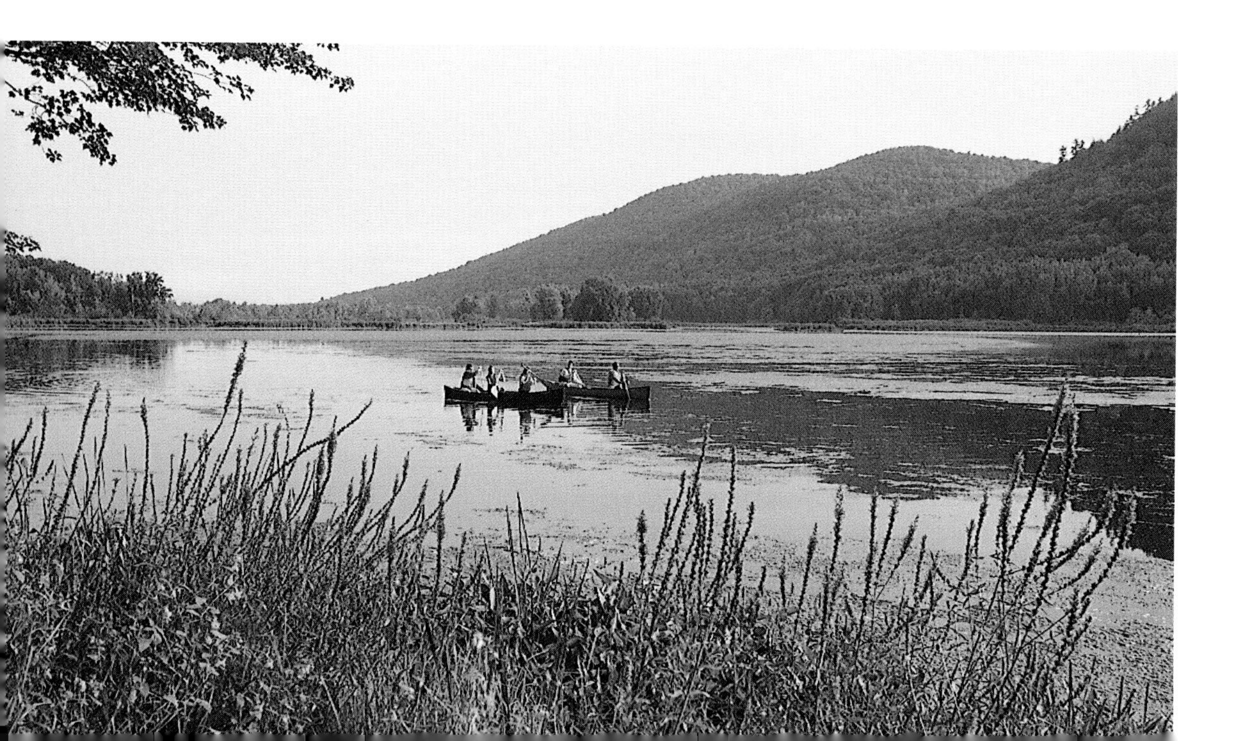

The old Chinese proverb says that the journey of a thousand miles begins with a single step. Know where you stand right now, have a vision of where you want to go, and, when you're ready, start putting one foot in front of the other. That's how a satisfying life is lived.

Managing Ourselves, Day by Day

OUR VALUES CAN provide the framework for a good and coherent life. To be happy and productive people, we also need to become conscious of the emotional energy behind our actions, and we need to view the world around us realistically and with appreciation. A crucial part of managing ourselves is learning to manage our habits of mind.

ACTING FROM LOVE; ACTING FROM FEAR

Love and fear are the basic human emotions: all the other emotions derive from these two. Anger is fear turned aggressive; envy is fear twisted by self-doubt; resentment is anger and envy combined and simmered well. Wanting something so badly it makes us crazy derives ultimately from fear of not having enough, and prejudice stems from fear of difference.

A simple and surprisingly powerful way of evaluating any action about which we're unsure is to ask whether it ultimately comes from love or from fear. (Analyzing the emotions that motivate others is interesting and often useful, but it's vastly more important to monitor our own impulses. This book is about achieving fulfillment, not power.)

Why is it important to understand the dynamics of emotion? Because, as we said above, emotions are our energy source, the hot, bubbling core of life. Emotion frequently drives action. When we act from love, in congruence with our values, we're the Olympic athletes of life; we move with power, grace, and efficiency toward our goals. Acting from love, we lose none of our momentum to defensiveness, resentment, shame, or desire to get even; all our energy flows toward accomplishment. And when we act out of passion—turbocharged love—we can change our destinies.

Fear is every bit as powerful as love, and it's the essence of stress. It's ultimately fear that triggers the fight, flight, or freeze response, and for a small, slow hominid on the veld, it was the key to survival. Fear has lost most of its biological value but lives on, and in all its many guises, it still triggers the hormone cascade that makes hearts pound, blood pressures rise, muscles tense, and stomachs knot. Why would anyone want to spend his or her time acting from fear?

> *"The mind is its own place, and in itself*
> *Can make a Heav'n of Hell, a Hell of Heav'n."*
> JOHN MILTON, *PARADISE LOST*

Of course, nobody gets to live without fear, and no one this side of full sainthood consistently acts from love. We don't get to be blissed-out all the time. Indeed, we need a balance of fear and love to survive. It's generally better, though, to have fear in the background and love in the foreground of our minds. And we can keep trying to improve the ratio of love to fear in our lives—to increase the amount of time we spend in a state of appreciation and to minimize the time we spend, shivering and alone, in the prisons fear builds for us.

Acting from love is often difficult, but knowing whether you're doing so is easy. Before you act, ask yourself, "Am I being generous, concerned, constructive, expansive, warm-hearted, appreciative, kind?" If the answer's yes, then even if things don't turn out the way you hope, you've been true to yourself and you've likely reinforced your values. When we act from love, we retain our self-respect, which makes us healthier and more resilient people. Acting from love ties us to others and makes us stronger, day by day.

There's a growing body of respectable research substantiating what we've always known in our hearts: love is good for us. And it does makes life easier. We operate with more certainty and ease when we're comfortable with our motives. It's better to avoid the burden of shame, the ache of regret, and the high price of defensiveness. We're more tranquil and ultimately more effective people if we try to act out of love, in accordance with our values, whenever we can.

Taking positive action for health—consciously improving the way we live—is a perfect example of the wisdom of acting from love. Too many people are only compelled to do something about their state of health by terror, and whether the revelation comes because of a health crisis, a test result, or an ominous diagnosis, when it comes from fear, it often comes too late.

If, however, we decide to take charge of our health as an act of love—love of family and friends, of independence, of life itself—we can change our lives at any time. When we act from love, we need not wait for fear.

SEEING THROUGH THE ILLUSION OF CONTROL

One of the most universal sources of human misery is the idea that we can control events, things, and other people. We convince ourselves that we should and can have control because we're afraid. The illusion of control is the clumsy armor we put on to battle our own terror. It only gets in the way.

In fact, we cannot control the world around us, and when we try we condemn ourselves to frustration. We most particularly cannot control other people: as any new parent can tell you, it's impossible to make even that most dependent of all humans, a newborn baby, do a single, solitary thing. Whatever control we seem to have over others is either strictly limited, and a function of their fear, or is actually their freely given cooperation in disguise. People will promise us control if they sense we want it, and may allow us to think we have it, but only as long as the arrangement suits them. If we hope to live happy and connected lives, we must recognize that everything we get from other people—everything—they give to us.

The antidote to a destructive obsession with control is self-management to reduce fear, and with it the need to deceive ourselves about how much power we really have. Among the many rewards of giving up the illusion of control is inner peace. Life is much more pleasant when you accept that you cannot *make* your kids get A's, or your colleagues toe the line, or the sun rise in the morning.

PRACTICING APPRECIATION

Another powerful habit of mind is the deliberate cultivation of an appreciative attitude, a vivid sense of the "rapture of life." This is impossible when you let yourself be infuriated or depressed by everything that doesn't go quite your way.

When you find yourself beginning to stew, rather than indulging the feeling, try stepping back from your habitual reaction pattern. First, ask yourself whether you have any control over what's bothering you. If the answer is no, then try to stop focusing on what's wrong and consciously turn your attention to whatever you can find to like or enjoy in the situation. You can even make a private game out of finding the funny side of frustrations and small disasters: try turning them into comic stories you can tell later. Or detach altogether and "go somewhere else" in your mind: practice withdrawing your attention and turning your thoughts to a pleasant memory or an absorbing task.

Such calming habits head off stress and subtly expand your view of things: the world isn't about you.

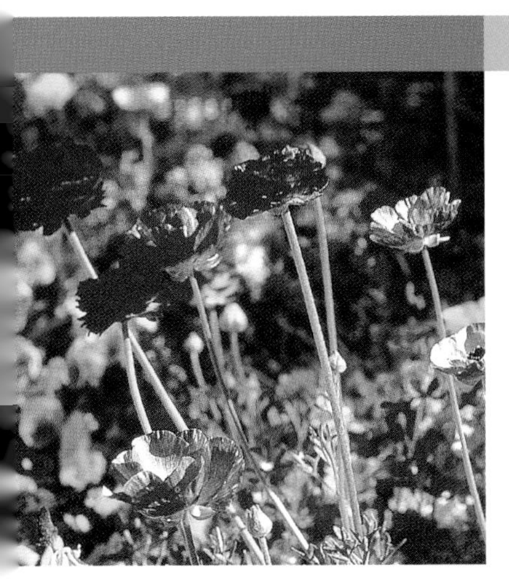

DAILY APPRECIATION RITUAL

HERE'S A ROUTINE TO increase mindfulness, thankfulness, and a positive awareness of the world around you, without taking a single minute from your busy schedule.

Every day, take note of three things that you enjoy. The glass of ice water you poured yourself after coming in out of the heat, a flower you noticed when you walked to lunch, a bird call, the sound of a child giggling, a favorite song on the radio—anything that gives you pleasure. Be sure to collect at least three good things in the course of the day. Then, when you get into bed at night, take a moment to remember and think about each of them. Summon up a feeling of appreciation for the fact that these things were there.

Micaela's Story—A Study in Resilience

As the average length of life increases, the psychological and spiritual challenges of age come into clearer focus. Old age is not for whiners: the longer we live, the more we're fated to lose. Living with zest to a great age is a matter of more than outstanding physical resilience and social support; it also requires mental, emotional, and spiritual resources gathered in the course of a lifetime. This is the true story of one woman's determination not simply to manage but to keep improving and learning until the very end.

When Micaela first came to Canyon Ranch in the Berkshires at an advanced age, she was as sharp as they come but sad and nearly overwhelmed. Her beloved husband of more than fifty years, David, was dying slowly, afflicted by dementia following a series of strokes and advanced prostate cancer. Micaela herself was having difficulty coping with glaucoma and arthritic joint disease; impaired depth perception, a halting gait, and a growing fear of falling had begun to affect her mobility and independence. Not surprisingly, when Micaela came to the ranch, she was clinically depressed. Life had pummeled her and she was reeling.

Giving up, however, had never been her way. When she was quite young, Micaela and David had fled Germany to escape the Nazi regime. After arriving in the United States in 1938, they saved enough in just two years to bring her parents, brothers, and sister over. Throughout the years that followed, she and David helped a number of other relatives get out of Europe.

She attended medical school and eventually became an associate professor at a prestigious university. She and David did not have children and rarely socialized: Micaela's busy, fulfilling life was devoted to her teaching and her practice, and to her husband and highly dependent relatives.

Now she felt that she had lost or was losing everything that had given her life meaning. Her parents were dead, her husband, who hadn't been able to recognize her for some years, was dying, and she was desperately afraid that soon her health problems would keep her from doing the work she loved. (She was still actively practicing and teaching with great satisfaction.)

Micaela, typically, did the courageous, hopeful thing by coming to Canyon Ranch. Even weighed down by a depression that made any action a struggle, this woman who had always been the one to help others came looking for the help she needed.

After a complete evaluation, the staff and Micaela agreed that her most immediate problem was stress-induced depression. Working with a psychologist, this proud, good soldier let go and began to express her grief over the cruel way her husband was dying. She was heartbroken about losing him and felt utterly helpless as his illness defied all her intelligence, caring, energy, and tenacity—the weapons with which she had faced her long life's many challenges. Surviving David's decline and death required that this aging woman develop a new way of understanding and of being.

As she wept and talked, allowing herself to open up and rely on her therapist, she began to recall the life she and David had shared, reliving the good times and satisfactions of their long partnership. As the feelings she'd pushed down in order to cope started to rise to the surface, Michaela's sense of emotional deadness began to lift and her spirit returned. Her therapist listened, validated her feelings, and encouraged her. She left the ranch still carrying great burdens but with renewed confidence in her ability to sustain them.

Over the next few years, Micaela suffered further losses—her only living sibling died, and her husband finally passed—and they hit her hard. She allowed herself to mourn, emerging with a sense of having done right by the dead and a new sense of connection. Many people loved her, and she was both surprised and heartened by the concern and support that poured in from friends, neighbors, colleagues, and patients. Many people came to David's funeral, and the realization that she was less alone than she had thought was a great help.

She returned to the ranch, determined to reclaim and refashion her life. In deep hypnosis, she was able to reexperience being knocked down on a city sidewalk by a running man, as well as a terrifying car accident decades before—incidents that had made her feel helpless. Examining these memories and her feelings about them helped her manage the exaggerated fear of falling that had limited her mobility more than her physical problems.

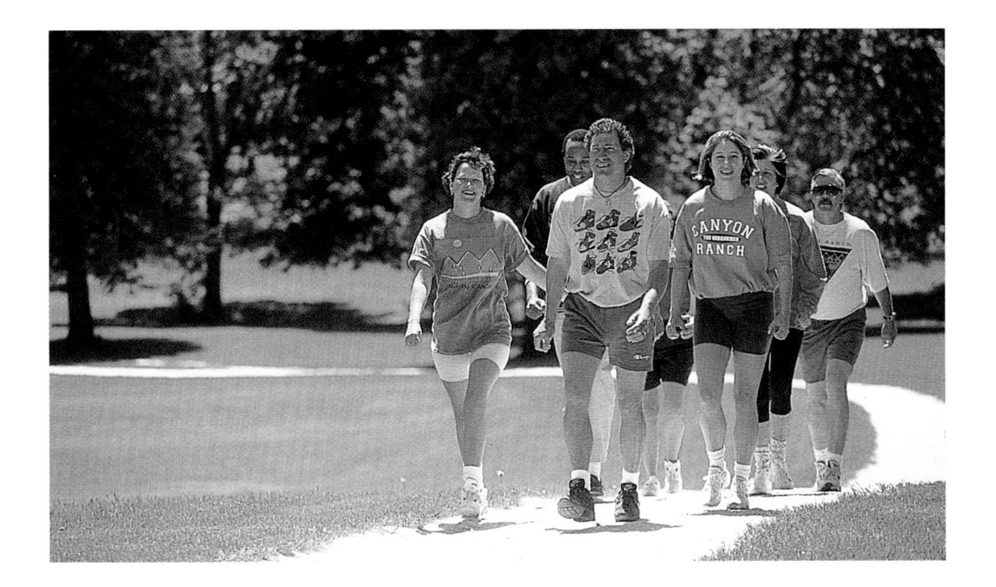

During her most recent visit to the Berkshires, Micaela was in vibrant good spirits. She is currently studying holistic healing and taking courses in nutrition and nutritional counseling, and she plans to integrate new ideas into her practice.

She has her down days, but on the whole Micaela is excited and enthusiastic about her studies and work, and about her life, which, for the very first time, is entirely her own. "My fun capacity was suppressed all these years," she reports, with a wicked glint in her eye.

She's irritated by an ageist society that keeps trying to pigeonhole her as "a little old lady who does great for her age," but judging from Micaela's story so far, there's little doubt that she'll keep fighting to be appreciated as the capable individual she is. "It's not how old you are, but how you are old," is her view.

She's essentially contented when she looks back on what was, and anticipates with pleasure and serenity what is to come. "I see where I'm going," Micaela says, "and I see a future for myself." She is inspired, once more, by possibilities.

Lessons from Life's Survivors

MICAELA, WHOSE STORY MIGHT be a pattern for living in congruence with personal values, has created her own well of strength. The way she has dealt with the hardest losses of her life illustrates one of the salient characteristics of people who live exceptionally long and useful lives: "flexibility in the face of loss." Anyone who lives to a great age has survived many losses, and there's a pattern to how these pioneers in time cope.

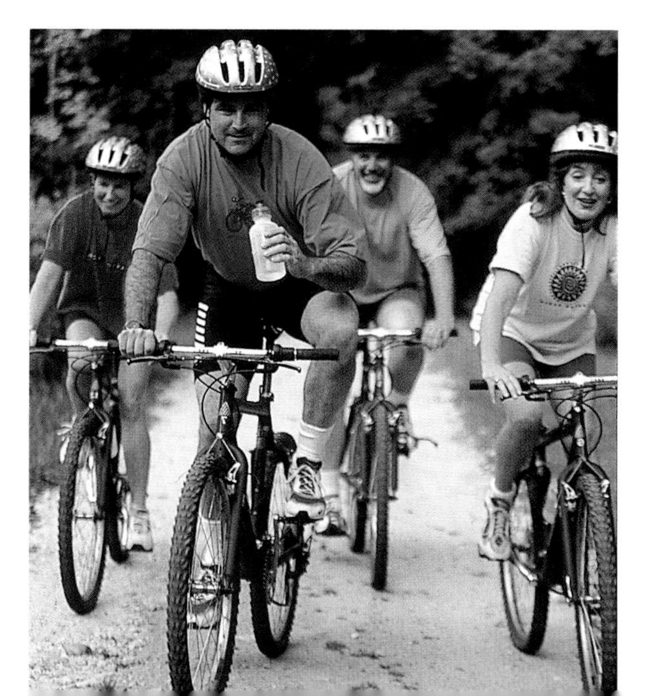

The first component is catharsis, the courage and willingness to share grief and pain. Many people prohibit themselves from expressing their sorrow with a self-devaluing prohibition: "I don't want to burden anyone else with my problems." On the surface, this familiar attitude seems selfless, even noble, but it isolates the mourner. The real sense of this statement is, "I don't value myself sufficiently to share heartache." No one with a weak sense of self lives to a great age, and everyone who grieves needs at least one trusted person who can serve as a witness to the loss. None of us can bear great pain alone without lasting damage.

The second thing that the healthy elderly do when confronted with loss is to manage their grief by not allowing it to overwhelm, or "flood" them. They mitigate sorrow by practicing appreciation—by recalling the good times gone by, the things they loved best about the people and things they've lost. Even in the midst of mourning, they feel the value of what they've had as much as the sorrow of losing it.

Third, they believe in a power beyond themselves. They value something that connects them to past and future generations. Faith offers a defined set of values and emphasizes their importance. A person who has faith and feels that he or she lives in accordance with it taps into an unfailing spring of comfort.

The last component of loss-resiliency is an appreciation of relationship: people who survive great loss and go on to live with joy are those who continue to create new relationships—to people, to the community, to arts and culture, to causes, to nature—throughout their lives. They connect and reconnect themselves to the world around them.

People like Micaela *choose* to value, and we can all learn from them. Living in accordance with our values gives life meaning, generates energy for transformation, and deepens our sense of who we are. It's how we create for ourselves a vital, unfolding sense of the cycle of life, and of our place in it.

Now and at the Hour of Our Deaths

IT MAY SEEM PECULIAR to invoke human mortality in a chapter on how to live well, and depressing you is certainly not the point. We live in a death-denying culture, in which we're all encouraged to pretend that the end will never come—for us, anyway.

It will. Believe it will, for the sake of your joy and fulfillment here on earth. You don't have forever. What you have is this moment.

Life holds no greater gift than inner peace, and to be truly at peace in the hour of our death is the best of all possible endings to our personal stories. Living in harmony with our values is the surest path to that happy ending.

3 GETTING FIT, LIVING FIT: *The Basics of Exercise Prescription*

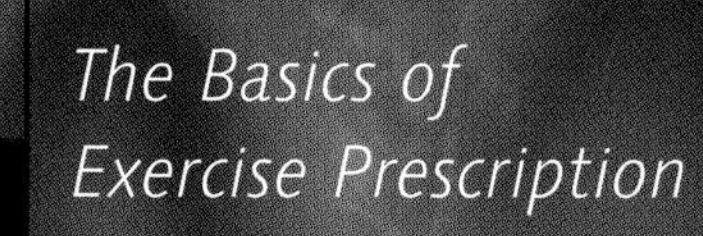

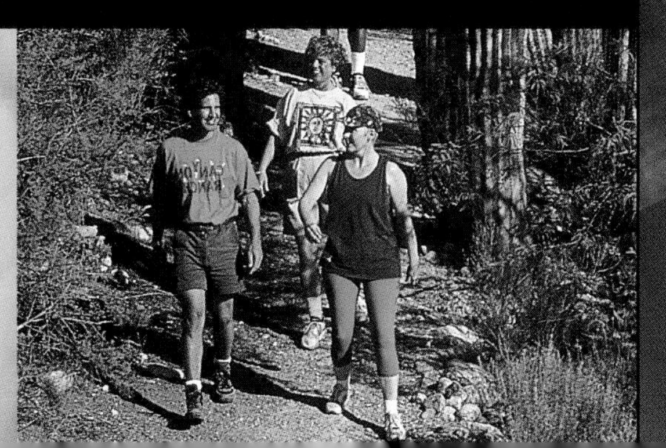

Susan came to Canyon Ranch to make some fundamental changes in her life. Not that there was much wrong with her life. She was in her late thirties, married with two children, and successful in her career; she was on happy terms with her destiny.

Nonetheless, there was one thing Susan wanted. She wanted to shape up.

Susan hadn't been athletic as a teenager, and her enthusiasm for exercise hadn't increased with age, though she gave it a go now and again. Over the course of some twenty years, she had joined a gym and gone a few times, bought equipment that she'd used for a week or two, walked around the high school track, jogged around the park. She had done a little bit of everything, though none of it for long.

She had never been overweight. On the other hand, she had never been as thin as she wanted to be and had never been toned. As the years passed, dropping those extra five or ten pounds had gotten harder. So when, one day, the scale hit a new high—13.5 pounds over her perfect-but-never-attained weight—she felt that it was time for drastic measures. Since she really didn't know what drastic measures were called for, she decided to consult an outside authority. And so she came to Canyon Ranch.

Tentatively, she tried a few aerobics classes, and, though she did sweat, she couldn't say she emotionally clicked with any of them. The fact was, group activity had never been Susan's thing, especially where working out was concerned.

Guided and encouraged by Canyon Ranch's staff, Susan struck out on a different tack. She swam a few laps in the pool. She strode along on the treadmill. She even hoisted some dumbbells and worked out on a series of strength-training machines.

And, to her surprise, she liked it.

Partially because she liked it, partially because she appreciated how she felt when she finished—pleased with herself, oxygen-flushed, simultaneously tired and alert—Susan kept at it through her week at Canyon Ranch. She learned more about strength training, and walked and ran on the treadmill, first a quarter mile, then nearly a half mile, and, a couple of days later, she ran a full half mile.

She found that no matter what exercise she did, she huffed and puffed less as the days went by; a trainer explained that her body was adapting to her new routine. To stay supple and injury-free, she took stretching classes. Traveling a bit further, she then tried chi gong, and found it both relaxing and stimulating.

By the end of the week, Susan had lost about two pounds. If Canyon Ranch had been a typical spa, this would have meant abject failure. But thanks to the guidance she received from Canyon Ranch exercise physiologists, nutritionists, and behavioral therapists, Susan knew that eating smart and exercising right would effect permanent change in her physique and in her life.

It was a beginning. Susan returned home full of great intentions, but after an initial burst of fevered exercise, the habits of a lifetime caught up and she slowed down. She didn't necessarily get up early to train before work. She didn't necessarily hurry to the gym at the end of the day. She didn't stick to eating smart and exercising right.

And she suffered for it. A month after leaving the ranch, those vanished pounds were back for a return engagement. Susan was annoyed with herself, but she had a leg up this go-round because of what she'd learned at the ranch; she knew what to do and she did it. She carved out a half hour here, an hour there, and she sometimes walked, sometimes biked, sometimes went to the gym, and kept at it. She finally committed to making exercise part of her life.

And it felt good. She felt fitter and healthier and slept better than she had since she was in school. She felt energized and, at last, in control.

A couple of months after she got home, Susan decided to weigh herself and found that she'd lost a grand total of five pounds. She'd also dropped two clothing sizes and acquired a healthy glow. After a lifetime of being a slave to the scale, she now understood, truly understood, that it no longer mattered, because she was strong and lean and was going to get stronger and leaner.

It had taken commitment and work and time, but she was there: exercise and healthful eating were part of her life. Susan was content.

Susan's story is far from the most dramatic in the Canyon Ranch annals. She didn't shed fifty or seventy or one hundred pounds or transform herself into a marathon runner or come to terms with a serious health issue, as so many guests have done over the years. Her conquest of flab and that last five pounds isn't the stuff of movie deals, but it possesses one sterling virtue: it's about real, attainable, positive life change. She had gained the tools she needed to live a longer and more satisfying life.

So let's continue, and see where it takes us.

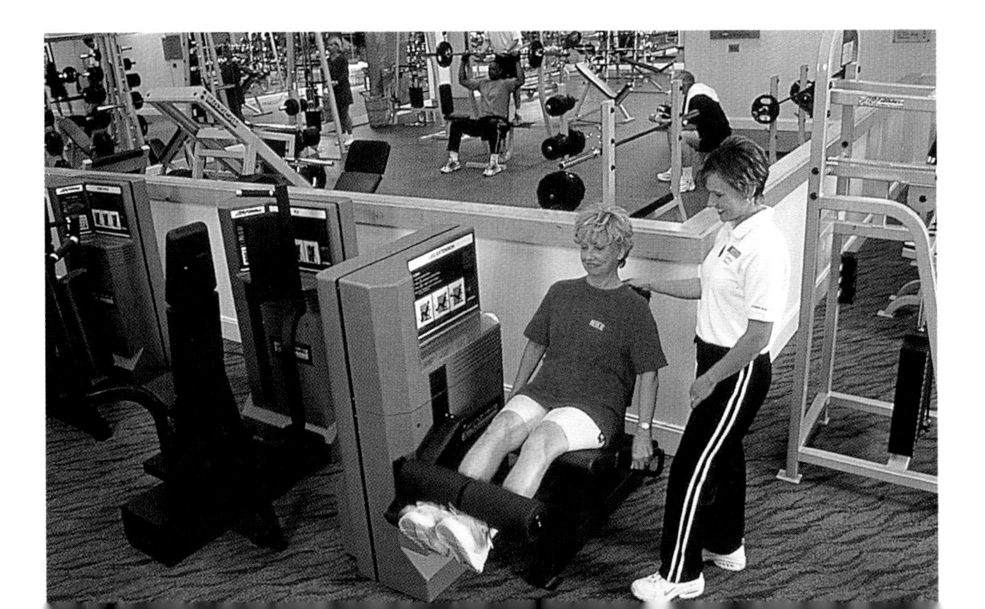

Fitness Matters

EXERCISE KEEPS YOU FIT, and being fit is a key component to safeguarding your prospects for optimal health, for taking the maximum advantage of your abilities—physical, intellectual, emotional—and enjoying your life to the fullest.

When you think about it, it's strange that we must make time to exercise. This is a need unique to just the past few generations in the industrialized countries of the world. Lack of exercise, and the afflictions it causes, affected only a wealthy few before the industrial revolution released much of humanity from physical toil. Since the invention of the steam engine, technological advances—mechanical, chemical, electronic—have tumbled forth and have allowed most of us to live without physical work. Cars, telephones, refrigerators, elevators, television, computers, all those shiny things we love so well, conspire to keep us seated most of our days.

Our bodies, however, were built to move, and without exercise they fall apart. With exercise, they flourish. It's almost that simple. "If we could put exercise into a pill, we would have our first great antiaging medication," Bob Butler, Pulitzer Prize winner and professor of geriatrics and adult development at Mount Sinai Medical Center, once told Congress.

There is no such pill. It takes will to get moving, but—this is a promise—once you get going, exercise becomes a habit and, eventually, on the best days, a delight, a daily escape from the noise of the world and the clatter of your mind.

Concentrate at the beginning on what you *do* like about working out, whatever that may be—the feeling of virtue, the freedom of propelling yourself through space, the pleasant tiredness afterward, the deep sleep. And keep at it. You can.

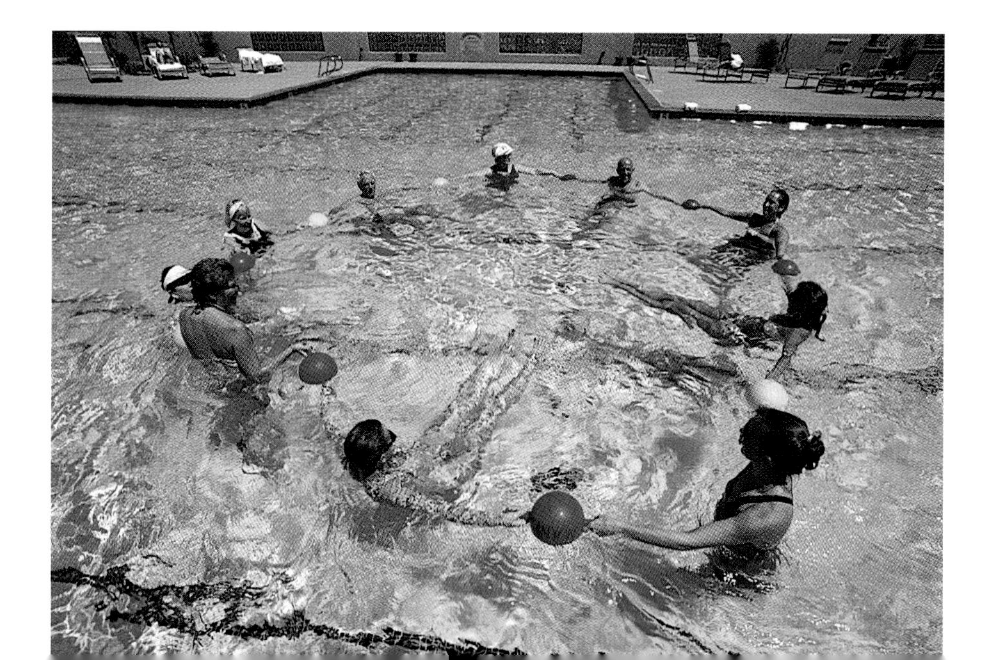

The Basics of Exercise Prescription

WHAT FOLLOWS IS A simple, versatile, well-rounded program that you can easily adapt to your needs and desires. We'll begin with what the Canyon Ranch experts call the Basics of Exercise Prescription. This chart describes three levels of fitness, and breaks training into four basic areas: cardiovascular, muscular, flexibility, and balance and agility. It also indicates body composition for each level.

The Basics of Exercise is not meant to be taken as rigidly prescriptive. Many paths to success—your own, personal definition of success—are possible. More important than following any or all of the programs is getting an idea of what it takes to achieve specific results. You need not reach the highest level to be healthy and happy. But as you read through it, take a few moments to consider where you belong, and where you'd like to belong, and then imagine yourself working to get there.

The levels are Basic Health, Fitness, and Performance. Each level imposes distinct demands and promises different results.

1. Cardiovascular fitness: Probably the most important element, it determines the ability of the heart, lungs, blood, blood vessels, and tissues to deliver and use oxygen. It also comes first because more people die from cardiovascular disease than from any other single cause. Everyday measures of cardiovascular fitness are your ability to walk, run, hike, and play.

2. Muscular strength and endurance: This refers to the capacity of your musculoskeletal system to exert force. Practically, it's your ability to lift and hold weight.

3. Flexibility: This is the measure of the body's range of motion. Flexibility is your ability to bend and twist without pain or injury.

4. Balance and agility: Balance and agility work together. Balance is your ability to maintain your position without falling; agility is your capacity to move gracefully. In other words, agility is balance in motion. Can you navigate a winding mountain trail, let alone along a tough, big-city street?

5. Body composition: The fifth component of fitness is a result of the efforts you put into the first four. Body composition measures your ratio of fat to lean (muscle, bone, and organ) tissue. Many people confuse thinness with fitness, but a thin person with little muscle has a lower life expectancy than a heavier individual with a high proportion of muscle to fat. Body composition changes over the long term and reflects the balance of exercise and nutrition in our lives.

The Basics of Exercise Prescription

	Basic Health Level	Fitness Level	Performance Level
Cardiovascular	Aerobic exercise (20 min., 3 times a week).	Aerobic exercise (40–60 min., 4 to 6 times a week).	Fitness-level training plus competition and/or interval training.
Muscular	Pilates work; Core 4* or equivalent program (1 set, 2 times a week) with challenging weight, 8–12 or 12–15 repetitions.	Pilates work; balanced whole-body free weights or machine (1–3 sets, 2–3 times a week), reaching "functional failure" in 8–12 repetitions.	Pilates work; fitness-level program plus ascending or descending pyramids; muscle endurance or power training.
Flexibility	2–4 specific stretches after activity (1 repetition of each, hold for 30 seconds).	6–10 whole-body stretches after activity and before competition (1–2 repetitions).	Fitness-level stretches plus yoga, Pilates work, and/or stretches with partner.
Balance and agility	"Act like a child": Balance on one foot, walk on the edge of the curb, "don't step on a crack."	Balance-ball training and recreational sports, including tennis, cycling, tai chi, social dance.	High-level sports including surf, ski, skate, martial arts; performance dance; agility drills.
Body composition	Men: Not less than 5%, not more than 25% body fat. Women: Not less than 14%, not more than 38% body fat.	Men: Not less than 12%, not more than 20% body fat. Women: Not less than 20%, not more than 30% body fat.	Men: Not less than 8%, not more than 15% body fat. Women: Not less than 17%, not more than 25% body fat.

* The Core 4 muscle groups are 1) chest and shoulders; 2) upper back; 3) upper legs (includes glutes, quads, and hamstrings); 4) abdominals. For the Core 4 program, see pages 62–63.

The Basics of Exercise Prescription, obviously, is just the bare bones of a fitness program; you'll fill in the details. But it can help you answer some crucial questions: Is my exercise program complete and well rounded? How fit am I? How do I get to the next level? You can use the Exercise Prescription to evaluate yourself.

Exercise and Age

AGE IS *NOT* AN excuse for being inactive. Period.

We're all getting older, and as time passes our bodies change. They can change for the better or for the worse—but change they will. What we do determines to a very great degree at what rate and in what ways our physical condition alters as we move through time.

Consider these facts:

1. The older we get, the more our lifestyle determines our health and well-being. In other words, the longer we live, the less genetics and chance have to do with how successfully we function and how well we feel.
2. After smoking, exercise is one of the most important determining factors for health—only sleep comes close—and of all types of exercise, strength training is the most effective in reversing the quintessential marker of age, frailty. On average, people lose about 30 percent of their strength between the ages of fifty and seventy, and another 30 percent per decade after seventy. Increased physical activity can halt and reverse these losses. In fact, strength training has been shown to substantially increase muscular strength and bone density in even very old, very frail residents of nursing homes, thereby radically increasing their mobility and quality of life.
3. A recent study showed that among seventy-five-year-olds, only 5 percent of men and *less than 1 percent of women* participated regularly in any sort of strength training.

What is wrong with this picture? Everything. With medical interventions and disease prevention prolonging life throughout the developing world, fact number 3 points to a humanitarian disaster—millions of very old, frail, and physically miserable people.

"If you tell me a person's age, and nothing else, you've told me nothing."

MICHAEL HEWITT, PH.D.,
CANYON RANCH EXERCISE PHYSIOLOGIST

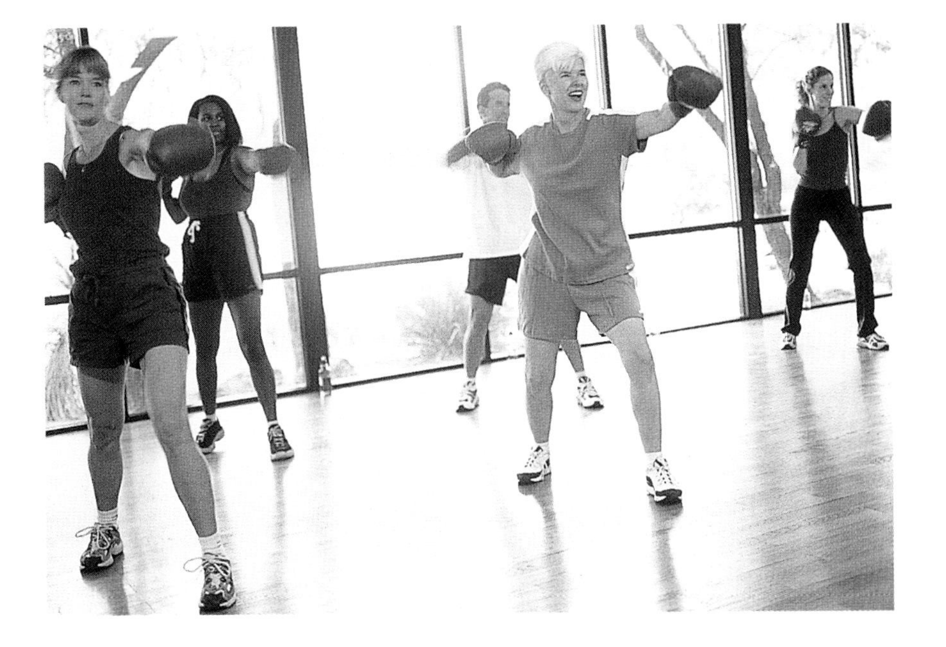

Fortunately, fact number 2 points to the solution: **it's never too late to start being physically active, and always too soon to quit.** Anyone can become moderately active today. Anyone who does will benefit. It's that simple. Advancing age itself is *never* a reason not to become physically active. In fact, it's the best reason to get moving. You have nothing to lose but your aches and pains.

It is, of course, a good idea for anyone who hasn't been active and who's just starting an exercise program that involves *vigorous* activity—sweaty, hard-breathing exercise—to have a medical assessment, and such an assessment is more important for older people. (Beginning a gentle walking or stretching program isn't going to hurt anyone who proceeds sensibly.) A good pre-exercise exam and evaluation will focus on identifying abilities and possible limitations. It's also advisable for an older person to have a bone density scan, a respiratory function test, and a cardiac stress test before starting on a program. The American College of Sports Medicine recommends cardiac treadmill stress testing (CST) for men over age forty and women

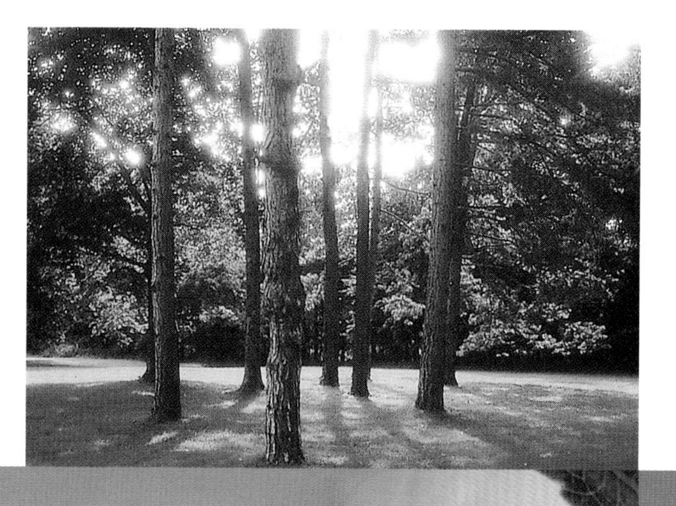

JUST ABOUT ANYONE can do some type of regular exercise, and proper physical activity helps alleviate many ailments and chronic conditions, but you should check with your doctor before increasing your level of physical activity if you have:

- a chronic disease or a high risk of getting one (if, for example, you're obese, smoke, or have a family history of chronic illness)
- chest pain or shortness of breath
- a heart that seems to flutter, pound, bump, or race
- a history of blood clots
- infection or fever, sores that won't heal, or unexplained weight loss
- continued pain or a limp after a fall
- swollen joints
- eye surgery or vision problems, or hip surgery
- new, undiagnosed symptoms of any kind

over age fifty, before starting vigorous exercise, and for all older high-risk patients with or without symptoms. People who are both over age sixty-five and sedentary should definitely obtain a CST before starting an exercise program.

The ideal, naturally, is the person who maintains a high level of physical activity throughout life. Our fitness role model ages slowly and has the great advantage of not having to start at retirement age from ground zero. Even the lifelong athlete, though, must gradually adjust her activities to the realities of less forgiving joints and tendons and slowly diminishing maximum function. She will probably feel some frustration at her narrowing choices. Ironically, the inactive person who discovers exercise late in life and makes rapid gains is likely to be more pleased with her degree of fitness than an older, lifelong athlete will be with hers. Such is life.

Safety precautions for older people are much the same as those for everyone else, but older people who have not been active for a while obviously need to be particularly aware of them.

- **If something really hurts, stop. This is the most important safety rule in exercise.** A familiar ache or a little day-after muscle soreness is one thing; actual pain is another. Always listen to pain, and obey its command to stop. Immediately.
- Be consistent. Exercising faithfully is always beneficial, but it becomes more important with the passing years, as muscles and connective tissues take longer to recover from unaccustomed exertion. A sudden burst of unusual activity—a four-hour tennis match or a massive session in the weight room—that would have cost you a little day-after stiffness when you were twenty-five will make you sore for a week at sixty-five. Older people can and do maintain high levels of athletic performance, but they don't do it in fits and starts.

WHEN ADRIAN CAME to came Canyon Ranch, she hadn't been able to get around without her wheelchair for ten years. In less than a week, she was up and walking.

A miracle? Not quite. Her recovered mobility certainly made a miraculous difference in her life, but all that had been keeping her in the chair was disuse. Her gluteus muscles were extremely weak, and her hip joints were stiff from inactivity but intact. Adrian's "miracle treatment" consisted of nothing more than neuromuscular therapy and carefully designed, intensive training in movement, balance, and strength.

Adrian had spent a decade of her life without walking because, in essence, the muscles in her hips had atrophied. If she hadn't decided to see if she could make a change, she would still be in the chair today, getting weaker. As it is, she's on her feet once more.

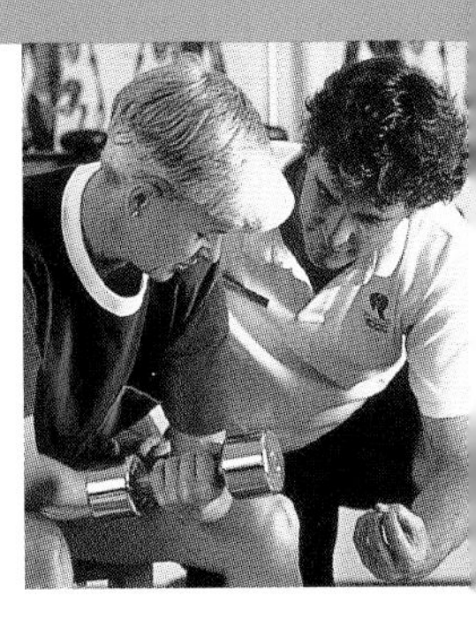

- Start slowly. Build up both intensity and length of exertion over time. Your body will adapt, and you will be able to do more if you are both patient *and* ambitious.
- Warm up with easy activity, and always stretch slowly and carefully after exercise. Flexibility is important, but you're not going limber up by pushing too hard too soon.
- Drink plenty of water, even before you feel thirsty, and keep drinking.
- Don't hold your breath when you strain: exhale on exertion; inhale on relaxation. This is especially important if you have high blood pressure.
- Don't use your pulse to monitor exertion if you take medication that regulates heartbeat, such as beta-blockers. The "talk test" (if you can chatter without interruption, speed up; if you can't finish a phrase without gasping, slow down) is simpler and more reliable.

Our final word to older readers: get going and keep going. Start slowly by walking or biking or swimming for a half hour or so daily, and gradually add light, high-repetition weight training, stretches, and balance practice. In other words, adapt our basic program to your needs and preferences. Keep adding bit by bit, branch out into other activities as you feel capable and interested. Listen to your body and never give up. Advancing age doesn't have to mean debility, and exercise is your ticket to continued well-being.

A Word About Personal Trainers

PERHAPS YOU'RE A DISCIPLINED type who prefers his own company and requires no motivation other than setting goals and sticking to them. Or maybe a good, hard look in the mirror every day is enough to get you moving. (Vanity is a wonderful motivator, and, within bounds, can be a very healthful sin.) Or maybe you've been so spooked by a health crisis that you get in motion and keep going.

If nothing motivates you sufficiently for the long haul, though, and you can afford the fees, you might consider hiring a personal trainer. A good trainer can be the best motivator in the world and a tremendous source of knowledge, advice, and help.

Realize, though, that anybody can call himself a trainer. There's no national licensing board, and while many trainers are qualified and knowledgeable, some are not. A "trainer" doesn't have to be certified by anybody to hang a whistle around his neck and advertise his services, so you need to be careful about whom you consult. The fact is that some exercises, especially in the weight room, can be dangerous unless executed correctly, and the most important part of a trainer's job is to ensure that you don't get hurt while trying to get healthier.

So how do you find the right trainer? As with so many things, nothing beats a personal reference. If you can find a trainer whom a friend uses and swears by, you're in luck.

Otherwise, look for a trainer who is certified by at least one of the nationally recognized organizations providing education and certification. Reputable groups include the American College of Sports Medicine (ACSM), the American Council on Exercise (ACE), the Aerobics Fitness Association of America (AFAA), the National Strength and Conditioning Association (NSCA), and the National Academy of Sports Medicine (NASM). Many personal trainers are certified by more than one of these organizations, which obligate their members to meet educational standards and to take continuing education courses. (Canyon Ranch requires that its trainers be certified by two nationally recognized organizations and have five years of experience.)

One final thought: once you decide to work with a trainer, don't be intimidated and don't be shy. He or she may be the expert, but it's your body, time, and money. If you're not comfortable with the exercises you're doing, if you're not enjoying the relationship, if you come to dread each session, then speak up and take charge. If you feel that you need a break from your trainer and want to work out alone, do it. And if you should change your mind after a day or week or six months, don't hesitate to sign up the trainer again.

Whatever works.

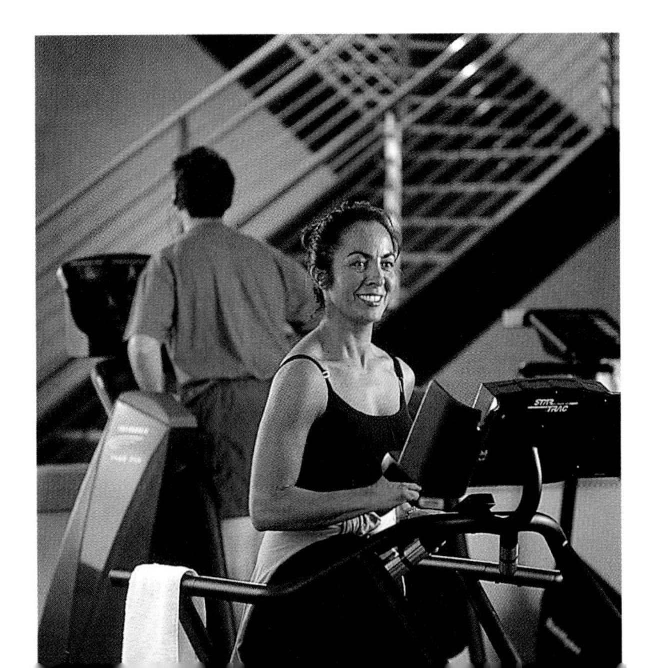

Exercise: Getting Down to It

BEFORE ANY WORKOUT, WARM up for a few minutes: walk, swing your arms, shake your hands and feet. Plunging into hard, flat-out exercise from a cold start is asking for soreness and even injury; a few minutes of mild, loosening-up activity before the main event can save you from a host of troubles. Athletes and dancers *never* start cold. A proper warm-up is also a pleasant, natural way to ease into more demanding activity.

I. CARDIOVASCULAR FITNESS

Aerobic exercise must stand as first among equals. Aerobic work strengthens and protects your heart and lungs, and, to put it bluntly, if your heart gives out or your lungs fail, you're dead.

The answer to your body's cardiovascular needs is nearly as obvious as the reason for attending to them. The Basics of Exercise Prescription chart indicates that just twenty minutes of cardio exercise three times a week is all that's required for basic aerobic fitness. Forty minutes of cardio four to six times a week will help you achieve the next aerobic level, the fitness level. To progress from there to the performance level requires longer and more intense aerobic work, plus other advanced training and competitive experience.

Once your doctor clears you to work out, you can, in time, reach whatever level you want, no matter what your age or prior experience. If you're so inclined, you can simply lace up your walking shoes, take yourself outside, hit the road, and do the time. That's exactly the ticket for many people: twenty minutes Monday,

SO YOU THINK THERE'S NO EXERCISE FOR YOU . . .

Cardio exercises requiring no equipment except shoes:

1. Walking
2. Racewalking
2. Running
3. Hiking

Aerobic exercises requiring equipment many people already own:

1. Cycling
2. Rollerblading
3. Jumping rope

Aerobic activities requiring elaborate equipment or special facilities or locales:

1. Stairclimbing
2. Elliptical walking/running
3. Spinning
4. Cross-country skiing
5. Vertical climbing
6. Treadmill running
7. Rowing
8. Recumbent cycling
9. Swimming

Wednesday, Friday, and they're done. Clockwork. That doesn't work for everyone, though. Most of us require more variety.

Boredom need not derail your fitness plan. Keep your routine fresh and fun by varying your activity. If you've had enough walking, hop on a bicycle, hit the cardio machines at the gym, jump in the pool, or go dancing.

Some aerobic activities cause you to pump vertically—like rock climbing—and others demand that you glide horizontally, like skating. And speaking of gliding, don't forget social dancing, from rock to rumba. Vigorous dancing is a fine workout and it's fun.

Finally, there's the whole realm of sports, from tossing the ball in the backyard to basketball to soccer to water polo to handball to surf kayaking to tennis and on and on. There *is* something out there for you.

Walking

Over the last decade or so, walking has become increasingly popular and appreciated. Some people—mostly runners—may still dismiss walking as a less-than-macho alternative to running, but, frankly, who cares?

Walking is great. Nearly everyone can do it without injury. Many inactive, injured, or postsurgical folks start out walking, often under doctor's orders, and eventually add more intense activities to their program, building on the base of fitness and enjoyment they've established by walking. It's true that walking takes longer to achieve the same cardiovasuclar effect as running or class-centered aerobic workouts, but it's convenient, safe, and unintimidating. If every American took what the Victorians called a daily constitutional, the overall health of the American population would begin to improve tomorrow.

Classes that can teach you to defend yourself while providing a good cardio workout:

1. Boxing
2. Kickboxing
2. Asian martial arts

Classes in which you can get a great workout while dancing:

1. Salsa-aerobics
2. Funkaerobics
3. Stepdancing

A comfortable exercise for people with joint pain and for pregnant women:

1. Swimming

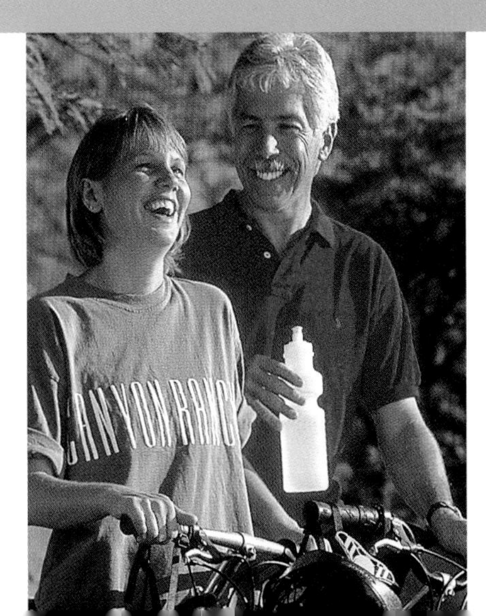

THE WALKING PROGRAM

We'll start with posture, because so much is centered on the spine. And of course you already know how to walk, but there's more to optimal walking than you may realize.

- Your eyes should be level, gazing forward except for occasional glances at the ground. Carrying the head forward puts strain on the neck, which can, in turn, lead to or aggravate back problems. Your head is heavy, and the best place for it is solidly atop your shoulders—neck long, chin parallel to the ground, crown to the sky.
- The chest should be up and open, with the breastbone leading. That means the shoulders should be slightly back and down, away from the ears. The arms should swing naturally and easily, from the shoulders.
- The abdominal muscles should be tight to support the lower back and spine. The hips are level and the pelvis is neutral, tilted neither to the back or front.
- The foot should strike with the heel leading and then roll forward through the ball and then off the toes.

Posture is important because it determines how much pressure you place on your back as you move through the world. The longer you can stand straight, the more protected your back is. That might sound a little counterintuitive—we tend to think that slouching is more comfortable—but good posture distributes weight and relieves strain. For more on posture, see Chapter 4.

LEVEL 1: Having stretched a bit and carefully adjusted your posture, walk at a slow, controlled, easy pace, somewhere between 1.5 to 2 miles an hour. The length of time you choose to walk is up to you: Basics of Exercise indicates that 20 minutes 3 times a week is what you need for basic health.

But how often or how long you exercise is not the most important topic at this point. Concentrate on technique and pace for the time being. If you are new to exercise and want a rough rule of appropriate exertion, use the talk test: adjust your pace so that you can't easily conduct a steady conversation, but don't go so fast that you can't finish a sentence.

LEVEL 2: To increase the intensity a bit, take everything from level 1 and build on it by altering arm movements and upper-body alignment slightly.

As you increase your pace to between 2 and 3.5 miles an hour, you can't keep your arms swinging long and straight without aggravating your shoulders. And if your pumping hands crossed your chest, they'd be moving in opposition to the forward direction of your stride.

Bend your elbows to 90 degrees and imagine a string in the center of your breastbone pulling you forward. Each time you swing your arm, your hand should reach up to just touch that string, without crossing the body's centerline. As each arm comes back down, drive the elbow back. This ongoing motion should describe a diagonal line up from the hip and back. The hands and arms remain relaxed to minimize wasteful expenditure of energy and constriction of blood vessels and to allow for a fluid motion that increases propulsion.

Tilt your upper body slightly forward from the hips so that you can more readily push off the ball and front of each foot. Your foot should land further in front than in level 1, and it should come down directly in front of your hip. When all this is in sync, you'll be able to increase your walking pace with reasonable effort. Even so, at the beginning and end of your walk, revert for a few minutes to the comfortable amble established in level 1. Always warm up and cool down.

LEVEL 3: At this strenuously aerobic level, focus on driving all your energy forward in one straight line, reaching a speed of around 5 miles an hour. To go that fast, you'll need to pump your arms harder and lengthen your stride until each heel naturally lands on the outer edge of an imaginary line drawn down the middle of your body.

The key to accomplishing this efficient, centered stride is to relax your hips a bit so the legs can move more freely. This adjustment can take some practice.

We're not, however, talking about anything as extreme as the odd-looking movements of racewalking. The racewalker's gait is peculiar because the body mechanics required to go much above 5 miles an hour without breaking into a jog are unusual. The racewalking stride is not a straight back-and-forth swing of the leg but a long oval that generates maximum power and speed; to achieve this motion, the racer's hips swing widely from side to side. You only have to loosen your hips a bit to achieve level 3.

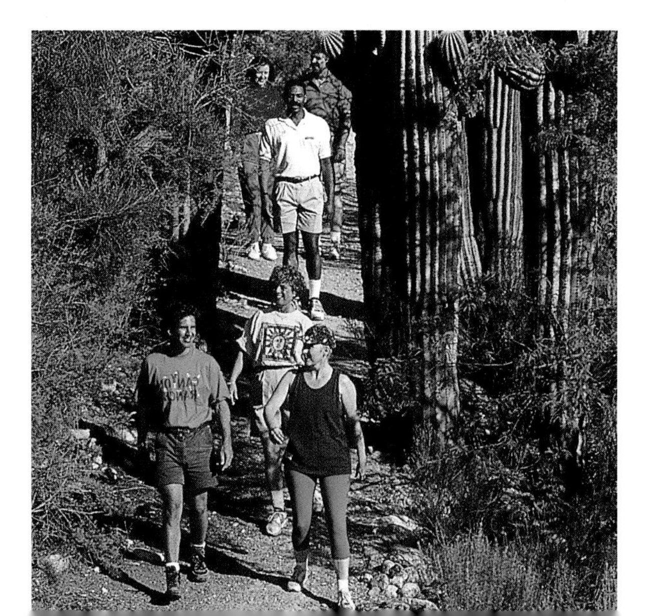

WALK ON!

Whatever your pace, form, or distance, nothing beats walking. You can do it virtually anywhere, wearing almost anything. You can walk indoors or out, uphill or downhill, in a straight line or around a track, in the city or the country, at home or when traveling. Walk to the post office or across a continent. No other activity fits so easily into daily life.

Even if walking is not your primary exercise, don't turn your nose up at it. When you're injured and can't go to the gym, when you're between meetings and don't have time to change clothes, when you can't do whatever you like best, you might still be able to walk.

And who knows? If you haven't walked for a while just for the sheer pleasure of it, you might rediscover an activity that allows you not only to exercise your legs and lungs but also to reconnect with the sights and sounds of the world about you. You can't ask much more from a workout.

II. STRENGTH TRAINING

Strength training, or strength conditioning, develops muscular strength and endurance. Increased strength gives you increased control over other physical activities and movements, helping you use your body safely and efficiently through a whole range of actions.

Strength training is now a substantial part of conditioning for almost every sport, and it's a vital component of any well-balanced fitness program. The weight room isn't just for football players any more. Track stars, for example, not only have tremendous aerobic capacity but are also extremely strong. The body is a system: everything works together.

WALKING OPPORTUNITIES

1. Walk your child to the bus or to school one morning a week instead of driving.
2. Walk to the corner store when you're just picking up a few things.
3. Get off the bus a stop or two early and walk the rest of the way to work.
4. Take the stairs.
5. Grab a quick yogurt or sandwich and spend the rest of your lunch hour walking—get some exercise and lose those office blues.
6. Be European: go for a relaxed stroll after dinner with a friend or partner.
7. Use the phone less at work. When you need to talk to the person down the hall, get up and go—a half dozen times a day, if possible. Your lower back will feel the difference.

The most common way of strengthening muscles is through weight training, either with free or machine-directed weights. Calisthenics, Pilates, and yoga, in which the body works against gravity, and pool exercises, in which the body works against the gentle resistance of water, also have substantial strengthening benefits. We shall concentrate here on weight training.

Most people who exercise regularly (90 percent by some estimates) lift weights, and most of us don't do it for our jobs, or, really, for our health. We do it because we like the way weight training makes us look. Well-toned muscles, and the lower percentage of body fat that comes with them, make us look young, healthy, and strong. There's not a thing wrong with vanity as motivation: as long as you build muscle safely and balance strength training with other types of exercise, you'll reap substantial health benefits from getting buffed.

Benefits of strength training:

1. Maintains and/or increases lean body mass
2. Manages weight
3. Increases bone density, which is particularly important in combating osteoporosis
4. Stops or reverses muscle atrophy, thereby reducing the effects of chronic problems such as arthritis and back pain
5. Supports and stabilizes joints, reducing risk of injury
6. Improves basal metabolic rate
7. Improves muscular coordination
8. Improves all aspects of daily movement

You may have heard of or witnessed a phenomenon called mall walking. Crowds of people meet to walk through air-conditioned shopping malls, sometimes for miles. Mall walking has become so popular that many malls open early to give walkers a clear field before the shoppers arrive. An interesting development is the reaction of mall bakeries, which have also begun opening early so they can entice the walkers with the aroma of cinnamon buns as they make their circuits. What could be more typically American than this counterproductive incentive to exercise?

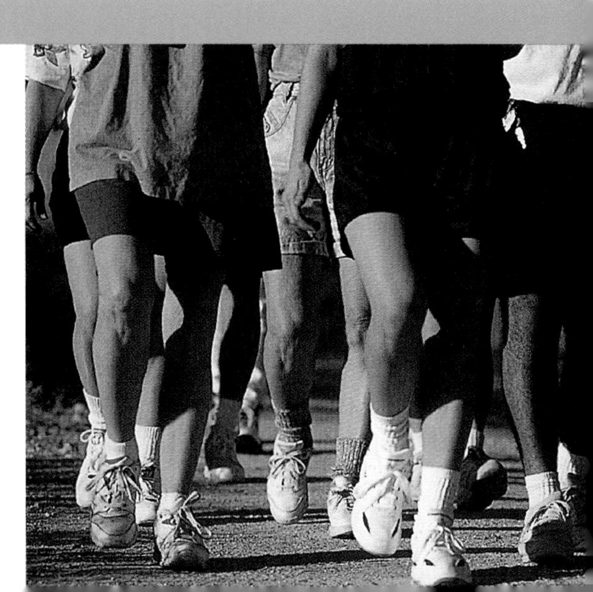

Amazing what a little vanity can do.

Weight training is also gratifyingly efficient. If you only lift weights one day a week, and do it with sufficient vigor, you'll see changes and you will benefit. Of course, we recommend that you strength train more often and get all the benefit you can.

Getting Started, Getting Strong

1. Start by warming up. Get some blood flowing in those muscles, loosen up the joints, raise your body temperature. Walk ten minutes, or jog or bike or row—whatever you prefer. It's best not to start lifting cold.

2. Consider wearing lifting gloves. They protect your hands and help you concentrate on the task, rather than on any discomfort from the grip.

3. Weight lifting isn't complicated. The movements should be done smoothly and deliberately. You can use either free weights—barbells and dumbbells—or strength-training machines. These machines, including those manufactured by Nautilus and Cybex, stack the weights and ensure that they will not move off their tracks, and feature seats and pads that put your body into the correct position. The machines are easier to use correctly than free weights, and, because their design counteracts the advantages of momentum, they're efficient.

   Experienced muscle men and women, however, prefer free weights for their greater versatility. Another advantage of free weights is that they're simple, and the same wherever you go. Once you've mastered proper lifting technique, you can work out anywhere—on the road or in your living room.

4. Before you begin a weight-lifting program, or before you add a new exercise or machine, have a professional show you how to do it and then have her check your form. Weight lifting is safe when done correctly.

5. After warming up, start your weight training session with two light sets of 10 repetitions each, one for your upper body (a chest press, for example), and one for your lower body (perhaps a leg press). A series of push-ups and squats will have the same effect.

6. Never forget to breathe. Our tendency is to tighten and hold our breath as we exert force, but working muscles need a constant flow of oxygen. Try to inhale and exhale normally no matter how much effort you expend. As you exert the greatest force, exhale; as you relax or return the weight to the starting position, inhale. You can breathe in the reverse order if you prefer: the important thing is to keep breathing and coordinate your effort with your breathing.

7. This point is key: the weight you lift should be heavy enough so that the point of muscular failure—that very distinct threshold at which your muscles can no longer raise or press the weight—occurs somewhere between 8 and 12 repetitions. Getting this right, obviously, requires trial and error. But never, ever, load on so much weight that you twist and jerk. If you can't pull or press a weight with proper form, you need to stop and take some weight off before you damage connective tissue and, possibly, a muscle. Tissues adapt over time as you challenge them; too great a challenge too soon is asking for trouble.
8. Lifting involves extending your limbs to their full reach before retracting them again. However, here's an important warning: when your arms or legs are extended, do not "lock" elbows or knees. Keep movement smooth. Locking—full extension of a joint—can result in damage.
9. Every now and again, whenever the mood strikes, change your routine. There are many ways to hit the same muscle groups: you needn't feel tied to any particular machine or move.

One addendum: Each of these exercises can be done at home with no more equipment than a bench (or couch, or chair) and some dumbbells. The addition of a barbell is useful, and of course you can go to the gym and find machines to substitute for free weights. Wherever and however you lift weights, do it right and your benefits are guaranteed.

Weight-Training Program

Any weight-training program consists of "reps" and "sets." A rep, short for repetition, is a complete stroke or action, from start to extension to return. A set is a number of reps, usually 8 to 12, that are completed in one continuous grouping.

Ideally, you'll lift at least twice a week, exercising the Core 4 muscle groups with three sets of 8 to 12 reps per exercise, increasing the weight if 12 reps don't take you to muscle failure. Rest for a minute or two between sets.

Of course, you're not limited to doing the minimum. If you want to, you can lift six days a week, alternating major muscle groups on a daily basis. (It's not advisable to work the same areas hard two days in a row: muscles need more than twenty-four hours to recuperate from intense effort.) For instance, you might work out your upper body on Monday, Wednesday, and Friday, and your lower body on Tuesday, Thursday, and Saturday.

A good set takes about one minute, so no matter how busy you are, you can make time for weight training if you make your mind up to do it.

The Core 4 Areas

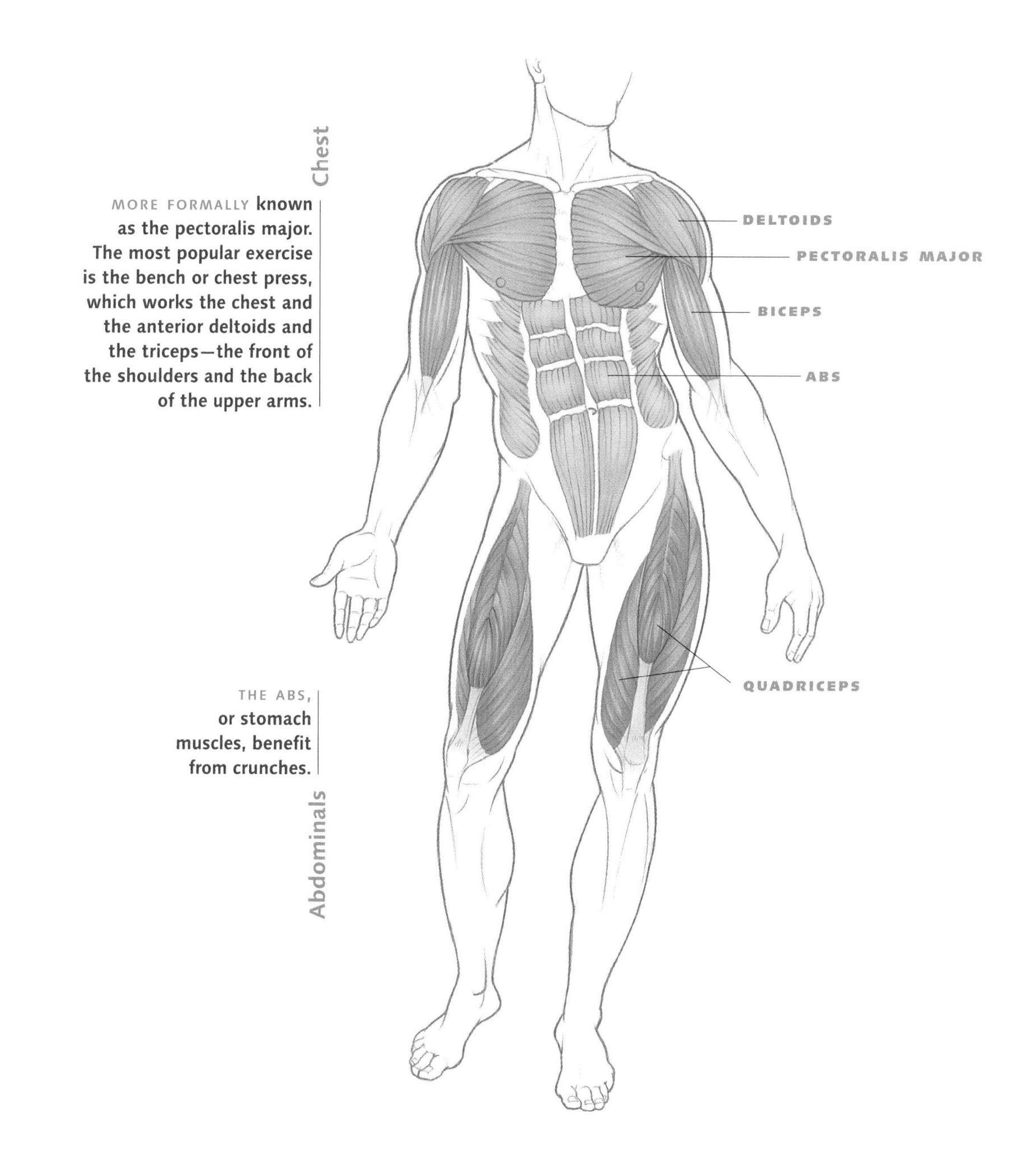

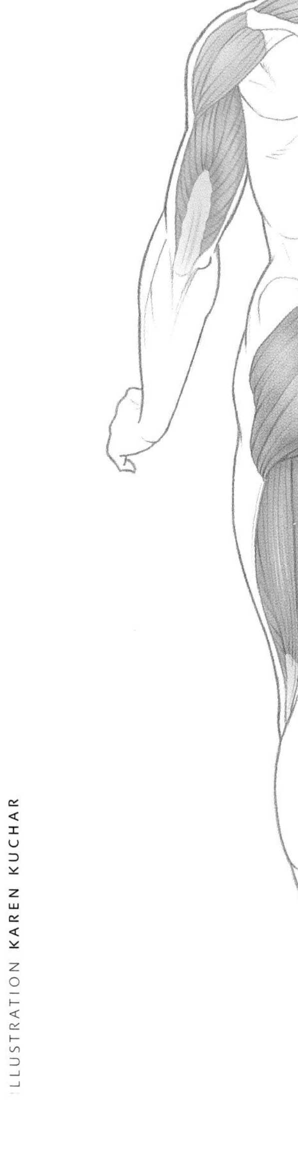

Upper back

THE LATISSIMUS dorsi, as well as the posterior deltoid (back of the shoulder).
The upper back can be worked with single-arm rows or pull-downs, among other exercises.

Upper legs

KNOWN PIECEMEAL as the gluteus maximus, quadriceps, and hamstrings;
in other words, the buttocks, thighs, and back of the thighs.
These can be worked simultaneously with exercises such as squats and lunges.

ILLUSTRATION KAREN KUCHAR

With each of our exercises, we will assume that you are using free weights. Most people who lift, particularly those working out at home, have access to dumbbells or a barbell rather than expensive strength-training machines. Wherever you work out, however, be sure to have a spotter—someone standing by to help you out—when you try something new. None of the exercises is complicated, though each movement must be done right.

1. CHEST AND SHOULDERS

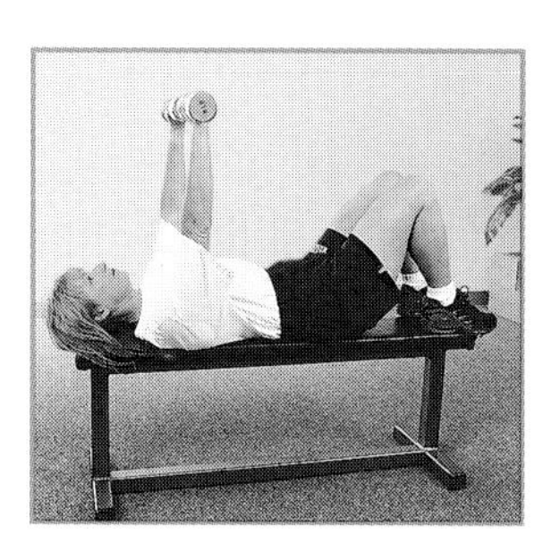

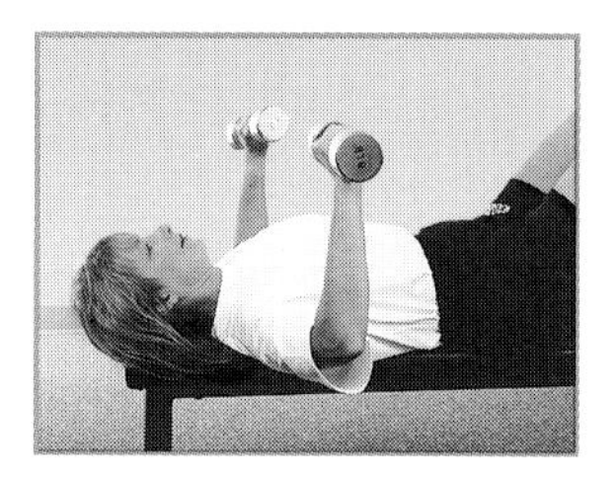

Bench Press

LIE back on a flat weight bench, with your feet flat on the bench and your head, upper back, and buttocks maintaining contact with the bench through the course of the exercise.

START with arms straight and dumbbells directly above your shoulder joints.

SLOWLY lower by bending the elbows until the upper arms are parallel to the floor. This half of the exercise, so frequently rushed as the "resting" phase on the way down to the working position, is just as important as the lifting phase, if you want to hit all the muscles in the target zone.

RAISE the weights straight up (back to starting position). When your arms are straight, the ends of the dumbbells should face each other.

STRAIGHT means straight—arms should begin and end perpendicular to your prone torso. Don't allow the weight to pull your arms toward your head or your heels.

KEEP the motion smooth and sure. Speed should be slow and controlled.

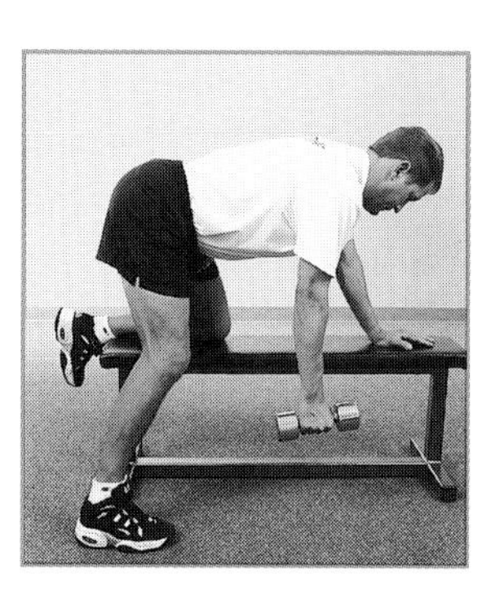

2. UPPER BACK

Single-Arm Row

PICK up a dumbbell with the right hand. Place the left knee and hand on the bench and the right foot solidly on the floor.

THE LEFT arm is straight and supports the upper body.

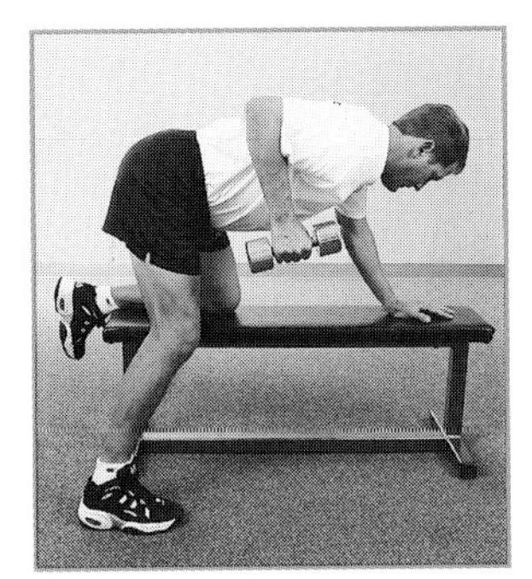

THE RIGHT arm hangs straight down toward the ground, while head, shoulders, and back are parallel to the bench.

KEEPING the body solid and immobile, lift the weight by first pulling the right shoulder blade toward the spine and then pulling the right elbow up and back, toward the ceiling. Lift the elbow as far as you can; the dumbbell should come up to chest level.

SLOWLY lower the weight.

DO ALL your reps on one side, then switch to the other side, mirroring the first position.

3.UPPER LEGS

Squat

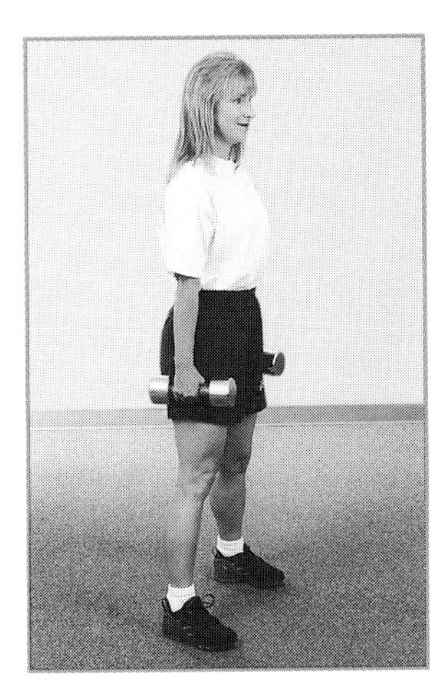

Note: If you're a beginner, you may do the exercise without weights; simply follow the form of the exercise until you feel strong enough to add them.

STANCE is everything. Place your feet slightly further apart than the width of your hips. Toes should be pointed either straight forward or slightly out, whichever is more comfortable.

BACK should be either flat or slightly arched.

CHEST is up and eyes focused.

HOLD dumbbells down by your sides.

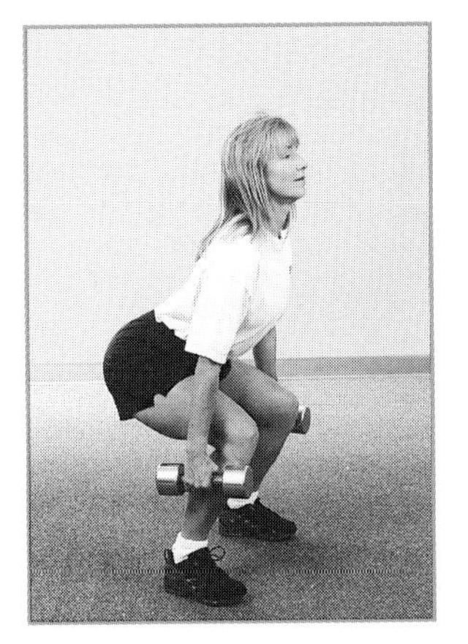

KEEPING back straight, head up, and heels on the floor, slowly lower your body by releasing your buttocks back and bending your knees. As you go down, check that your knees remain directly over your toes.

KEEP bending until knees reach a 90 degree angle, with thighs close to parallel to the floor. Keep the back tight and heels firmly planted so you don't come too far forward.

AS SOON as your knees are at a 90 degree angle, begin to rise slowly, keeping your back firm and tight, head level, and chest up.

AT THE top, make sure your hips are level and that you straighten up fully.

A SMALL modification makes the squat slightly easier: place a flat bench behind you, positioning it so that your buttocks will tap it when you reach the lowest point, providing you with both a checkpoint and a momentary rest before you straighten up. If you wish, you can also stop short of the 90-degree knee bend.

4. ABDOMINALS

There are a dozen variations of the abdominal crunch, each designed to hit a slightly different area. We'll concentrate on three basic crunches.

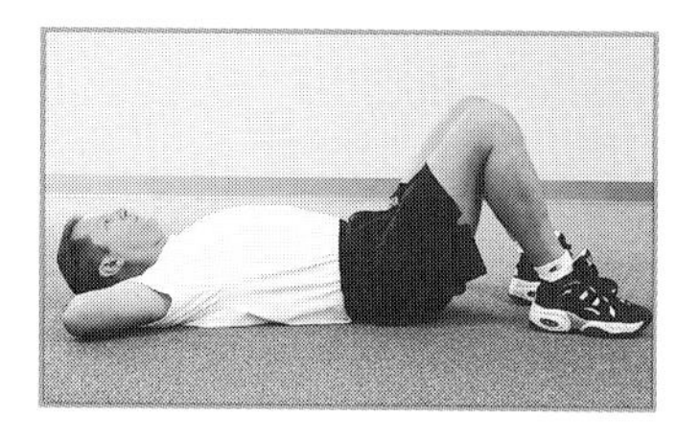

Crunch 1

LYING on your back, hands behind your head, and knees bent at a comfortable angle, make sure your lower back and the soles of your feet are in contact with the floor. Keep them pressed to the floor throughout the exercise. Do not *pull* your head up and forward with your hands—they're behind your head for balance and to ease the load on the neck.

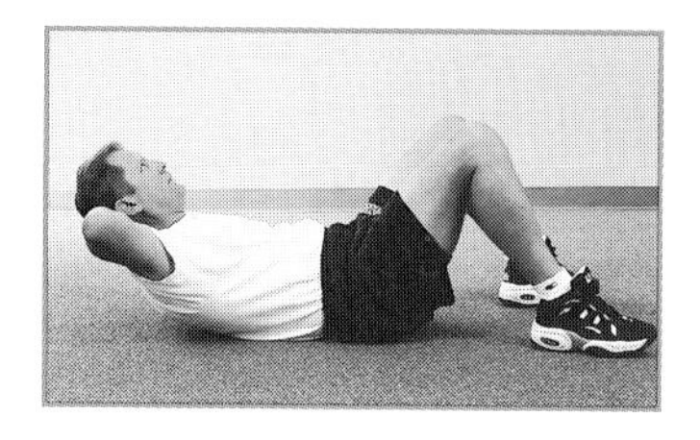

LEADING with your rib cage, eyes fixed on the ceiling, move your ribs and upper body toward your pelvis, slowly and evenly.

KEEP abs tight.

WHEN you're up as far as you can go without pulling on your neck, slowly lower.

REPEAT. Because this exercise does not use weights, you can repeat as many times as you like.

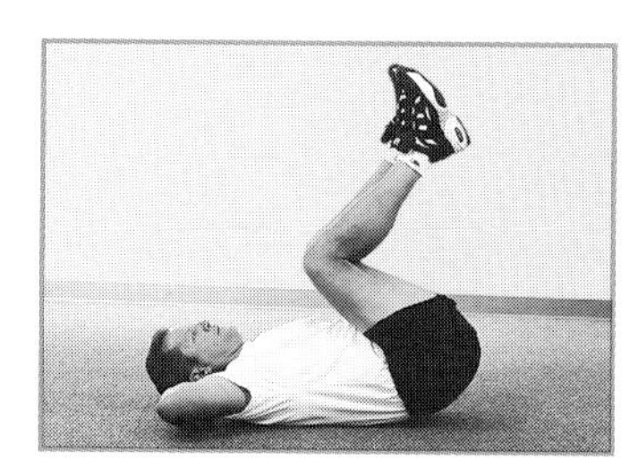

Crunch 2 (often referred to as a reverse crunch)

KEEP your head, neck, and shoulders on the floor and tilt your pelvis up.

CURL the pelvis and hips toward your rib cage.

WHEN you're as far as you can go without breaking form or feeling discomfort, lower the buttocks back to the floor. Keep feet in the air between crunches.

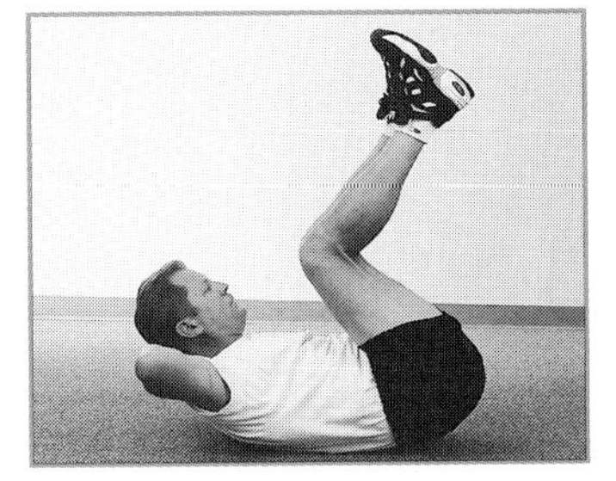

Crunch 3

THIS, essentially a combination of 1 and 2, is the most difficult crunch of the three. Before you begin, put the hands behind the head and lift the pelvis off the floor, feet high and knees slightly bent.

LIFT head and shoulders off the floor while pulling the pelvis up and the knees toward your elbows, concentrating on keeping the neck relaxed and the abs tight.

SLOWLY lower your shoulders, head, and buttocks to the floor. Keep feet in the air between crunches.

The Core 4 exercise group is that simple, and it works. This however, is just the beginning of the possibilities of the weight room.

If you reach a point at which you feel your routine is too easy, you have a number of options. You can increase the weight, increase the number of reps, or add new exercises to your routine. It's helpful to have a full arsenal of strength-training exercises at your disposal. When you get tired of one, you can switch to another.

Unfortunately, when most beginners try to use weights, they are introduced to every machine in the gym by an instructor or friend who runs them through a long, complicated routine and then hands them a clipboard and a piece of paper filled

YOU'RE FEMALE, AND you have no desire to look like Arnold Schwarzenegger. Should you stay out of the gym?

Not if you'd like to be stronger, tighter, and better proportioned, all of which lifting can do for you. And don't worry about your muscles getting unattractively bulky. You'd either have to take dangerous and illegal anabolic steroids or work out five or six hours a day to even come close to looking like a guy: women can get very strong but don't have the right hormonal mix for monster muscles.

Weight work will not make you less flexible, either, unless you neglect your stretching. The legendary inflexibility of bodybuilders is to some extent a myth; some world-class lifters can do splits. "Musclebound" lifters are those whose entire exercise lives are devoted to making muscle.

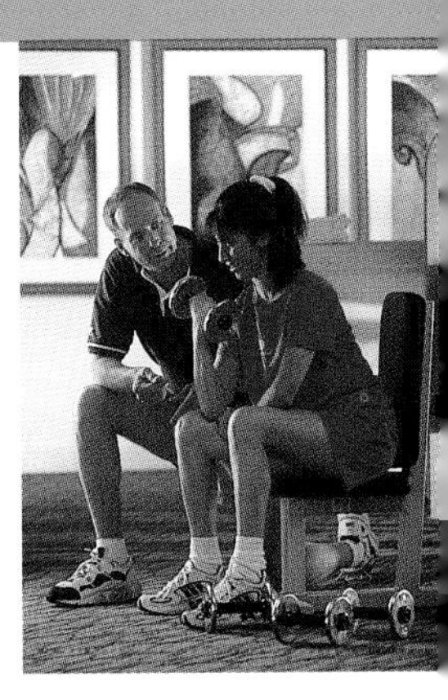

with tiny boxes to keep track of it all. This overwhelming and confusing approach stacks the deck against the beginner. We strongly suggest that you take the opposite path—start with just a few essential moves. When you're confident and motivated, enlarge your strength repertoire. Here's a nice set of four additional weight-lifting exercises to supplement the Core 4:

1. SHOULDERS

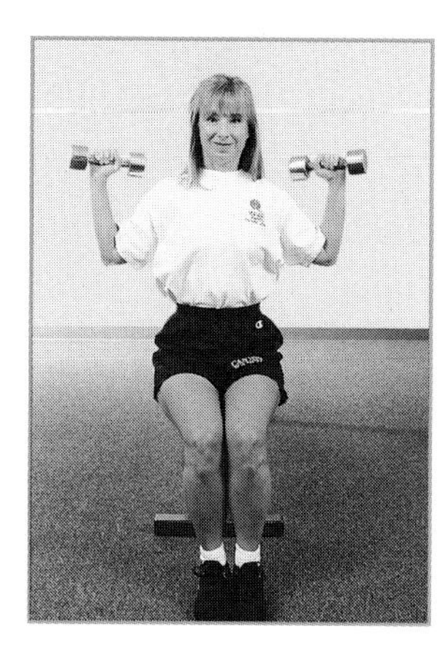

Overhead Press

This works the deltoids (the shoulders), triceps (the back of the upper arms), and the trapezius (the lower neck and upper middle back).

SIT on a bench or sturdy chair, feet flat on the floor, with dumbbells gripped in your hands, arms raised, elbows bent, weights beside your shoulders, palms facing front. A mirror is helpful to be sure that you are, and stay, square.

KEEP the back straight as you press the dumbbells directly overhead.

AVOID raising the weights behind your head: keep the exercise in front of you, where you can maintain physical and visual control.

SLOWLY bring the weights back down to the starting position and begin again.

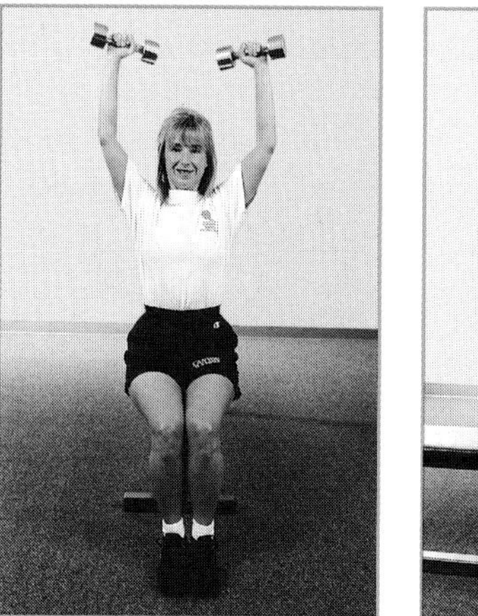

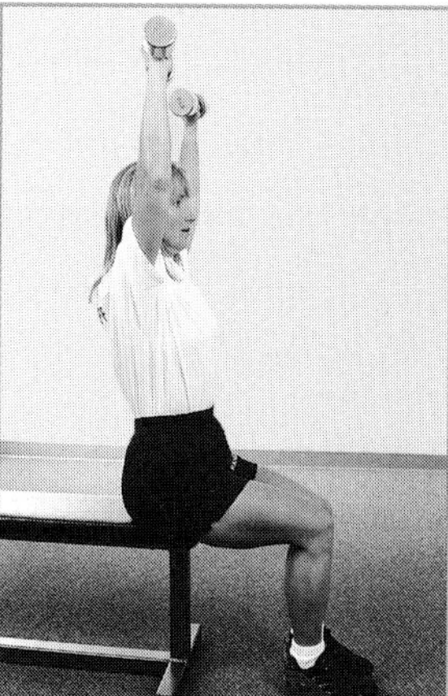

2. ARMS

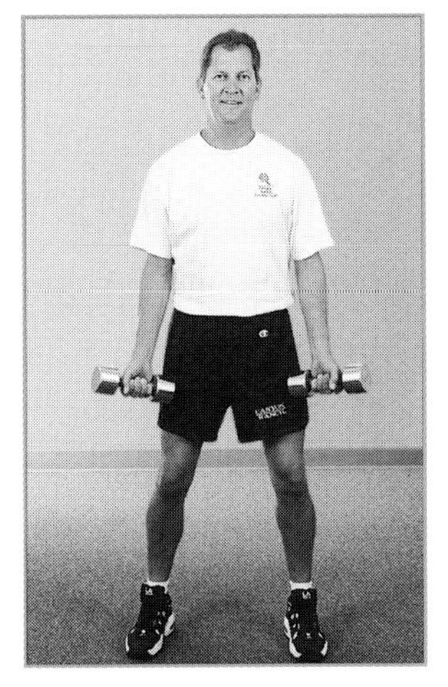

Biceps Curl

Some people—actually, some men—would let the rest of their bodies shrivel up and fade away as long as they had big biceps (those muscles in the front of the upper arm). While we can't condone this fixation, it is important to exercise the upper arm. It's simple, too.

STAND straight, feet hip width or further apart, knees slightly bent.

DUMBBELLS rest beside your legs, palms facing front.

CAREFULLY, deliberately, bend your elbows, lifting the weights toward your upper chest and shoulders. Keep everything but the lower arms immobile.

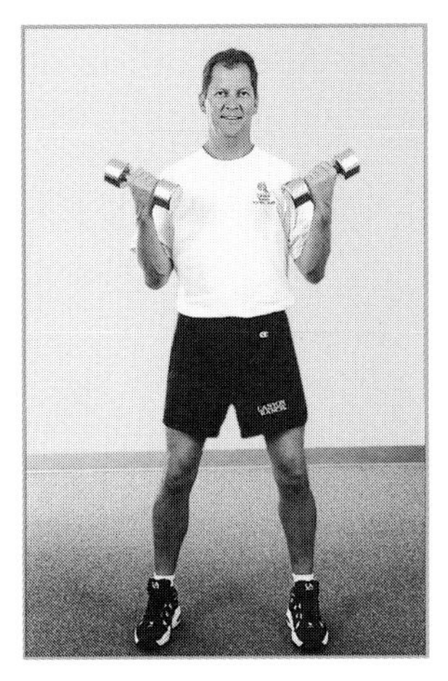

AS YOU lift, keep your elbows tight against your body—this forces the biceps to do the work. Be sure not to *swing* the weights up or down—if you let momentum and gravity help you with the movement, you won't build as much strength.

AN EASIER alternative is to lean your back against a wall, knees slightly bent, holding the dumbbells at rest on your quadriceps, palms facing out. Be sure your back maintains contact with the wall as you bend your elbows and raise and lower the dumbbells.

YET another option: Alternate your lifts, using first your left arm, then your right, and so on. This method may help you maintain your balance and will reduce the chance of your back arching as you lift. Do not *jerk* the weights—your wrists and elbows will pay the price if you do.

3. TRICEPS

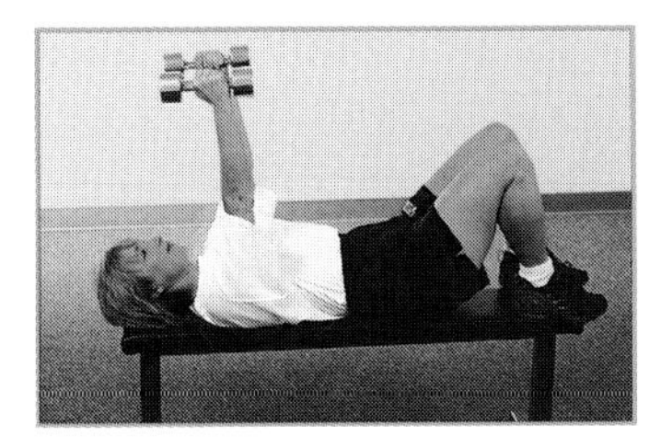

Triceps Press

LIE back on the bench with feet flat.

HOLDING a dumbbell in each hand, lift the weights directly over the shoulders. Arms are straight and palms face in.

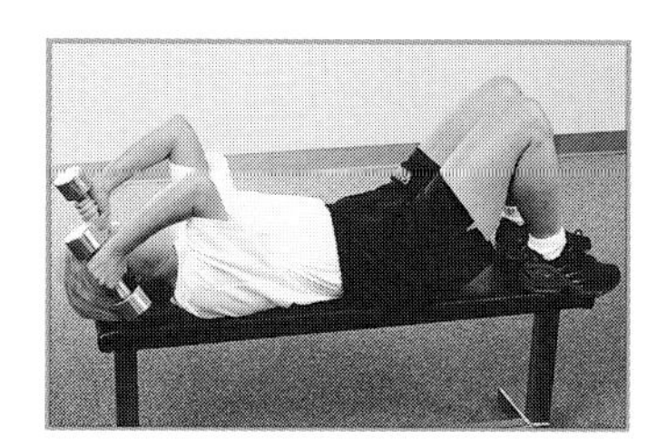

KEEP your upper arms still and nearly perpendicular to your body while you slowly lower the weights to either side of your head by bending the elbows.

STRAIGHTEN arms back up to the starting position.

4. BACK

Back Extension

This move targets several key muscles—the spinal erectors (lower back), gluteus maximus (buttocks), and hamstrings (back of the thighs).

Note: If you have a disk problem in your back, don't do this. See Chapter 4 for exercises for sore or weak backs.

LIE facedown on the floor. Bend your elbows and rest your forehead on the backs of your hands.

AS ONE piece, in a unified action, lift your head, arms, and chest, as well as your legs and feet, off the floor.

LEGS stay straight, eyes down, elbows remain out to the sides. The back is slightly arched.

HOLD this position for two to five seconds, then carefully lower your body to the floor. Don't collapse on the ground. Instead, touch lightly, then repeat.

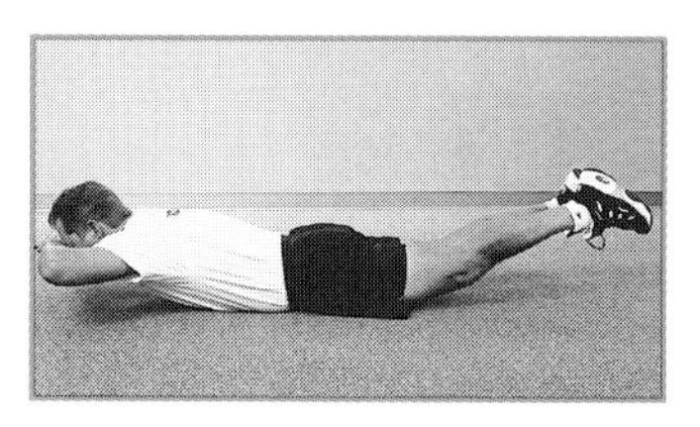

AN EASIER version starts with arms and legs reaching out on the floor as you lie facedown. Lift one arm and the opposite leg off the floor simultaneously while lifting the face off the floor and looking down. (Do *not* crane the neck.) Hold for two to five seconds. Keeping the head up and neck parallel to the floor, lower the arm and leg and repeat with the other arm and leg. Do 8–12 repetitions.

These, along with the Core 4, are eight of the most popular strength-training exercises. Do these every other day and you'll have the bases covered. As with anything else, what you get out of a workout is what you put into it. The more you do in the weight room, the more changes you'll see and feel.

There are hundreds more weight-training moves, using both free weights and machines. If you have access to both free weights and machines, try them all and see what you like best. Explore. Have fun. Keep pumping.

Other Strength-Training Techniques

Weight training isn't the only way to get stronger; other techniques are also extremely effective.

1. Tubing. In tubing, you use simple elastic cords resembling surgical tubes to provide resistance as you go through a series of specially designed movements. The more you pull, the more resistance you get. The circumference and density of the tube determine the starting level of resistance.

2. Water work. Water is heavy, and as we move through it, we contend with gentle but encompassing resistance. Exercise in the water is a great way to build muscle with virtually no chance of damage from impact or sudden strain. (It also improves balance.) Special equipment—water dumbbells, flotation devices, and paddles—may help you get the results you'd like.

3. Gravity-based body movements (calisthenics). These include push-ups, pull-ups, squats, and crunches—a sequence that works the entire Core 4. In these exercises, which you undoubtedly remember from PE or camp, the body itself is the weight lifted. Calisthenics might seem out of date, displaced by gleaming metal machines with exotic names. The fact is that they're still challenging exercises, with the advantage of perfect simplicity. Calisthenics aren't wildly amusing, and they certainly aren't glamorous, but they can give you a thorough workout using no equipment at all. Keep them in mind, particularly when you travel.

III. FLEXIBILITY

Maximizing flexibility makes everyday physical activities easier and more pleasurable. It also contributes to a general sense of well-being: flexibility work is a vital component of stress-reduction plans. A more flexible body is a more comfortable body, and we feel better emotionally when our muscles are relaxed and our joints bend freely. Because stretching reduces tension in the muscles, it leaves the body feeling more relaxed. This state of relaxation is not merely pleasant: relieving tension in the neck, for instance, relaxes tight shoulders and helps alleviate tenacious pain in the lower back. If you have a few minutes, you can loosen and relax your entire body.

Flexibility is the area of physical training in which you'll see the most rapid improvement once you start to work. You can work on flexibility every day, throughout the day. At your desk, in front of the TV, standing in line, you can stretch. You don't need a special place, or clothes, or equipment to become more flexible. You won't even have to work up a sweat.

Achieving flexibility means stretching, and stretching exercises come in many forms. Stretching is good for everyone, but it's crucial for people who are just beginning to get into shape. If you're flexible, you can avoid many types of injury: the more easily the body adapts to unexpected or difficult movements, the less trauma it suffers.

Stretching Program

Here's a well-rounded selection of favorite stretches from Canyon Ranch, divided for convenience into standing and floor versions of the same routine. Either version will leave you stretched from top to toe. We recommend stretching immediately **after** all exercise sessions, while muscles are still warm. Stretching at other times when you are warm—when you get up in the morning or after a warm bath, for example—can also be beneficial.

Do not bounce, and do not force the stretch. Forcing can cause injury. Hold each stretch for ten to thirty seconds. Relax the muscle group being stretched and "breathe into" the stretch, taking your stretch further with each exhalation, if possible. As stretches become easy, increase your range of motion. Hold each stretch to the point of **slight discomfort only**—no more.

STANDING STRETCHES

1. Calves

STAND upright facing a wall four or five steps away.

PUT hands on the wall and bend the left knee, keeping the right leg straight and right heel planted.

LEAN into the wall, keeping the right heel down and feet parallel. Try to lean as a "plank," keeping head, neck, spine, pelvis, and right leg in line.

HOLD, then switch sides and repeat.

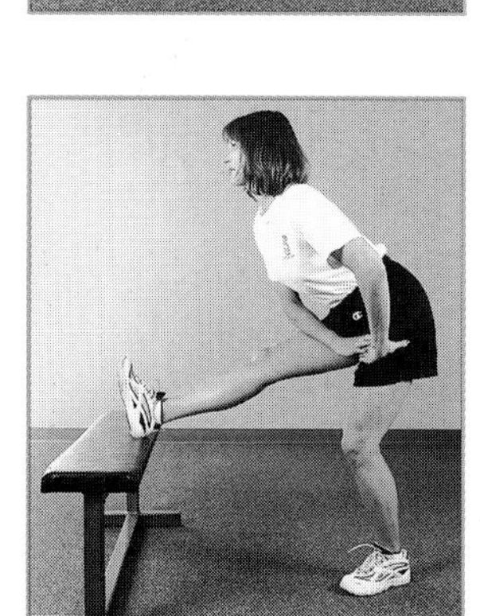

2. Hamstrings

STANDING upright, place the right foot on a low step or bench.

PLACE your hands on the left thigh. Keeping your back straight, bring your chest toward the right thigh.

HOLD.

SWITCH and repeat.

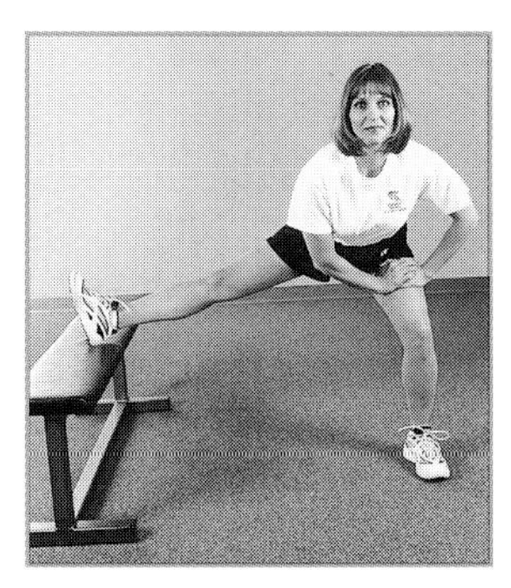

3. Hip adductors

START with the right foot on a bench or step. Turn your whole trunk, from the hips, to the left.

EXHALE, flex the standing leg so the knee is bent, push hips back, bending forward slightly at the hips. You should feel the stretch on the inside of the right thigh.

SWITCH and repeat.

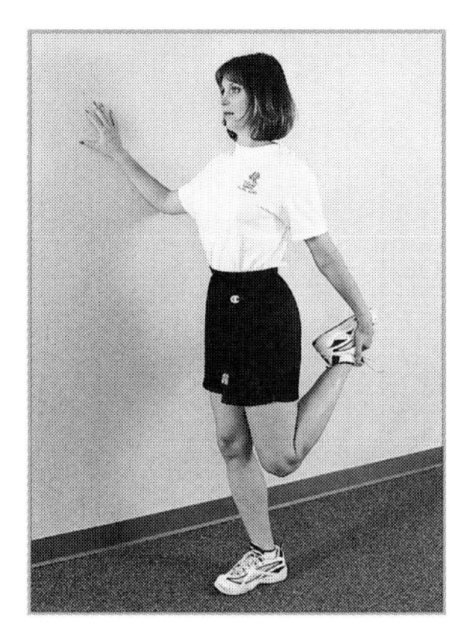

4. Quadriceps

STAND upright with right hand against the wall for support.

BEND the left knee and raise the left foot behind you, toward the buttocks.

BEND the right leg slightly and keep the knees in line with one another.

EXHALE, and reach down behind you, grasping the left foot or ankle.

SWITCH and repeat.

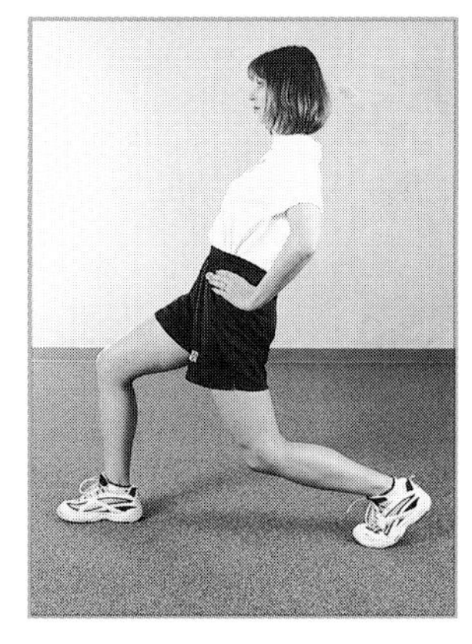

5. Hip flexors

STAND upright, right foot in front and left foot about two feet back, heel lifted.

KEEPING knees pointed forward, bend both knees.

PLACE hands on your hips.

EXHALE, then gently and slowly lean back while pushing the hips forward.

SWITCH and repeat.

6. Lower back

STAND upright with your legs straight and your hands on your thighs.

BEND both knees and lean forward from the hips.

EXHALE, and round up the back while tucking your tailbone under the pelvis.

LOOK down at your navel, then return to a flat-back position before standing upright.

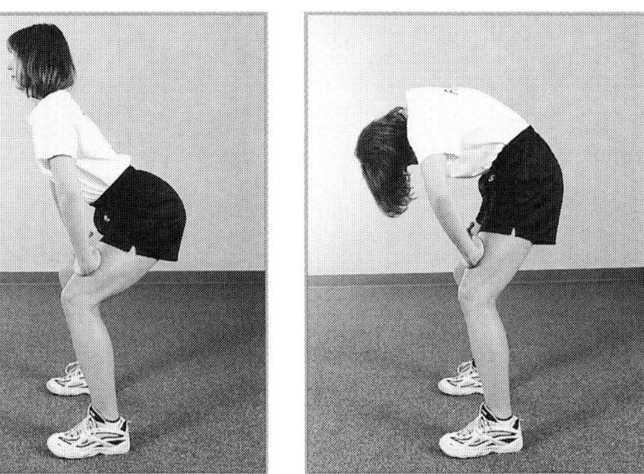

7. Sides of trunk

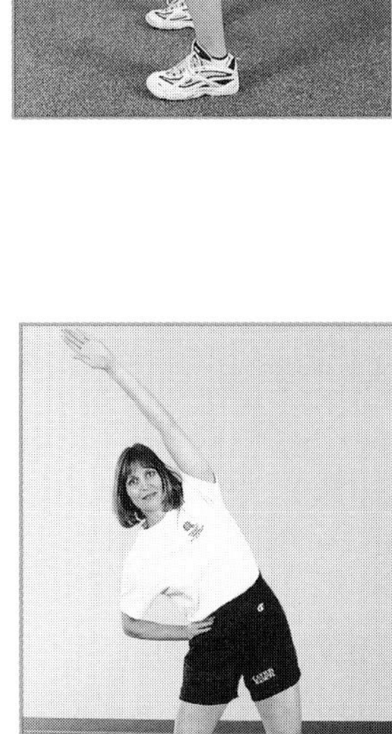

STAND upright with your feet slightly apart.

REACH the left arm straight up.

PLACE the right hand on the right hip and bend the whole upper body to the right. Drop the right ear toward the right shoulder.

CONTINUE reaching long with the left arm as the body curves to the right. Hold.

REPEAT on other side.

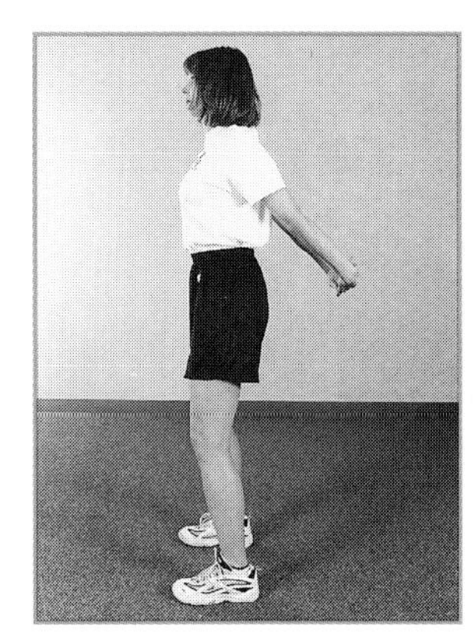

8. Chest

STAND upright with your feet slightly apart and hands interlocking behind you.

EXHALE, straighten, and lift your arms, keeping your head and chest up, maintaining good posture.

KEEP lifting until you feel a stretch in the shoulders, chest, and the front of the arms.

9. Chest

STAND upright with your hands behind your head.

EXHALE and pull your elbows back. Keep your head neutral; don't allow the hands to push it forward.

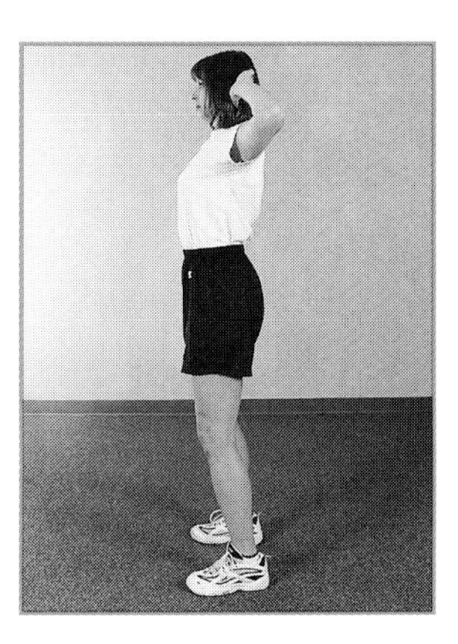

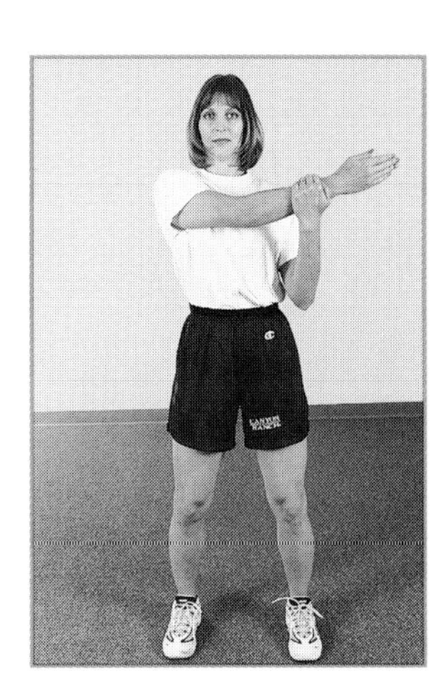

10. Shoulders

STAND upright. Take the right arm straight across the body with the palm facing back.

USE the left hand to gently press the arm further back into the body.

KEEP the right shoulder down.

REPEAT with the other arm.

11. Triceps

STAND with feet hip width apart and knees slightly bent.

PLACE the left hand behind your neck, reaching the hand toward your opposite shoulder, elbow pointing up.

PLACE the right hand on the flexed elbow and slowly pull the elbow across and behind your head until you feel a stretch in the triceps.

EXHALE and gently bend your trunk to the right until you feel the stretch down the left side of your body.

HOLD.

SWITCH and repeat.

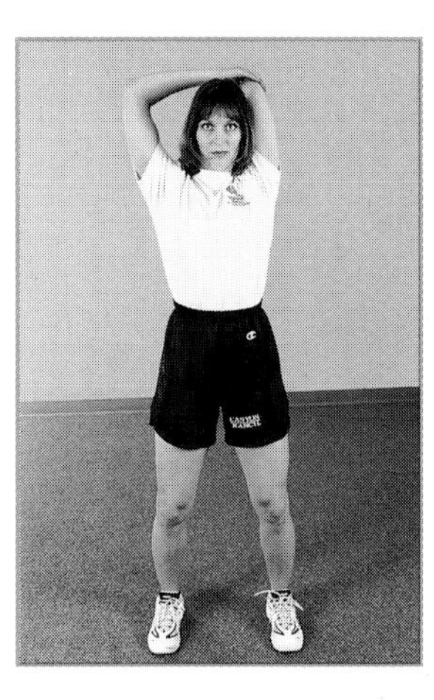

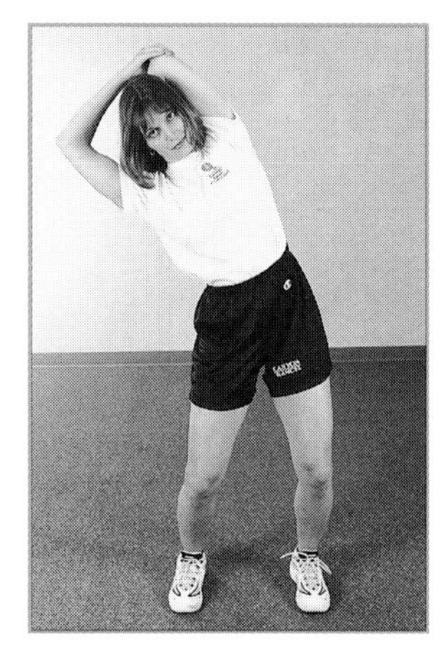

12. Neck

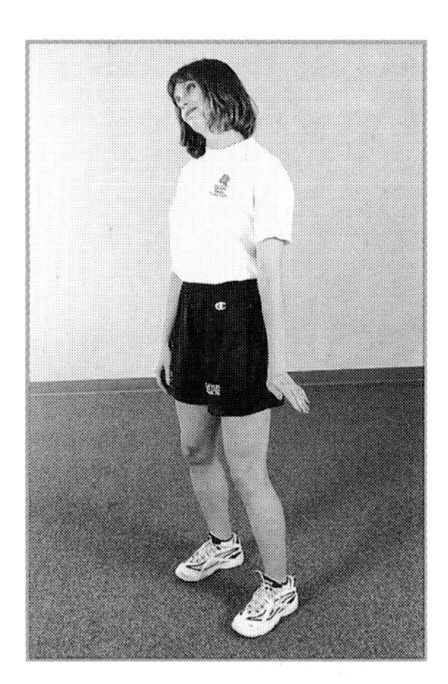

BEGIN from a standing position, arms hanging loose by your sides.

EXHALE as you slowly tilt your head to the right—right ear dropping toward right shoulder—while pushing the palm of the left hand toward the floor. Hold.

SLOWLY rotate your head straight forward, exhaling again. Hold.

SLOWLY continue rotating the head as you exhale until your left ear is dropped toward your left shoulder.

PUSH the right palm to the floor. Hold.

Do not rotate your head backward.

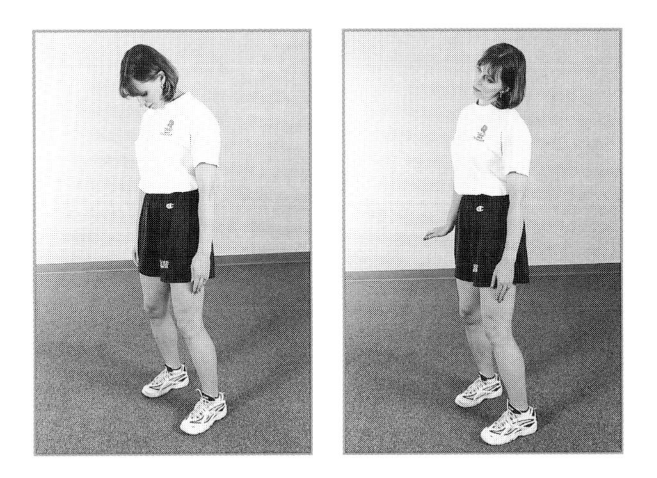

FLOOR STRETCHES

People who are less flexible may be more comfortable doing their stretching on the floor. A mat and a towel or stretch strap come in handy for these.

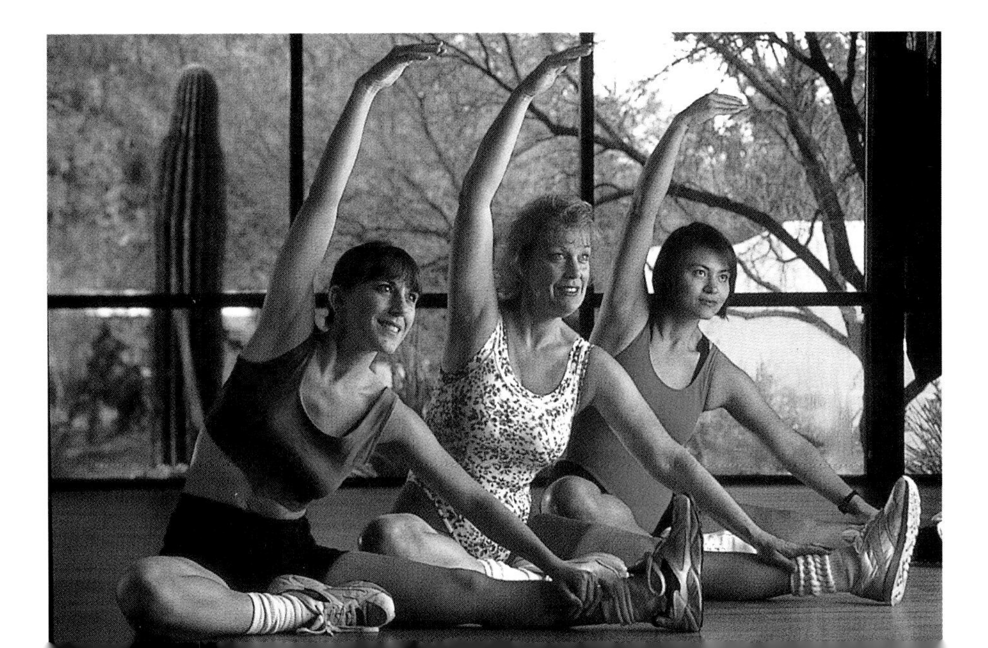

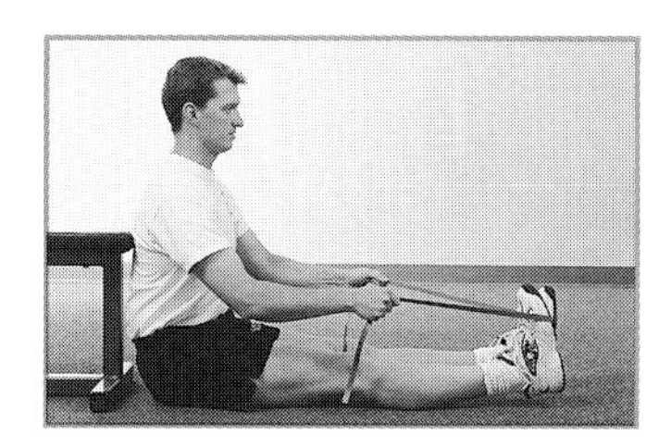

1. Calves

SIT upright on the floor with back against a wall or bench, legs straight out in front of you.

IF YOU can't reach the bottom of your foot with your hand (and most people can't), loop a towel or stretch strap around the ball of the right foot.

KEEPING your spine long and upright, exhale while gently pulling the toes toward you, leg straight, heel on the floor.

SWITCH and repeat.

ALTERNATIVE: Lift your foot a few inches off the floor for a more intense stretch.

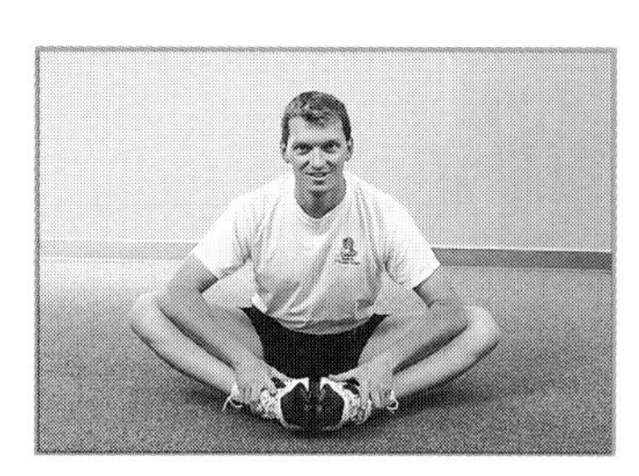

2. Hip adductors

SIT upright on the floor.

BEND your knees and bring the soles of your feet together, at the same time pulling the heels toward the groin.

PLACE your elbows on the inside of your thighs.

EXHALE and slowly press your thighs toward the floor, knees outward.

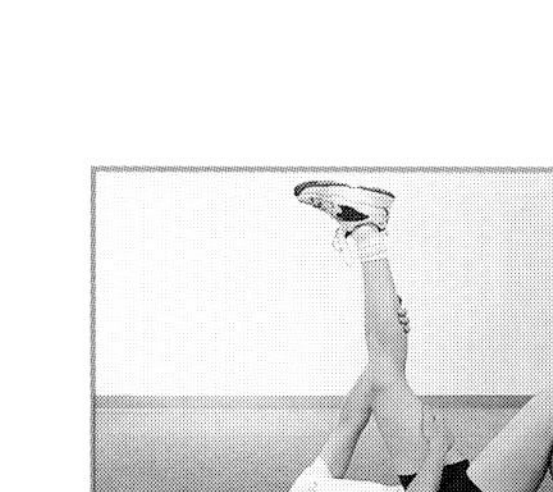

3. Hamstrings

LIE on your back with knees bent and feet flat on the floor.

RAISE the left leg, aiming the foot toward the ceiling. Loop a stretch strap behind the ankle or hold the back of the leg while keeping your shoulders, neck, and head on the floor. Keep the tailbone and lower back flattened to the floor.

STRAIGHTEN the knee without locking the joint.

PULL until you feel mild tension in the back of the thigh and hold.

RELEASE left leg, putting the foot flat on the floor, and repeat on the other side.

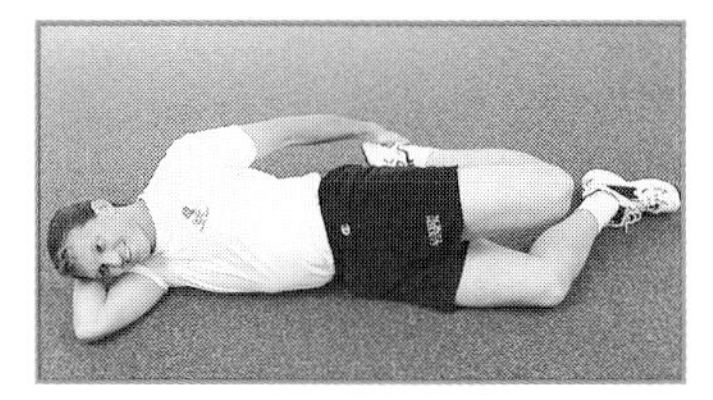

4. Quadriceps

LIE on your right side.

BEND your left knee and swing your left arm back to grasp your ankle behind you. (Use a strap if you can't reach the foot.)

KEEP the right leg bent to help you balance. Push your left leg out against your hand to intensify the stretch without straining the knee.

SWITCH.

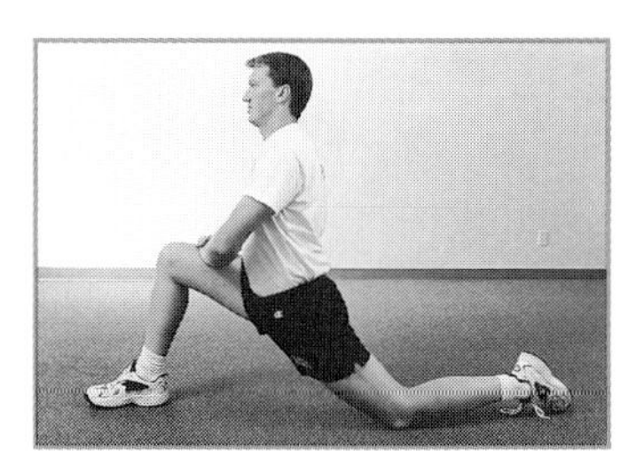

5. Hip flexors

KNEEL on the floor.

PLACE the right foot on the floor in front of you. Toes point forward and the heel is planted.

BEND into the right knee, pushing the right hip forward.

PLACE your hands on your thighs or on the ground.

DON'T let the right knee go further forward than the toes.

SWITCH.

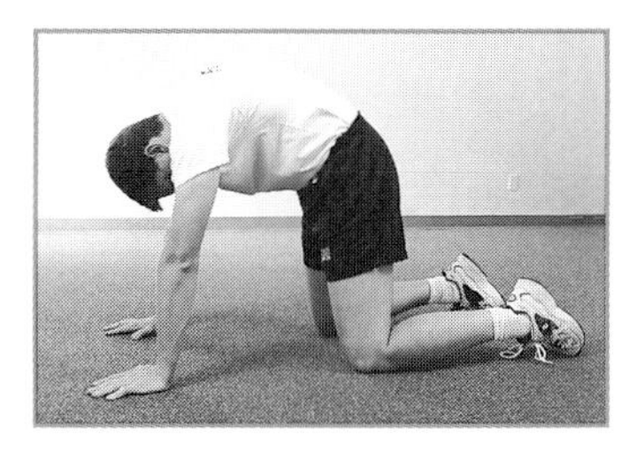

6. Lower back

KNEEL on all fours with your toes pointing backward.

EXHALE, then contract the abdominals and round the back up. Hold.

RELAX the abs and return to a flat-back position.

Note: Keep shoulders down and back (away from the ears) throughout sequence.

Alternative: **LIE** flat on your back with knees bent, feet on the ground.

PULL one knee and then the other to the chest.

HUG them as tightly as you can without causing knee pain. Hold.

RELEASE. Lower one foot at a time back to the starting position.

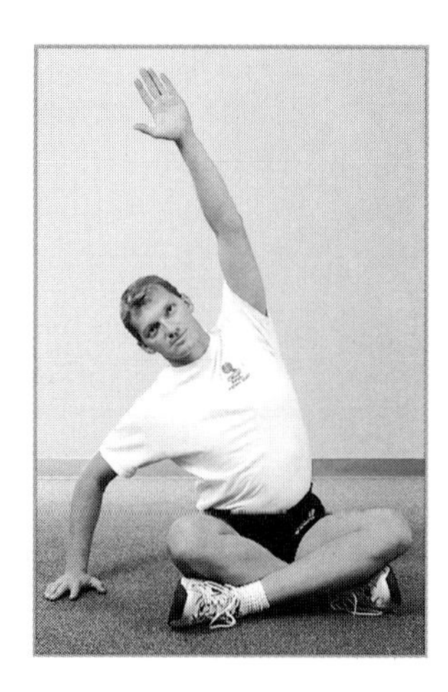

7. Sides of trunk

SIT upright on the floor with your legs crossed.

REACH your left hand to the ceiling, lengthening your left side.

EXHALE and bring your right hand to the floor while leaning your body to the right side and continuing to reach your left arm long.

KEEP both buttocks flat on the floor.

SWITCH.

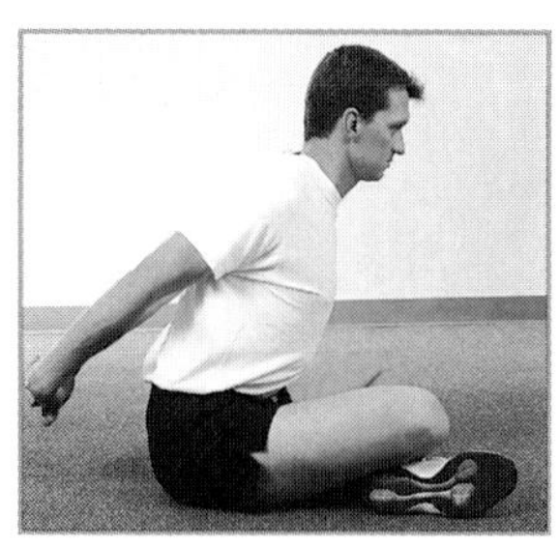

8. Chest

SIT upright with arms straight behind you and fingers interlocked.

LIFT hands toward the ceiling, leaning forward from the hips as necessary.

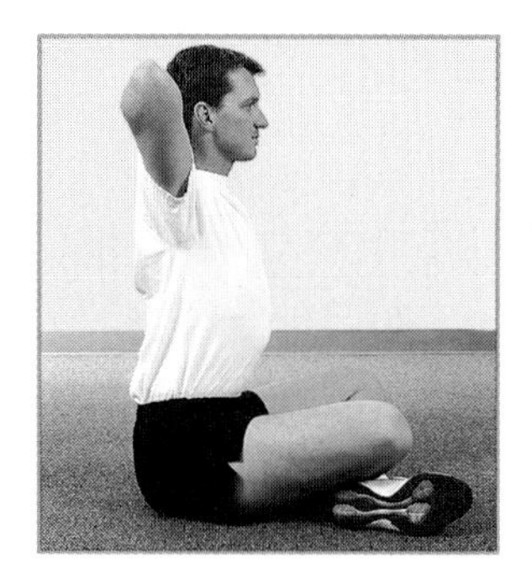

9. Chest

SIT upright with your hands behind your head. You may lean forward from the hips if that's more comfortable.

EXHALE and pull your elbows back.

DO NOT allow the head to move forward.

10. Shoulders

TAKE the right arm straight across the body with the palm facing back.

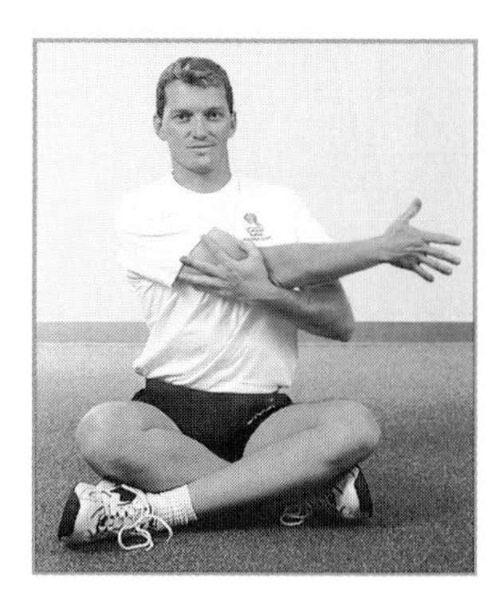

USE the left hand to gently press the arm further back into the body.

KEEP the right shoulder down.

REPEAT with the other arm.

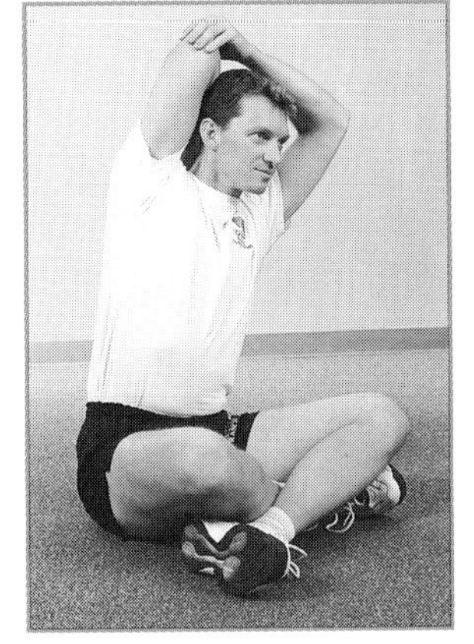

11. Triceps

SIT upright with the right arm flexed and raised overhead.

PLACE the right hand behind your neck, reaching the hand toward your opposite shoulder, elbow pointing up.

PLACE the left hand on the flexed elbow and slowly pull the elbow across and behind your head until you feel a stretch in the triceps.

EXHALE and gently bend your trunk to the left until you feel the stretch down the right side of your body. Keep the neck neutral.

HOLD.

SWITCH and repeat.

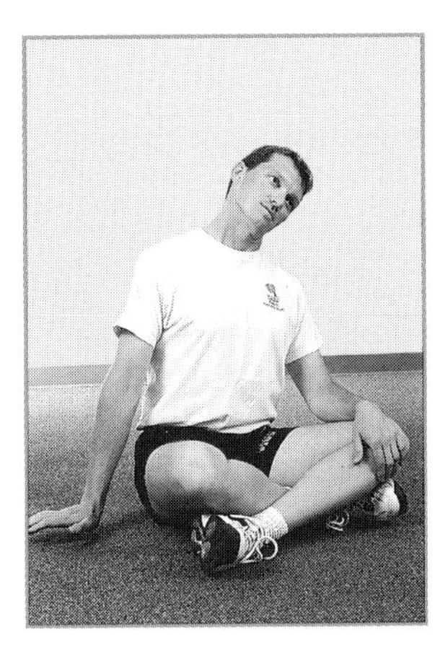

12. Neck

SIT in a comfortable position, arms by your sides.

EXHALE as you slowly tilt your head to left side—left ear dropping toward left shoulder—while pushing the palm of the right hand toward the floor. Hold.

SLOWLY rotate your head straight forward as you exhale. Hold.

SLOWLY continue rotating the head as you exhale until your right ear is dropped toward your right shoulder.

PUSH the left palm to the floor. Hold.

Do not rotate the head back.

Do either the floor or standing routine regularly and you'll find yourself very well stretched indeed.

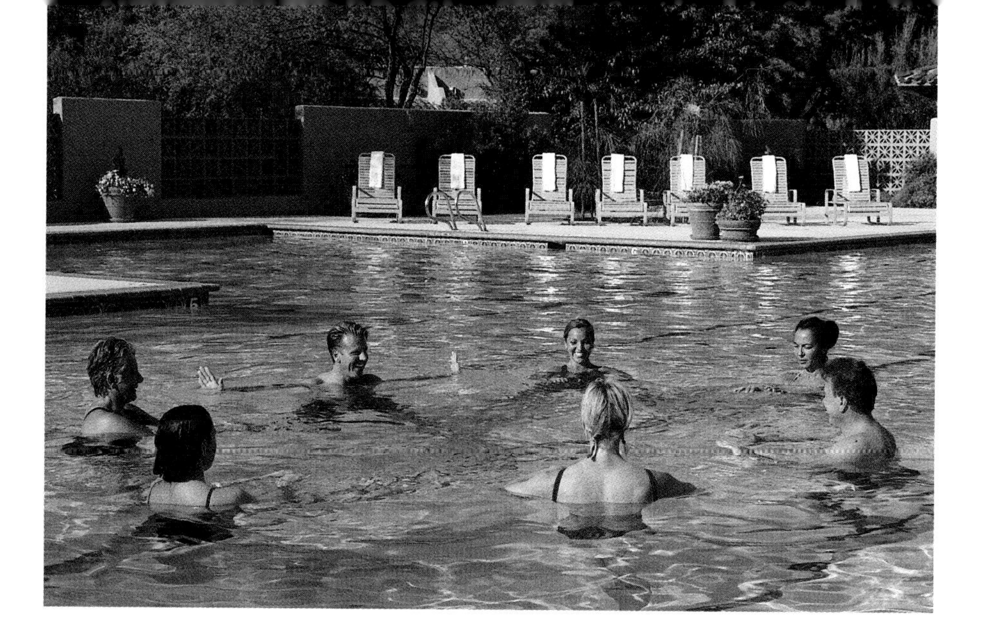

IV. BALANCE AND AGILITY

Agility is balance in motion, but our discussion of balance will take us into the large and important subject of movement therapy, which we address in depth in Chapter 5. For the moment, we'll just talk about agility, which in many ways is the final measure of all-round fitness. To be agile, your heart and lungs must work efficiently, your muscles must be strong, your whole body must be supple, and your balance must be fine-tuned. When you're agile, you have it all.

Agility is Michael Jordan twisting and hanging mid-jump to drop the ball in. It's Venus Williams diving for an impossible backhand and making it. It's Mikhail Baryshnikov leaping, turning, and landing on his mark. It's something we're all too content to sit and admire in professionals, when we'd do well to be cultivating it in ourselves. Each of us can improve the grace, power, and certainty with which we move through space, and we should, because agility makes us graceful and surefooted, whether we're hiking, charging along a crowded sidewalk, or swinging the kids up onto the monkey bars.

As our lives grow ever more rushed, we become less agile. Instead of riding a real bike—exercising our agility as well as our legs—we use a recumbent bike at the gym. (Anybody who falls off a recumbent bike has balance issues of a very serious nature indeed.) Instead of running cross-country (or cross-city), we opt for the more convenient treadmill in the climate-controlled gym. This is often a good choice because of the reduced impact, but what we miss is the valuable challenge the real world presents to our agility.

As we lose our agile edge, we grow less adaptable and more awkward and prone to accident. At the same time, we also become less graceful. The saddest part of agility erosion, however, is that we begin to feel less pleasure in our physicality.

The most effective way to put more agility practice into your life is, quite simply, to act more like the child you once were.

1. Substitute recreation—softball or tennis, dance lessons or a boxing class—for a nose-to-the-grindstone workout whenever you can.

2. Do the original activity rather than the gym imitation of it whenever possible. Ride your bike, climb a steep trail instead of slogging on the stairclimber, help a friend move and skip a session in the weight room.

3. Practice agility daily in small ways, by doing things kids do all the time, just for the fun of it. Try tying your shoes or putting on your stockings while standing on one foot and then the other. Walk on lines in the sidewalk or on curbs. Notice the patterns on the ground wherever you walk and challenge yourself to do something with them. (Remember "Don't step on a crack"?) Balance on one foot while you brush your teeth, and on the other while you floss. Have a little innocent fun with your body again.

What agility practice boils down to is remembering how to play. Race the dog or jump a rope and you might discover, or rediscover, something exciting and fresh about yourself—the child you never thought you'd meet again.

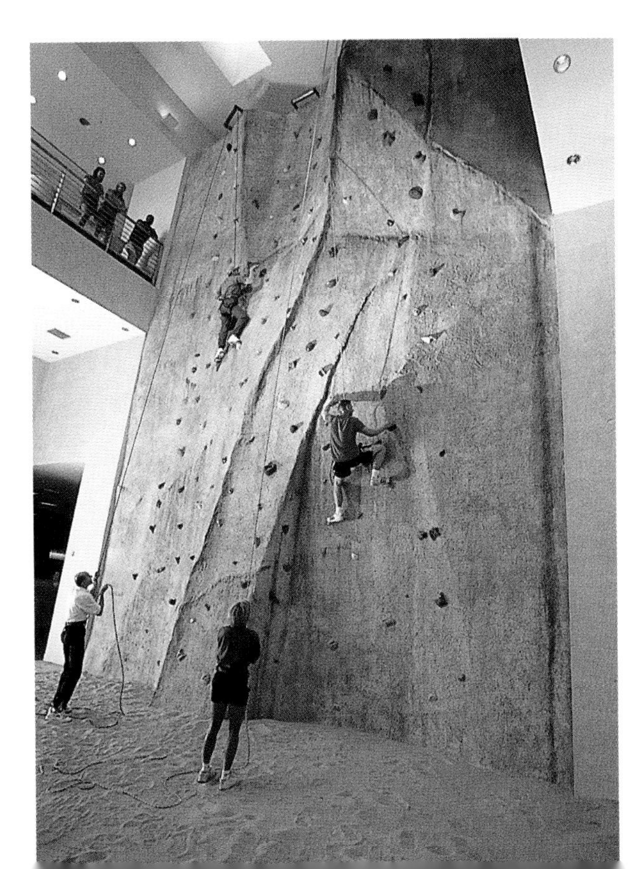

Motivation: Creating the Exercise Habit

ALL THE KNOWLEDGE, good intentions, and equipment in the world won't do you a bit of good if you don't keep at it. Here are strategies that work for many folks; try them and see what helps you stay moving.

1. Set realistic goals. Decide on a training schedule that you have the time, ability, and energy to follow. Few people stick to an exercise regimen that soaks up all their free time—especially when they're just starting out. Be ambitious, but don't punish yourself; the goal is to make exercise part of your life forever. Gym rats—those folks who seem to live in their workout clothes—have developed both their physiques and their appetites for physical accomplishment over a period of years. All appearances to the contrary, they actually weren't born in crosstrainers, so don't be intimidated. You might eventually *be* one of those impressively focused people.
2. Seek out activities that you enjoy. If you get bored with one thing, do something else. There's a world of possibility out there.
3. Be honest with yourself. If you go to the gym for an hour and spend two thirds of the time chatting, you're only getting twenty minutes of exercise. That's okay if twenty minutes is all you planned on, but don't pretend to yourself that you put in sixty hard minutes. On the other hand, don't beat yourself up when you're too tired to work out. Canyon Ranch exercise physiologists advise people to use the Five-Minute Rule: if you feel that you're really too exhausted to do your workout, then just do it for five minutes. If, at the end of that time, you're still tired, then stop. You need rest. But do give it five minutes to see whether exercise might revive you. Most times, getting started is much harder than continuing.

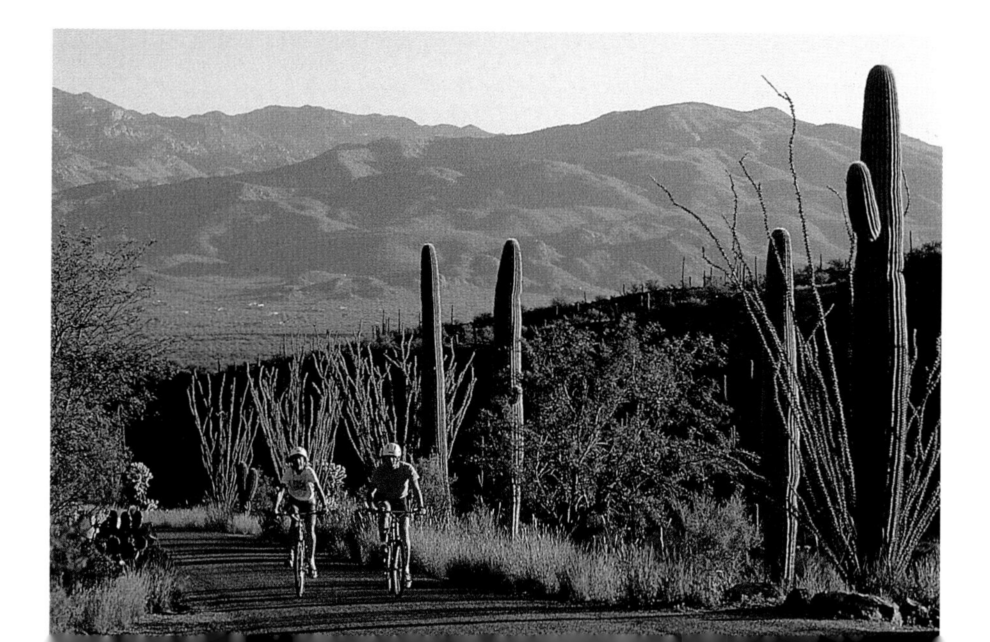

The Five-Minute Rule, by the way, works in all areas of life. The next time you face a task you dread, tell yourself that you're going to do it for just five minutes and then you can stop. You'll probably keep going and get it done and off your mind.

4. Keep yourself entertained by listening to music or books on tape while you work out. Alternatively, you can try to concentrate on something pleasurable—plan a vacation or a menu, reminisce about the past, or dream about the future. Your body's working, so let your mind run free.

5. Recruit a workout partner, someone you like whose level of fitness is similar to your own. Your mutually agreed-upon schedule can help keep both of you on track: it's much harder to skip a workout if it means disappointing a friend.

6. Keep track of your training. Achievement is keenly motivating. If you remain aware of your routine and your progress, mile by mile, exercise by exercise, machine by machine, it'll be that much easier to stick to your personal commitment. Keep a notebook or a chart. Better yet, get a yearlong poster calendar and give yourself a gold star every time you exercise (even on those five-minute days—hey, you tried, and even five minutes cranks up your metabolism). A line of gold stars satisfies the good child in each of us, and you may be able to see patterns in your regimen that might not become clear to you otherwise.

   You might also want to review and plan your training on the first of each month. This is how it works: you walk fifteen miles a week in January. Reviewing in February, you decide you like your progress and want to keep it up, maybe raising the bar to twenty miles a week. As March rolls around, it occurs to you that you're going to the Caribbean at the end of the month, and while all this walking has been good for your legs, you're looking a little skinny on top. This review will alert you to do some weight work in time for the beach. (One of the pleasures of getting in shape is showing it off. And why not? You've earned it.)

7. Set goals, and reward yourself generously. Set a goal at the beginning of each month and decide that if you hit your mark, you'll get yourself some small treat: a nice new pair of sweatpants, a baseball cap, a sports watch. It doesn't have to be a big deal, and it shouldn't be something you can't live without. The idea is simply to give yourself a definite, concrete reward for a job well done.

The last word on fitness: Canyon Ranch doesn't endorse any brand of workout gear, but we do heartily endorse the famous slogan of one shoe manufacturer: just do it. That's straight from our exercise physiologists to you. Don't worry about doing everything, instantly. Just do *something,* and build from there.

All the programs and diagrams and schedules in the world mean nothing if you don't get started. Our exercise program works, but only if you do, too. Start today.

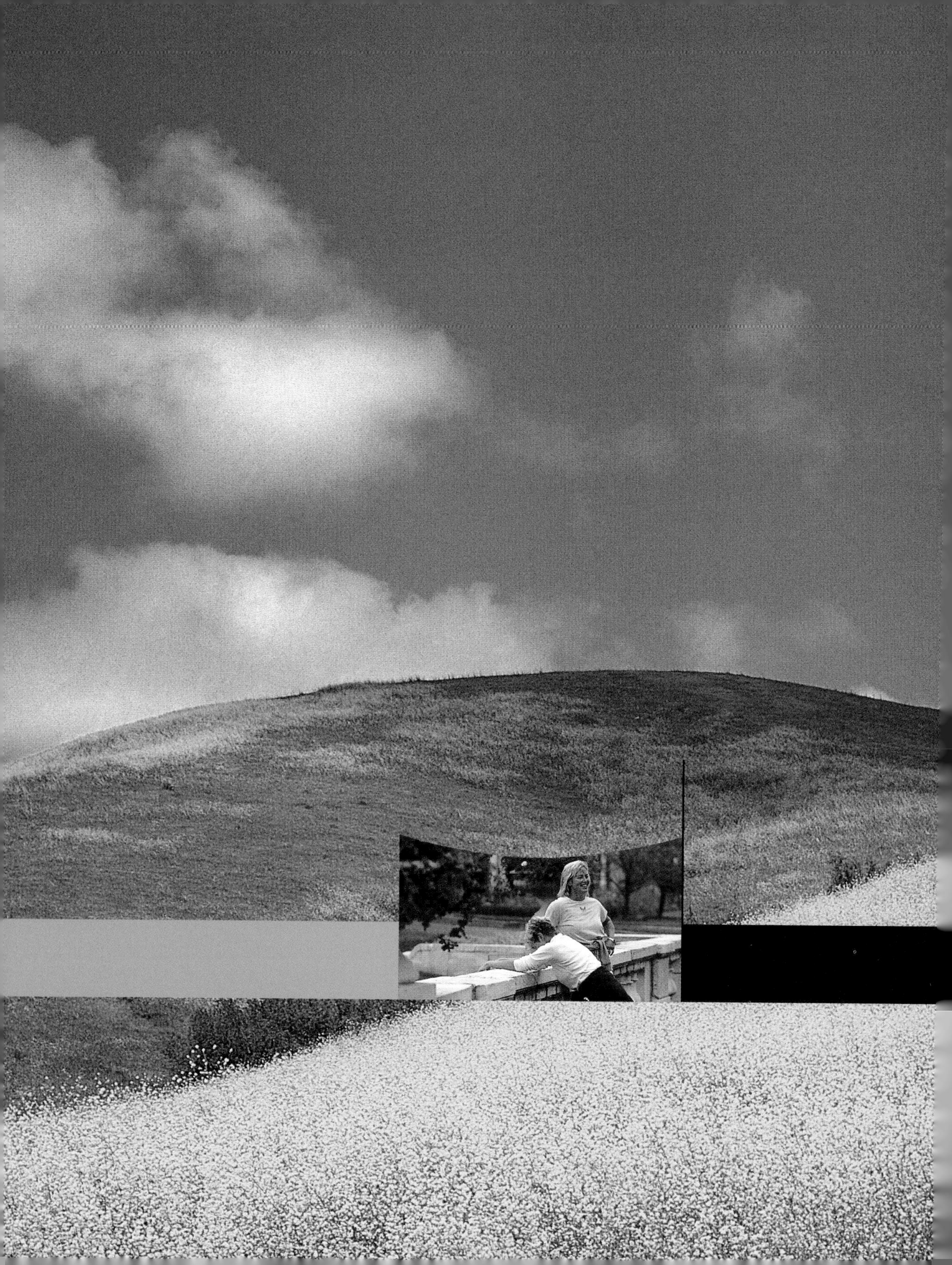

4 THE STRONG AND FLEXIBLE FRAME: *Musculoskeletal Wellness*

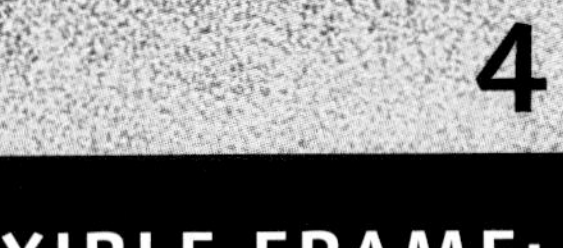

Do you hurt? Is pain in your back, shoulder, or knee keeping you from exercising, or, for that matter, doing much of anything with real enjoyment? If so, you're hardly alone: 73 percent of Americans between the ages of fifty-one and sixty-one report suffering from one or more chronic musculoskeletal problems that stop them from doing what they want to do—an appalling statistic when you consider the loss not only of fitness and health but of joy in life that these numbers suggest.

The purpose of this chapter is to empower you to take care of the most common injuries yourself, and to show you how to avoid reinjury or new injury later on. When it comes to your musculoskeletal frame, your framework of bone, muscle, and connective tissue, an ounce of prevention really is worth a pound of cure. More, actually, since there *are* no medical cures for many ailments arising from long-term mechanical damage.

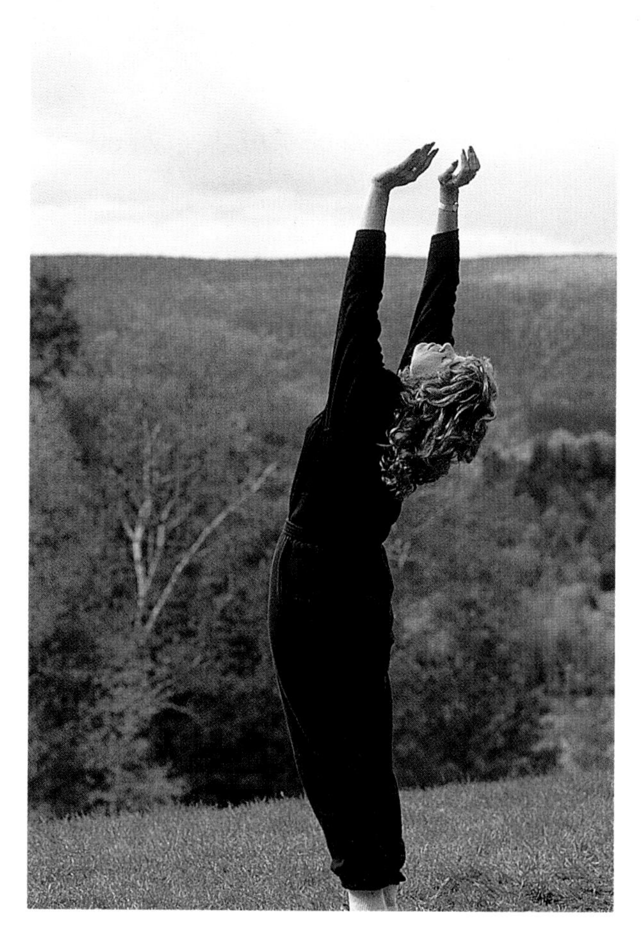

"Take care of your body. If it wears out, you won't have anywhere to live."

MEL ZUCKERMAN

Injury to the musculoskeletal system occurs in two ways. The first is sudden trauma—unforeseeable injury sustained, for example, in car wrecks, bad tackles, and skiing accidents. We can't prevent sudden trauma, but it's a relatively uncommon cause of long-term debility.

The other major cause of injury is a very different matter. Low-level repetitive stresses can, over time, cause enormous damage to the musculoskeletal frame, damage that can be prevented. Abuses like running too far on hard surfaces, typing day after day with bad technique, or simply sitting with poor posture not only cause significant mechanical stress; they also set the body up for further damage by weakening its structure. The critical principle here is that small changes in function (what we do) lead to changes in structure (the shape and substance of our bodies) over the long run.

Joints are the focus of concern in both types of injury. Our joints take most of the strain of impact and misuse: in the human body, as in most other mechanisms, contacts between moving parts take the wear and tear. And our joints are where we feel the pain of most musculoskeletal damage.

If you understand how your body works, however, you can effectively address injuries with corrective exercises and protect yourself from further damage.

Breaking the Cycle of Damage

AFTER SUFFERING AN injury, whether sudden and traumatic or low-level and long term, prospects for recovery quickly fade if you don't take proper care. You can find yourself plunged into a cycle dominated by pain:

1. Pain
2. Avoidance of use
3. Deconditioning
4. Loss of strength, flexibility, and function
5. Greater vulnerability
6. Further injury or tissue damage
7. More pain

This cycle seriously affects the lives of tens of millions of people, but it is not inevitable.

For many of us, accustomed as we are to relying on physicians to "fix" us, the idea of vigorous, conscious self-care is a radical departure, and it's important to understand its limits.

1. If you have a traumatic injury, or think you do, or if you suffer constant, unremitting pain, then by all means go to the doctor. Pain that never lets up may be caused by something other than mechanical injury—tumor, fracture, and infection must be ruled out. At the very least, you need a clear diagnosis.

2. If you diligently attempt to heal yourself through exercise and other treatments, but you don't see significant improvement by the third or fourth week, see a physician. Your problem, again, may not be purely mechanical, and may require medical intervention.

3. If you have severe osteoporosis, or are recovering from surgery, a recent accident, or an acute infection, or if you are pregnant, you should not attempt to treat yourself except under the direct supervision of your doctor.

4. If you experience numbness or tingling between the elbow and fingertips, or below the knee, see your doctor.

Most aches and pains don't require medical attention, however, and the traditional medical approach, focused as it is on acute problems in single body systems or parts, won't do much for them in the long run. Caring for your frame is something only you can do. Take it slow, do it carefully, give yourself time to rest, keep building, listen to your body, and stick with it. With patience, knowledge, attentiveness, and determination, you *can* work miracles for yourself.

Before you can begin to heal yourself, you need to know the difference between the feel of work and pain. If you have been very sedentary, the sensations of muscle work, day-after muscle soreness, and the hurts-so-good pull of stretching may be only distant memories. Most of us, though, instinctively know the difference between the pleasant ache of use and the shrill warning that is pain. If you pay attention to your body as you move, you'll recover that intuitive feel for the difference. If you feel mild soreness a day or so after working, it's probably harmless discomfort. Tingling, burning, or intensification of a familiar pain, however, are signs that something is wrong.

The Parts That Hurt

THE MOST COMMONLY reported and troublesome injuries to the human frame affect the lower back, the knees, the neck, and the shoulders, in that order.

THE BACK

The lower back is the hands-down king of pain. There's nothing wrong with the construction of our lumbar region: nature doesn't do bad design. The trouble is how we live, what we do to our backs. We use them in disastrous ways—sitting, slumped, on our tailbones day after day; picking up heavy loads as if we were cranes, as opposed to forklifts; and standing still on hard surfaces for hours at a time. For our backs to be healthy, our spines must be correctly aligned, and much of what we do as modern *Homo sapiens* might have been deliberately designed to distort the gracefully curving column of the healthy spine.

Add the abuse we put our lower backs through to the extraordinary structural complexity of the region, every intricate cranny of which is packed with pain receptors, and you have the more than seventy distinct causes of back pain recognized (but mostly not well understood) by medicine.

Back Pain Facts

1. Eight of every ten adults will suffer significant lower back pain at some time.
2. While most sufferers will recover from their first bout of back pain within a few months, for fully 90 percent of them this is just the beginning of recurrent trouble. Most back pain recurs, often with increasing frequency and severity.
3. Thirty-three percent of all people with back pain eventually develop sciatica, a painful impingement on (squeezing of) the main nerves supplying the thighs, lower legs, and feet.
4. Back pain is the leading cause of absenteeism from work in the United States. Seven million people are at home (or in the hospital) because of their backs on any given day.

Back Pain Fallacies

1. *An MRI (magnetic resonance imaging) scan can always pinpoint the cause of back pain.* Wrong. An MRI scan can reveal bulging disks and narrowed channels but cannot show pain. In fact, up to 60 percent of people with abnormal MRI scans of the back have no pain. At the same time, patients in acute pain often have normal MRIs. The cause of much back pain is nerve irritation, and nerves are so small that an MRI cannot distinguish a normal-acting nerve from an irritated one. In addition, MRIs only furnish images of body structures when the body is horizontal and at rest.
2. *Lower back pain always gets worse over time if it's untreated.* Some does and some doesn't. Many people are needlessly distressed to learn they have degenerative disk disease, when all this really means is that they're getting older. Degenerative disk disease is a natural part of aging and often does not correlate with pain—back pain is *not* an inevitable part of getting older. In fact, the peak years for back pain are between the ages of twenty-five and forty-nine.

3. *Bed rest is the best thing for all back pain*. Not true. Studies have shown that bed rest actually slows healing and increases loss of normal function in the spine.

4. *Strengthening the abdominal muscles always helps the lower back*. False. Many exercises for the abdominals put more stress on the spine. The key to reducing back strain is for *all* the muscles affecting the spine to work as a strong, supple, stable team. In fact, research suggests that the endurance—not the absolute strength—of the muscles of the lower back is a very good predictor of a pain-free back.

5. *Most back pain is "mental."* No. Only a small number of cases are relieved by psychological treatment. Some people do react to stress by holding tension in their neck, shoulders, fingers, and toes. Since most paths to the brain lead through the spine, this tension may be communicated to the muscles of the lower back, causing spasm. For these individuals, coming to terms with whatever's bothering them can relieve their physical symptoms. Most back pain, however, has a purely mechanical cause.

6. *Short-term treatments work*. Rarely. Most back pain results from our habitual posture and movements, and it tends to persist until we change the way we sit, stand, bend, and lift—even the way we sleep. Therapies like massage and chiropractic cannot change the twenty-four-hour-a-day stress we put on our lower spine and usually provide only temporary relief. These pain-relieving treatments can be extremely valuable, however, in conjunction with an appropriate exercise program.

7. *Surgical solutions to back pain are successful in most cases*. They aren't. The lower back is complicated and diagnosis is tricky, which makes surgery a questionable solution in many cases. Even when the diagnosis is unproblematic and surgery is clearly warranted, a technically successful operation can still fail to relieve symptoms. The best surgeon in the world cannot help a patient who doesn't faithfully carry out the prescribed postoperative course of exercise designed to strengthen, coordinate, and lengthen the muscles that support the spine—which, of course, is further insulted by the trauma of surgery. Back patients must improve their body mechanics and posture, or they are likely to end up with the same problems as before, plus a scar.

OUR PROGRAMS for spinal care and rehabilitation are based on the work of Robin A. McKenzie, pioneering physiotherapist and author of *7 Steps to a Pain-Free Life, Treat Your Own Back,* and *Treat Your Own Neck,* plus many technical works.

And Now, the Good News About Your Aching Back

Generally speaking, the prognosis is good for people with back pain who are committed to helping themselves. Be intelligently aggressive. Listen and learn as you train, and keep (carefully) trying new things, until you hit on the precise regimen that works best for you.

The basic strategy here, as with all the musculoskeletal self-help programs that follow, is simple: first restore normal range of motion, then strengthen . . . but don't stop working on range of motion.

LOWER BACK TEST

If you have low back pain when you bend, or when you sit for long periods of time, try this assessment:

Stand with legs straight and bend forward as if to touch your toes—you need not touch them.

Straighten up again and repeat 10 to 20 times without stopping.

If your usual symptoms are increased at any point by this movement, stop. You need to try the Spine Stretch (Extension), use a lumbar roll behind your lower back when you sit, and break up long periods of sitting with a few minutes of walking.

The Spine Stretch (Extension) allows joints and soft tissues that have been pushed out of alignment to relax back into their healthful natural curve, and it's a very important first step in the treatment of acute low back pain. It also can be used to treat stiffness of the lower back and to prevent low back pain from occurring or returning. (If you have experience with yoga, please note that this is *not* the same posture as the Cobra. The arms lift the upper body in this exercise—the back and abdomen should not be tensed—and the emphasis here is maximum relaxation, or sag, of the lower back, pelvis, and belly.)

Should the Spine Stretch (Extension) increase your symptoms after several repetitions (as opposed to causing a feeling of "work" in the back, which is normal), stop. Try the Spine Stretch (Flexion) instead.

However, if this Extension stretch does not relieve your pain but causes it to centralize—to move *toward* the central part of the lower back—that's a good sign and you should keep doing the stretch. *Centralization of symptoms is improvement.* Conversely, if the stretch makes your lower back feel better but causes a new symptom, or more symptoms, in your hips or legs, stop. Symptoms that move *away* from the lower back are a sign that an exercise is not helping you.

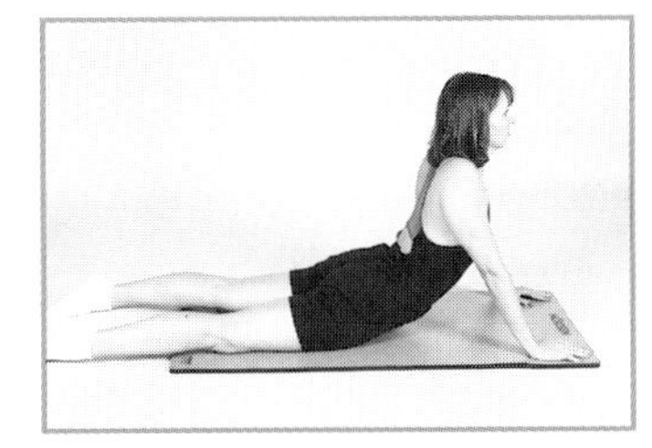

Spine Stretch (Extension)

LIE facedown on the floor.

PUT your hands flat on the floor, directly under the shoulders, in push-up position.

STRAIGHTEN your elbows and push the top half of your body up as far as the pain permits, keeping your pelvis, hips, and legs limp and relaxed.

HOLD for only a second or two, deliberately letting your pelvis sag, then lower yourself to the starting position.

PERFORM this movement 10 times per session, trying to straighten your arms a little more each time you come up—once again, as your symptoms permit. Even when you are able to straighten your arms, remember each time to let the hips sag for a second or two—this is the most important part of the exercise. You may maintain the sag longer if the pain is reducing or centralizing.

The "hold" in this exercise is very short for a reason: injured tissues should be stretched for very short periods to begin with. A stretch might feel good while you're in it, but your back might feel worse when you come back down to the floor. The short hold permits you to monitor your symptoms constantly. Your spine decides its course of treatment, and you must listen to it carefully if you want to live pain-free.

To treat pain or stiffness, do sessions of approximately 10 reps each, 8 or 10 sessions a day, spreading them evenly. For maintenance and prevention, do 2 sets of 10 reps a day.

If the toe-touch test above does not summon up your back pain, if the Spine Stretch (Extension) increases your symptoms, or, especially, if your lower back hurts more when you stand than when you sit, then try the Spine Stretch (Flexion). Your pain may be caused by an exaggeration (as opposed to a collapse) of the lumbar curve, and your back will benefit from being stretched the other way.

POSTURE TIPS FOR SITTING

WHETHER IN A CAR or a plane or at the theater, you will inevitably have to deal with a horrible seat. Even most "good" seats—supposedly ergonomic office chairs and car seats—have lumbar curves that are cosmetic and totally inadequate. Be prepared.

- **When you're traveling or heading out to the theater, a restaurant, or a ball game, carry a substantial lumbar roll with you. A small backpack or purse stuffed behind your lower back, or even your arm, bent behind you, can help in a pinch. (Some of the best lumbar rolls available are various models of the Original McKenzie Lumbar Roll, available from OPTP Conservative Care Specialists, PO Box 47009, Minneapolis, MN 55447-0009; 800-367-7393.)**
- **Place your feet flat on the floor to equalize and square your body. Your tailbone should touch the back of the seat. Keeping knees and hips aligned helps reduce strain on the lower back from the hips and pelvis.**

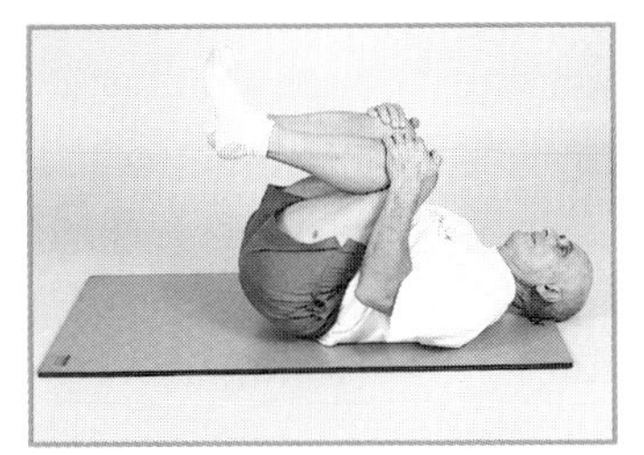

Spine Stretch (Flexion)

LIE on your back with your knees bent and your feet flat on the floor or bed. Bring both knees up toward your chest.

PLACE both hands on your knees and gently but firmly pull the knees as close to the chest as your symptoms permit.

MAINTAIN the stretch for a second or two, then return to the starting position.

EACH time you repeat the movement, try to pull the knees a little closer to the chest, as pain permits.

DO 6 to 10 repetitions per session, 3 or 4 sessions a day.

Work on the Spine Stretches until they're easy and you're clear of pain; everyone heals at a different pace, so it's up to you to monitor your progress. (If you find yourself relapsing, check on your seated posture during the day—it's probably the culprit.) Only when you've reached this point is it time to start other stretches and strengthening exercises.

Once your symptoms have been completely gone for one to two days and the Spine Stretches have become easy, you can begin to stretch muscles and other tissues that connect to the lower spine. Tightness and asymmetry in the hamstrings, buttocks, hips, and groin can pull the spine out of line: lengthening and aligning these tissues is the next step in healing your back.

Note: You should not feel pain in the lower back with any of these stretches and exercises. If you do feel pain, stop, and go back to doing Spine Stretches only.

Our model for most of these exercises, Canyon Ranch program coordinator Ralph Summa, turned seventy the week these pictures were taken.

Eliminating this pressure, in turn, helps you maintain proper posture.

- **Concentrate on keeping your head where it belongs—back and centered on your shoulders—and the rest of your spine will follow. Avoid a head-forward position with the chin jutting forward. Good posture is aligned but not stiff.**
- **If you do get stuck without lumbar support in a bad seat for more than twenty minutes or so, you have no choice but to scoot toward the front and maintain a very upright posture without leaning against the back at all. Clearly, this only works for a relatively short time—a spell in a restaurant or waiting room, for instance. In addition, if you find that your feet don't reach the floor, then try to find something—a book, a briefcase—to place under your feet.**
- **Get up and walk around as often as you can.**

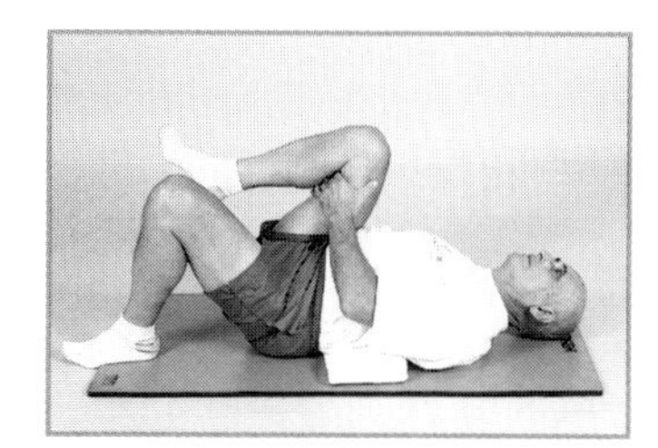

Hamstring Stretch

LIE on your back with a rolled or folded towel under the small of your back.

FLEX the right hip to 90 degrees and place both hands behind the thigh, at a comfortable distance below the knee. Keep the right knee bent.

BEND the left knee, if necessary, but keep head and shoulders on the floor.

KEEP the elbows straight while straightening the right knee until you feel a stretch in the back of the right leg. (The leg does not have to fully straighten.)

FOR an additional calf stretch, flex the right foot toward your shin.

HOLD for 15 seconds. Repeat 2–3 times.

SWITCH legs and repeat.

Buttocks (or Arrow) Stretch

This stretch lengthens the piriformis, a relatively small muscle in the buttocks that tends to clench in response to nerve irritation originating in the lower back. If the first version hurts your knees, do version 2.

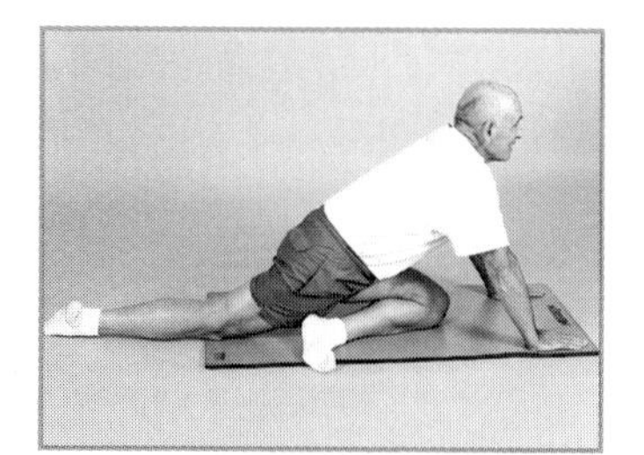

Version 1

START on hands and knees.

SLIDE the left knee toward the right hand. Raise the right knee over the left foot and place it on the floor next to the outside edge of the left foot. The left foot is now pointing to the right.

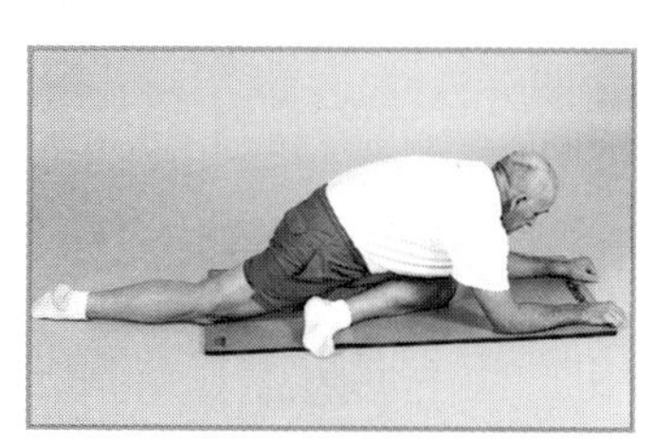

SLIDE the right leg out behind you, keeping the hips level.

GRADUALLY sink down until you feel a stretch in the left buttock. You can then rest on the forearms.

HOLD for 30 seconds.

COME up slowly and switch sides to stretch the right buttock.

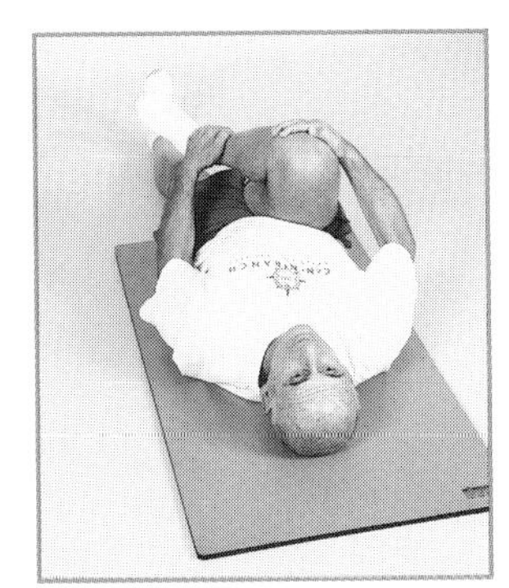

Version 2

START lying on the back.

GRASP the right leg with the left hand over the ankle and the right hand around the outside of the knee.

PULL the right leg toward the left shoulder until you feel a stretch in the right buttock.

HOLD for 30 seconds. Repeat, then switch to opposite side.

Hip Adductor Stretch

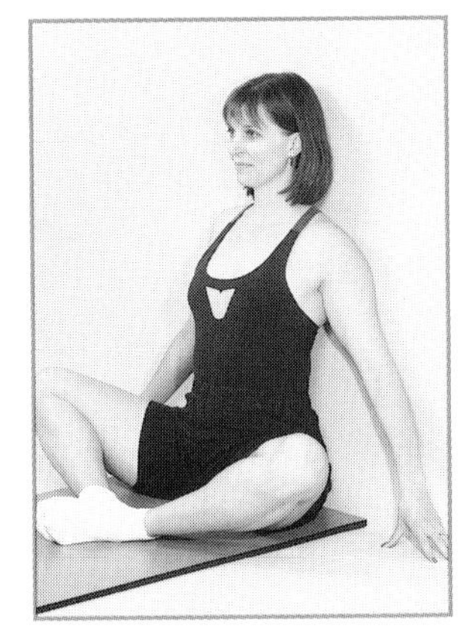

SIT on the floor with your back up against a wall, maintaining a neutral lumbar curve. If you have trouble doing this, sit on a pillow.

PLACE the soles of the feet together, with the knees pointing outward.

PUT the hands on the floor behind the hips to assist in lifting and arching the spine.

ARCH the spine.

HOLD for 10 seconds. Repeat 3–4 times.

Kneeling Hip Flexor Stretch

This muscle on the front of the hip connects to the lower spine and tightens with prolonged sitting. Note: It is easy to become too aggressive on this stretch and to feel sore afterward. You want to avoid this: think "light, gentle, and sustained" as you do this stretch.

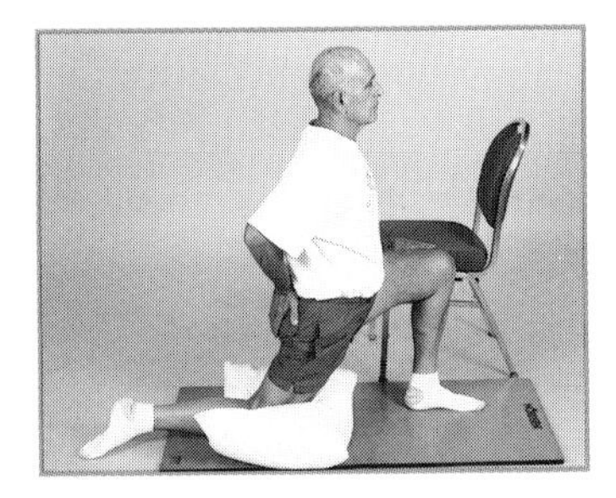

TO STRETCH the right hip flexor, kneel with the right knee and the left foot on the floor. The left hip and knee are both bent to 90 degrees. A pillow under the right knee may help make you comfortable.

HOLD onto a chair with the left hand for balance. Position the right leg so that the right foot is pointed slightly outward.

PULL in the stomach and contract the right buttock. Do not arch the back at any point—keep the trunk in a straight line.

PUT the right hand on the buttock to make sure the muscle is tight.

KEEP shoulders square and positioned over the hips, and use the left leg to pull the body forward. Follow the forward movement with the right hip until you feel a mild stretch in the front of the right hip and thigh.

HOLD for 30 seconds. Repeat 2–3 times.

SWITCH to the other side and repeat.

Strength Work for a Healthy Spine

Once you're limber and free of pain, you can begin working on two moves that will improve your everyday function and protect your lower back. Start doing these exercises gently, while continuing your stretching program and carefully monitoring your back. Continuing to stretch is important for two reasons: 1) you want to maintain length and continue to improve your habitual posture, and 2) you can use the stretches to gauge the effect of your strength work. If the Spine Stretch (Extension), in particular, becomes more difficult, or if you feel that your symptoms are recurring, then stop the strength exercises for a while and stick to assiduous stretching.

Remember: it took time for your back problems to develop. Have some patience about fixing them.

The Bridge

This exercise promotes spine strength and stability.

Version 1

LIE on your back with hands at your sides, knees bent, and feet flat and hip width apart. The knees should be close together but not touching.

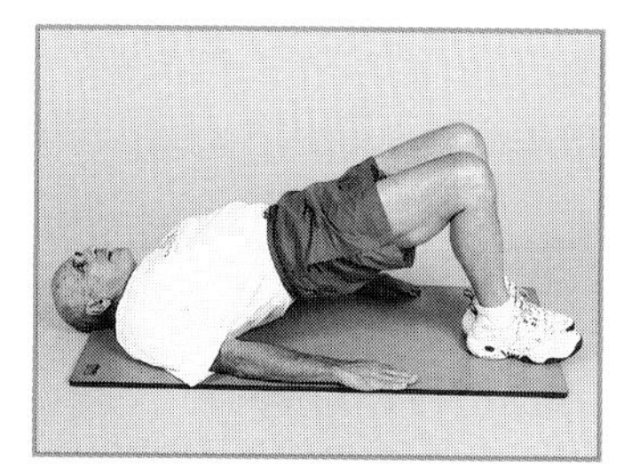

FLATTEN the back to the floor by tightening the abs and tucking the tailbone under.

WHILE maintaining this tilt, lift the buttocks straight up, as far off the ground as you can. Do not arch the back, and keep the hips level. Think of your body as a plank from knee to shoulder.

SQUEEZE the buttocks tight.

HOLD for 10–20 seconds.

LOWER yourself back to the floor, keeping the buttocks tight and trying to roll the spine down gradually from the shoulders, feeling the vertebrae touch down sequentially. The tailbone touches last.

RELEASE the squeeze in the buttocks only when the tailbone is on the ground.

REPEAT 3–10 times.

Version 2

If version 1 becomes easy:

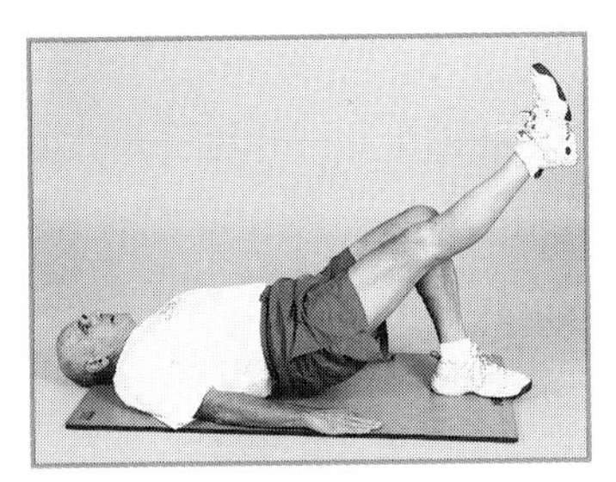

AT THE top of the bridge position, lift one foot off the floor, straightening the knee and reaching the leg long. Keep hips and knees level. Hold for 5–15 seconds.

RETURN foot to the floor.

CONTINUE to hold the position while repeating with the other leg.

ROLL BACK down (as in version 1).

Version 3

If version 2 becomes easy:

GET ready for the Bridge, but with the right leg already straight. Lift up into position with just the left leg for support, keeping hips and knees level, right leg extended and off the floor. Your body is like a plank from shoulder to ankle.

HOLD at the top for 5–10 seconds, lower with control, and repeat on the other side.

Squats

Done correctly, squats strengthen and promote integration of the buttocks, quads, hamstrings, and spine extensors. They also reinforce the correct method for bending and lifting: lifting with your legs won't protect your lower back if you dutifully bend your knees but still stoop forward from the waist.

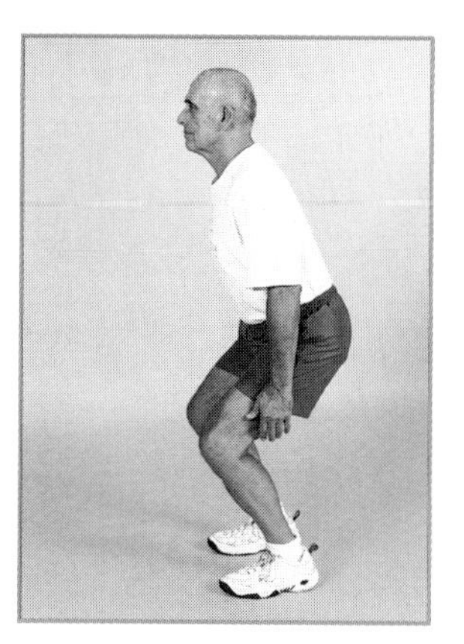

Note: don't do squats if they make your knees hurt.

STAND with feet hip width apart, toes pointing slightly out.

WITH back slightly arched, eyes focused straight ahead and chest up, push the buttocks back and squat until you reach a sitting or near-sitting position. Keep your weight on your heels—which stay solidly planted—to reduce pressure on the knees.

CHECK to be sure that knees are bending directly over the toes. Both knees and toes must point slightly outward. Avoid a knock-kneed position—which can stress the joints—by pretending you have a balloon or soccer ball between your knees. Face a mirror and check your form.

RISE from the squat position smoothly, keeping chest up.

STRAIGHTEN up fully at the top and squeeze buttocks before beginning next repetition.

REPEAT 6–15 times.

Back Maintenance

Let's say you've healed your back—bravo! Will you have to do an hour of stretches and exercises every day forever?

No, but you will need to do a streamlined, customized selection of these stretches and exercises regularly—unless you want to become reacquainted with your old friend pain. The exact regimen that keeps you symptom-free is something only you can determine. For many people, just ten minutes a day of a sequence that suits their backs is enough maintenance. Since only you know how your back feels, and what makes it feel better, only you can determine your best maintenance regimen. Your body will tell you what's the least you can do, if you listen.

SORE KNEES

Any aging weekend warrior will tell you that the knee is a very badly designed joint, and if you don't watch out, he'll tell you more than you ever wanted to know about *his* knees in particular. The knee comes just after the lower back in number of complaints, and it's perfectly true that it did not evolve for the purpose of playing full-court basketball—which is hardly the same thing as being badly designed.

The knee is the largest joint in the body, and while it can't compare with the lower back in complexity, it's more complicated than it appears. Further, we tend to subject our knees to a tremendous variety of stresses without adequate conditioning. Result: pain, decreased mobility, and frustrating limitations.

The most common type of knee pain is what the experts call patellofemoral. This umbrella term covers a number of conditions in which pain is centered on the interface of the kneecap (patella) and the head of the thighbone (femur). Such pain can be either primary (caused right there) or secondary (caused by other mechanical problems in the knee).

Interestingly, a recent seven-year study concluded that the best single predictor of this type of knee pain is weakness of the quadriceps (the large muscle of the front of the thigh). The upside of this finding is that strengthening the quads—and balancing the strength of some of the other muscles that attach to the knee—can stabilize the joint and significantly relieve pain. Strong, balanced muscles share the load, taking strain off the joint itself.

Strengthening both hip adductors and abductors helps equalize the tension exerted on the knee by muscles on the inner (or big toe) side and outer (little toe) side of the thigh. Women are particularly susceptible to knee problems caused by unbalanced development of the thigh muscles, probably because their hips are wider, causing the thighbones to slant in more toward the knees. This angle may make their knee joints more vulnerable than men's.

The trick here is to strengthen the thigh muscles without putting strain on the knee. You'll start your program with three exercises that work the muscles while keeping the joint still.

IF YOU THINK you've "torn something" in your knee, then perhaps you have, and if you haven't seen a doctor, what are you waiting for? There's a well-defined protocol for dealing with traumatic meniscus and ligament injuries, but it's beyond the scope of this chapter.

Hip Adductor Squeeze

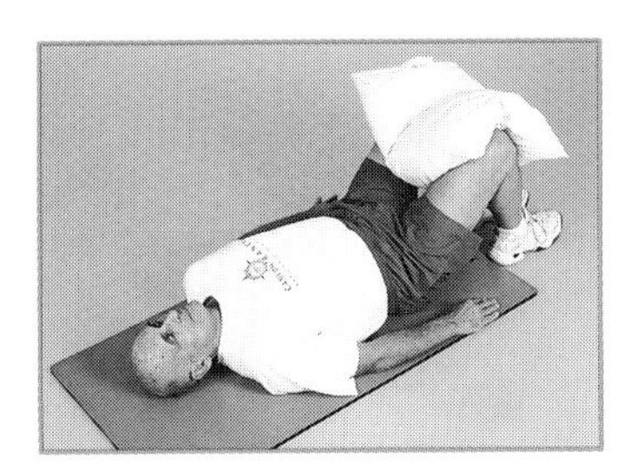

LIE on your back, feet flat on the floor, knees bent to 90 degrees, with a large, folded pillow between the knees.

SQUEEZE knees together, hard!

HOLD 5 seconds, breathing normally.

REPEAT 10 times, 1–2 times a day.

Note: This exercise can also be done with the legs stretched out straight on the floor.

Hip Abductor Squeeze

This exercise works the muscles on the outside of the thigh while keeping the knee still.

SIT down on the floor next to a wall and lean back, comfortably supporting the upper body with your arms.

BEND the knee closest to the wall while keeping the other leg straight.

PUT a pillow between the bent knee and the wall.

PUSH into the wall firmly and hold 5 seconds, breathing normally.

REPEAT 10 times, 1–2 times a day.

Quad-Strengthening Straight-Leg Raise

To work the right quadriceps:

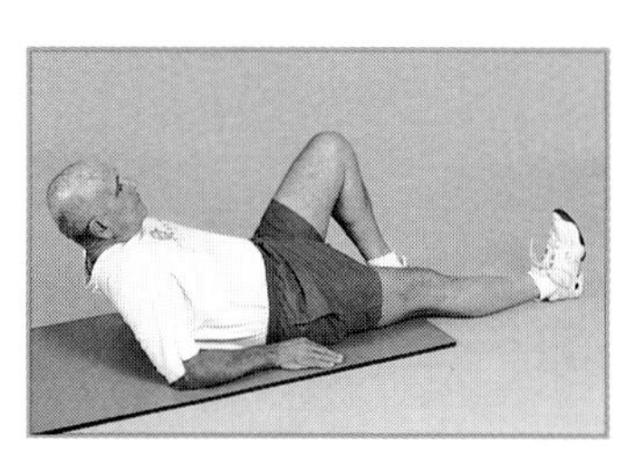

LYING back and resting comfortably on the elbows, bend the left leg, resting the sole of the left foot on the ground.

STRAIGHTEN the right leg and tighten the muscle on the front of the right thigh, as if to tense the kneecap. Be sure that the right foot points straight up.

SLOWLY lift the right leg 12–15 inches from the floor, keeping the knee locked and the leg very straight.

HOLD 2 seconds. Repeat 10–15 times, 2–3 times a day.

WHEN this becomes easy, you can add ankle weights or sit up straighter.

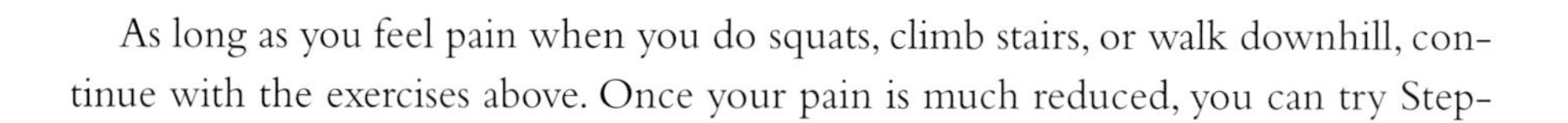

As long as you feel pain when you do squats, climb stairs, or walk downhill, continue with the exercises above. Once your pain is much reduced, you can try Step-

Ups and the Half Squat, in which you bend the joint while strengthening it. These exercises, which help improve muscle coordination in the legs, utilize a low, solid step or platform four to six inches high. (Most stairs have too high a rise for these exercises. Check the height first.) A thick phone book or two works well. Note: when these exercises become easy, add hand weights—don't add height to the platform.

Forward Step-Up

STAND with the foot of your sore leg resting on the step in front of you and your other foot on the floor.

STRAIGHTEN the knee and stand up on the step or platform. Move slowly—2–3 seconds to go up, and 2–3 seconds to get down.

RETURN. Keep the working foot on the step. You can touch a wall or chair back lightly for balance. Avoid pushing with the other leg.

REPEAT 6–15 times, twice a day.

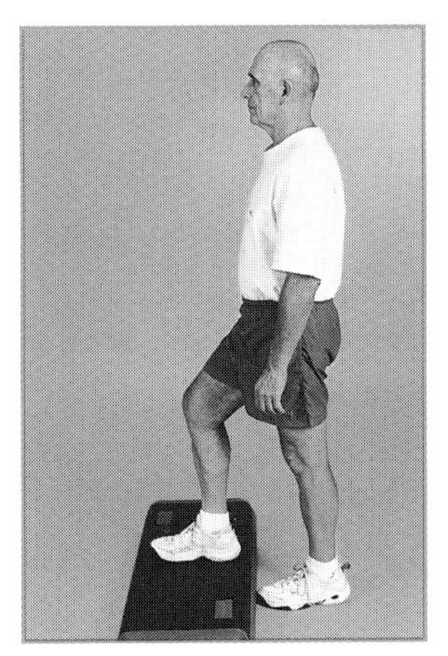

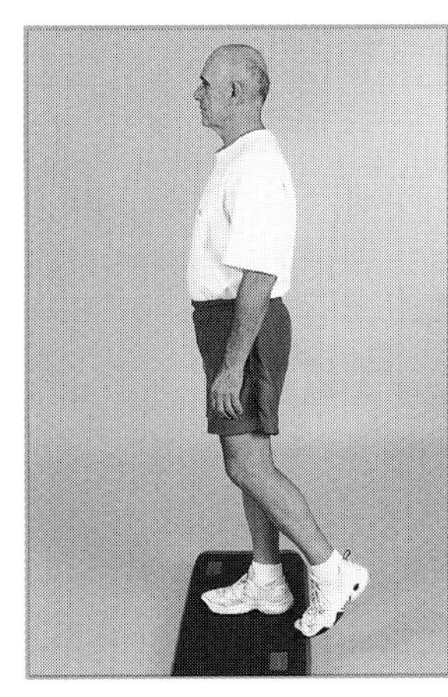

Lateral Step-Up

STAND beside the step, with the foot of the sore leg resting on it.

STRAIGHTEN the knee and stand up on the step or platform. Your body weight should shift sideways, from your good leg to your bad leg, as you move.

RETURN, gently shifting your weight back to the good leg. This helps develop lateral stability.

REPEAT 6–15 times, twice a day.

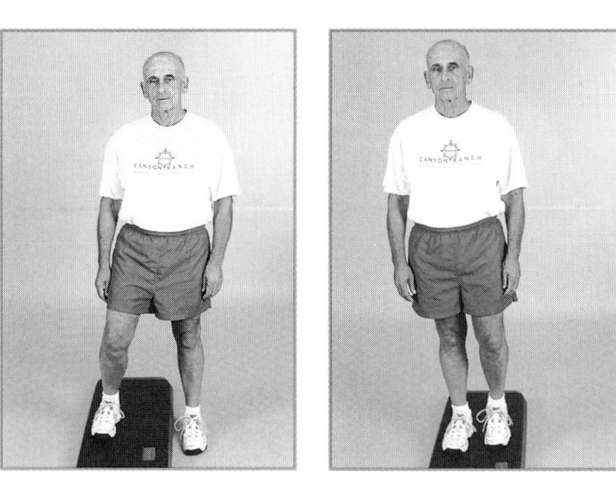

Retro Step-Up (not illustrated)

You may need a lower step for this variation. This is usually the hardest of the three step-ups. If it hurts, stop.

STAND on the step, feet together.

SLOWLY step down and forwards with the good leg.

THEN—keeping the foot of the sore leg on the step—step back up, very slowly.

REPEAT 6 to 15 times, twice a day.

Half Squat

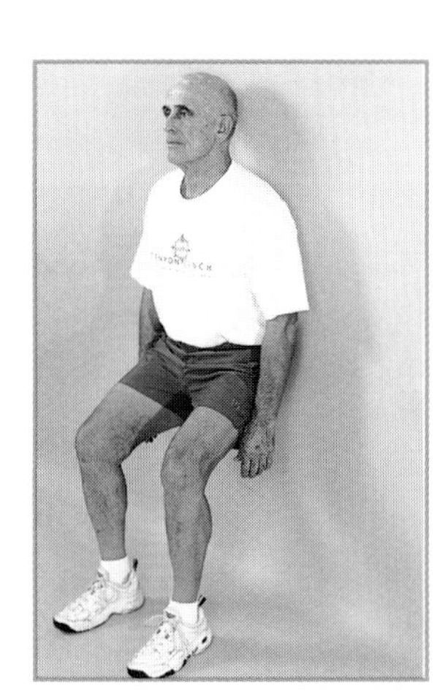

START with your back against a solid wall, feet hip width apart and 12–18 inches in front of you.

SLIDE down the wall until knees are at no more than a 75 degree angle (counting straight knees as 0 and sitting as 90 degrees).

HOLD for 10 seconds.

RETURN.

REPEAT 6–10 times, twice a day.

Note: Do not bend knees enough to cause pain.

A PAIN IN THE NECK

Since the neck is part of the spine, the first three words here are *alignment, alignment,* and *alignment.*

Your head is a heavy object—look at the work babies do to lift it—and it belongs squarely on your shoulders, not jutting out or hanging in front of your chest: leading with the chin is as bad for an accountant as for a prizefighter. Many of us, however, carry our heads too far forward, eventually causing serious structural changes—and pain in the neck, head, and shoulders.

The most important thing you can do for your neck is to develop an acute awareness of the position of your head in all your activities.

Five top ways to make your neck hurt and develop an unattractive and eventually debilitating stoop:

1. Read in bed, flat on your back, with pillows behind your head and your book on your chest.
2. Watch TV in the same position.
3. Don't get glasses, or, if you have them, don't wear them. Cultivate the habit of leaning forward and peering into your computer monitor, or at whatever's in front of you.
4. When you do upper body training or lift anything heavy, jut your chin forward. In this way, you increase the strain of your hangdog posture by the load on your arms.
5. Never stretch or change position while working. This ensures fatigue, soreness, and loss of flexibility.

If, however, you'd like to improve the flexibility and comfort of your neck muscles, reduce your incidence of tension headache, and improve your posture, try the following.

Head Retraction in Sitting

To correct the habitual posture of your neck while sitting, you must first learn how to retract the head, which can feel quite odd at first.

SIT on a chair or stool and look straight forward. Relax completely. Your head will protrude a little.

MOVE your head slowly but steadily backward until it's pulled back as far as you can manage. Keep your chin tucked down and in and eyes forward (do not *tilt* the head back). This movement lengthens the back of your neck.

IF DOING several repetitions results in increased symptoms, stop.

YOU can push your chin with your fingers for the greatest possible retraction.

A FEELING of stretching in the back of the neck is normal. Hold for 1–2 seconds.

RELAX for a few seconds and repeat.

FOR neck pain, do 10–15 repetitions every 2 or 3 hours. To improve posture and prevent pain, do 10 repetitions 3 times a day, striving to achieve a comfortably erect carriage of the head, slightly in front of the fully retracted position.

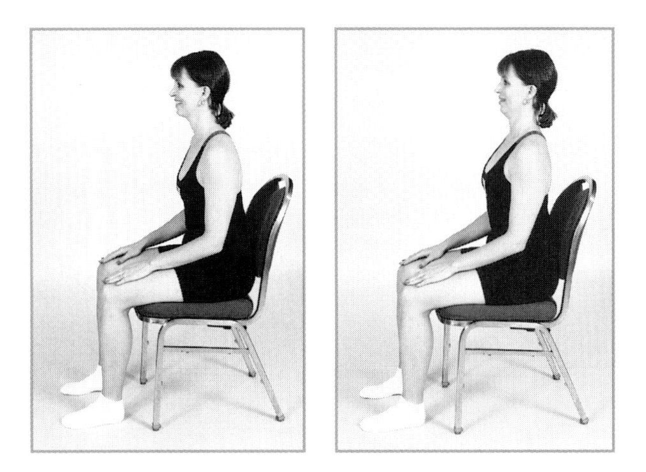

SHOULDER PAIN

The first thing you must do, if a shoulder hurts, is to be sure that the pain is not originating in your neck.

Check by paying attention to your shoulder pain as you move your head back and forth, slowly, in every direction ten or twenty times—chin to chest, looking up and down, turning from side to side and bending to either side (ear to shoulder). If any neck movement changes your shoulder symptoms either for better or worse, the problem is not in the shoulder itself, and the following assessments and exercises probably won't help. Consult a doctor, or try the neck tips in the previous section.

If, on the other hand, neck movement has no effect on your shoulder symptoms, then the problem is in the joint itself, and you can start corrective exercises.

First you need to determine whether there's swelling in the joint. Stand up and perform the following movements with both arms, noticing when and where pain occurs.

Let your arms hang straight down at your sides. Keeping them straight, palms toward the body, slowly raise both arms out to the side and up until you're pointing straight to the ceiling.

Lower, and do the same thing toward the front. Lift the arms up in front of you until you're pointing at the ceiling.

If, with either movement, you feel your symptoms increase or you experience a "catching" sensation at the top of the shoulder as your arm reaches the top of the movement, or if the top of your shoulder is sore to the touch, you have inflammation in the joint and need to treat it with ice massage for a few days before beginning the exercises below. Lightly rub the sore area with ice for ten minutes or so, three times a day, for three to four days. (You can use an ice cube directly on the skin, but keep it moving. Hold it with a cloth to catch drips.) Ice massage reduces inflammation and swelling, which makes more room inside the joint for things to move.

If, on the other hand, when you perform the assessment, the shoulder hurts more or less in the same way through the whole movement, or symptoms increase when your arm is about halfway up and then decrease as you go higher, you can begin strengthening and stabilizing the rotator cuff complex with the following exercises.

It's also important to avoid overhead weight work (such as military presses and lat pull-downs) and exercises that take the elbows behind the body (such as chest presses and dips) while a sore shoulder is healing. *All* movement should be done below the threshold of pain, and icing the sore joint after exercise is helpful.

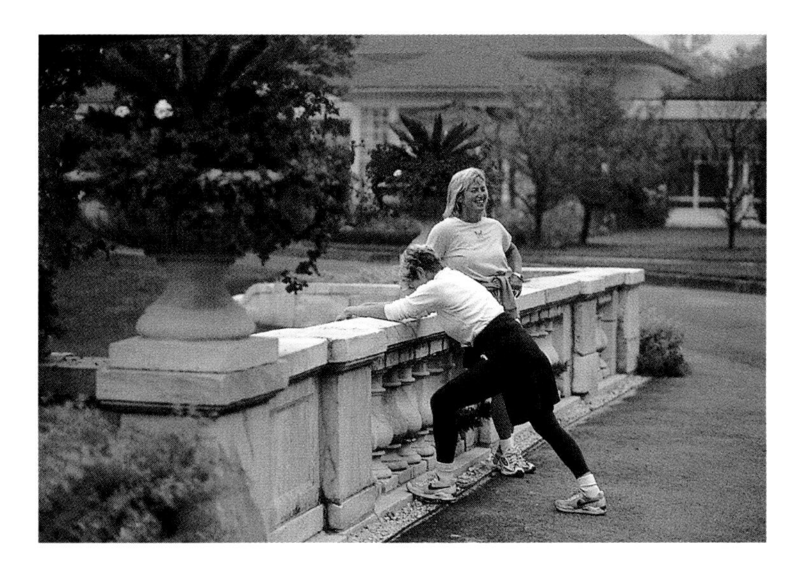

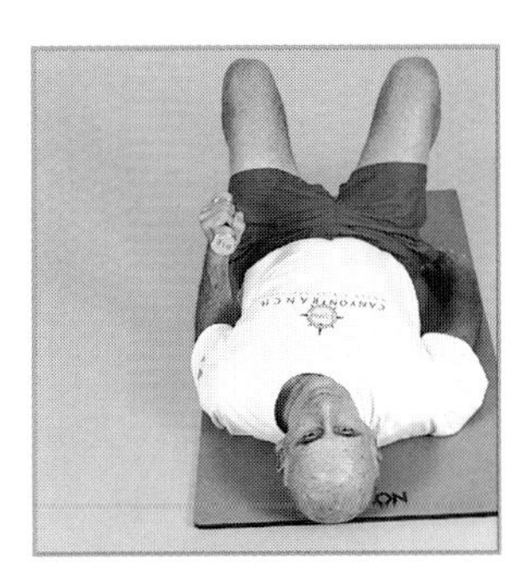

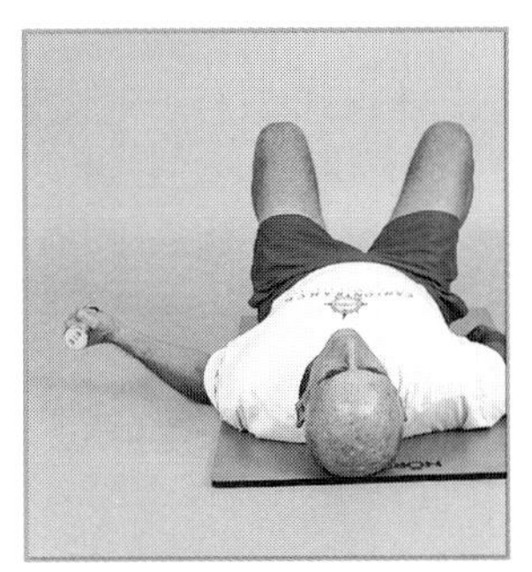

Internal Shoulder Rotation

LYING on your back on the floor, hold a 2 to 5 pound weight with the upper arm resting on the floor, close to the body. The elbow is bent at a right angle, and the forearm is vertical.

KEEPING the upper arm and elbow resting on the floor, slowly lower hand and forearm toward the floor, keeping a 90 degree bend in the elbow. Allow the hand to get as close to the floor as possible without pain. Raise the forearm back to the vertical starting position.

DO 2 sets of 10–20 repetitions each; reduce when symptoms diminish.

External Shoulder Rotation

This exercise is more difficult, and often more beneficial, than the Internal Rotation. Use a lighter weight if necessary—many repetitions with a light weight and proper form are the key. You should not feel pain in the shoulder.

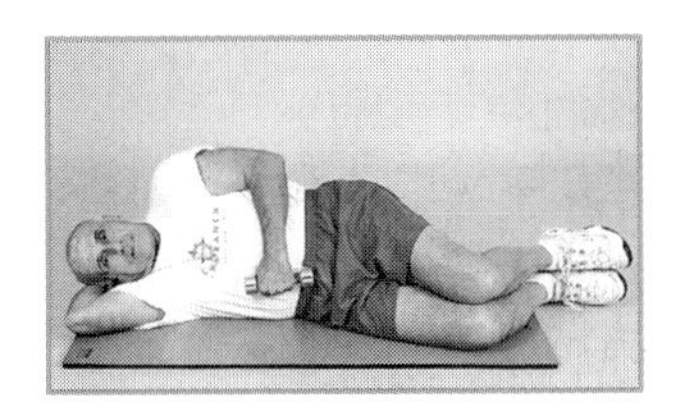

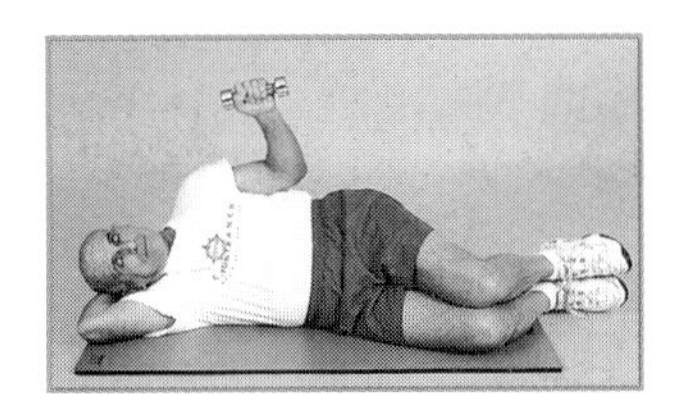

LIE on the floor on your good side, your good arm bent to comfortably support your head.

WITH your upper (sore) arm close to your side, hold a 1 to 3 pound weight, letting it rest across your waist, elbow bent 90 degrees.

SLOWLY raise the weight up until the hand is pointed at the ceiling, or as high as you can manage. Keep the upper arm close to your side.

LOWER back to the waist.

DO 2 sets of 10–20 repetitions 1 or 2 times a day.

Codman's (Pendulum) Exercise (described for a sore right shoulder)

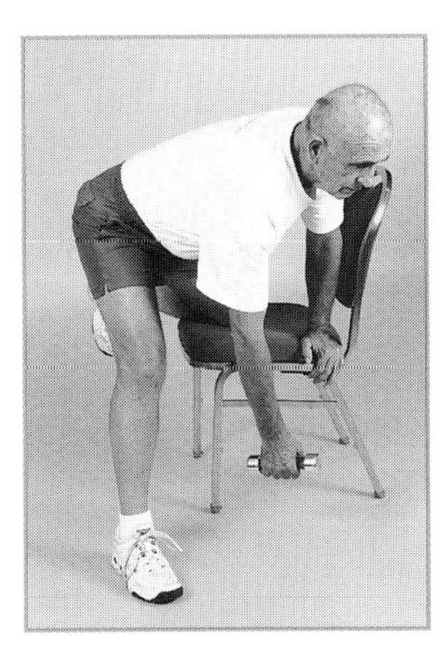

KNEEL with the left knee on a bench or chair, supporting your upper body with your left arm. Keep lower back contracted and slightly arched.

LET the right arm hang loose and straight, and hold a 3 to 5 pound weight. The arm, neck, and shoulder should all be relaxed. Keep the head neutral.

AS the weight pulls the arm straight down, slowly make small, *relaxed* circles from the shoulder, 20 clockwise, then 20 counterclockwise. Let momentum move the arm.

DO this exercise, which effectively stretches the whole shoulder capsule and posterior muscles, several times a day.

Taking Charge of Your Aches and Pains

THOUGH THIS CHAPTER'S focus is on injury and damage prevention, the payoff for taking care of your frame can be much greater than just relieving or avoiding pain—as important as that is. Employing better body mechanics and getting more exercise will also make you stronger, more flexible, and better coordinated—in short, more physically adept. And that means you can have much more fun. You can, with luck and perseverance, get back to doing the things you enjoy, and go on to discover new ones.

The satisfaction of successfully treating your own muscle-joint health is incalculable. Not having to depend on others to fix you—knowing how to fix yourself, and doing it—feels wonderful. Freedom from pain and limitation is great; achieving that freedom yourself is better still.

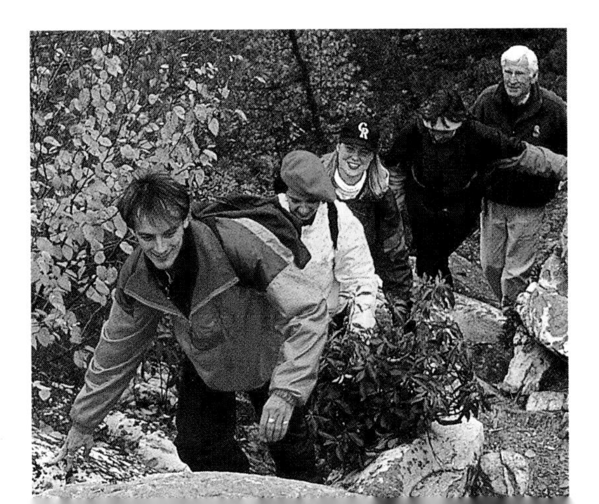

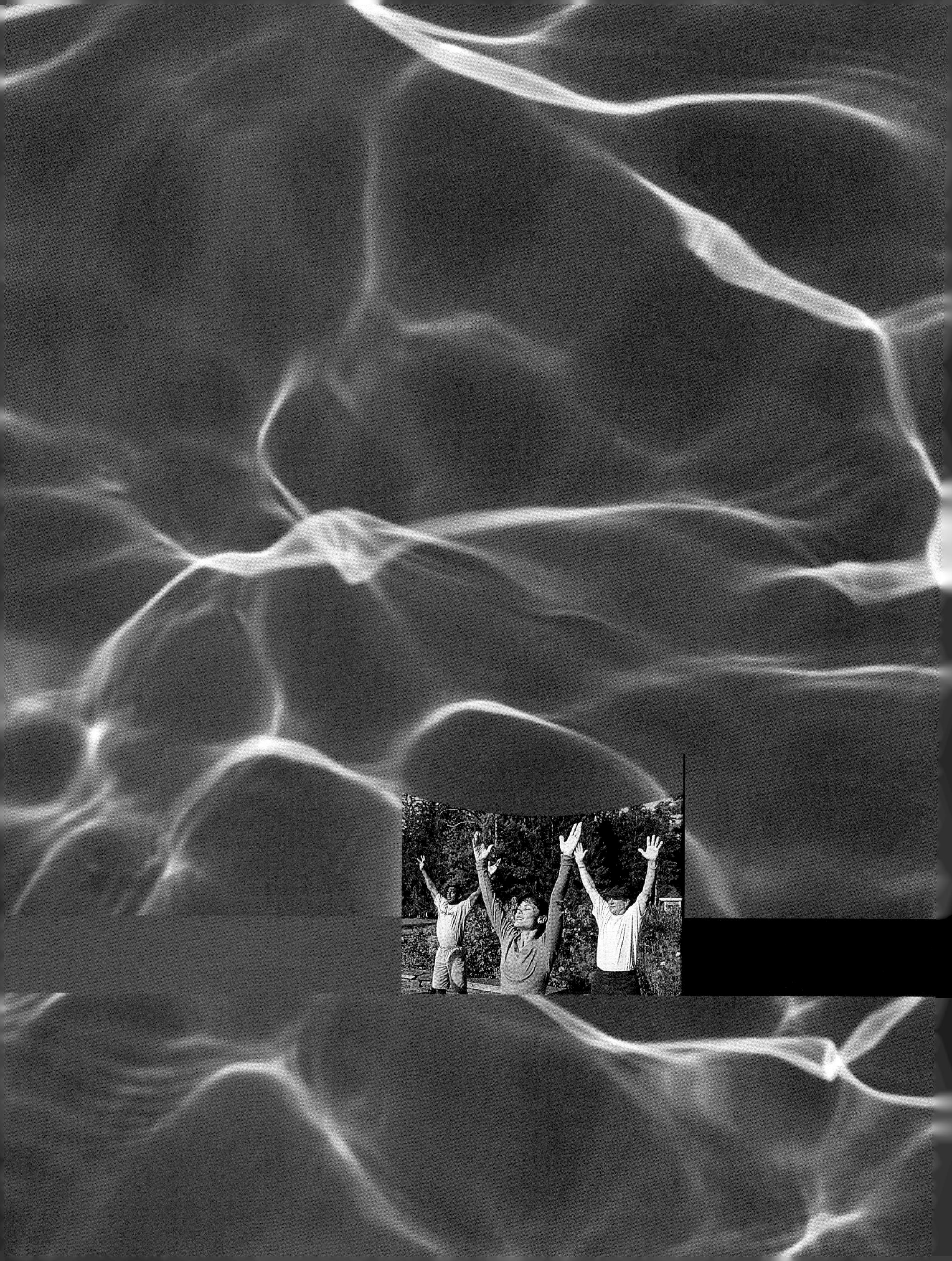

5 BALANCE AND MOVEMENT: *An Essential Component of Fitness*

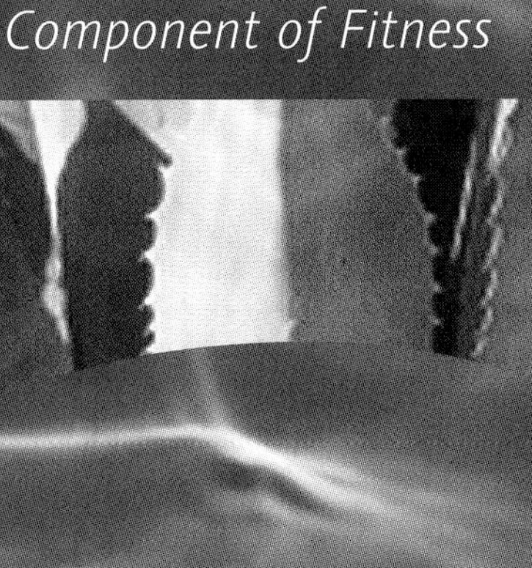

Balance and agility—which is balance in motion—together make up one of the four essential components of fitness. Balance is an integral part of our physical being and a powerful metaphor. If our lives are in balance, all is well.

Movement therapies from yoga to chi gong to Pilates focus on restoration and cultivation of physical balance, stability, and symmetry. Not coincidentally, they also tend to address the body-mind connection with greater directness than most physical disciplines. This is the area of physical training where personal integration is closest to the surface, and for many people movement work is the most satisfying and intuitive path to fitness.

Physical balance is a dynamic state, requiring continual adjustment. Picture a child who's just learning to ride a bicycle: she makes constant, deliberate corrections. As she continues to ride, her corrections become more subtle and less conscious as neuromuscular patterns establish themselves.

We're born with an innate sense of balance, and an innate drive to perfect it. Babies and young children, those incomparable athletes, work at balance all day long.

Unfortunately, balance begins to erode as soon as we stop moving. Somewhere in early adulthood, most of us stop playing, and our spontaneous movements become inhibited. This is usually a slow process, because healthy patterns are hardwired into our systems. It takes years of being told to sit still, behave, stop tilting that chair, and for heaven's sake get down from there, before we finally settle into our recliners and let it all go.

Reclaiming balance increases our sense of physical buoyancy, lightness, and ease. Good balance contributes to what the experts call "felt sense," knowing how to carry your body through space. Improve something as basic and simple as your sense of balance, and you may find that you can move through the day, and through life, with more freedom and grace than you thought possible.

Stability is the other side of balance. While balance allows you, for example, to position yourself so you can reach over a railing to pick something up, stability plants your lower body so you don't topple over when you reach down. In general, you must stabilize one part of your body to mobilize another.

Stability, like balance, goes fast when we don't use it, and with balance and stability go coordination and agility; once they're gone, we fall. That's the bad news. The good news is that with surprisingly little work, even very frail, very old people can regain the balance and stability that prevent falls.

For a younger person, balance and stability practice improves athletic performance and reinforces body symmetry. Ideally, the body is arranged around a vertical axis as perfect as Leonardo da Vinci's famous drawing of the ideally proportioned man. In maintaining or improving the symmetry of our bodies, our relationship to gravity is key.

"The way you move your body is the way you move through life."

ASIAN SAYING

Why Movement Therapy?

OUR QUALITY OF MOVEMENT and postural alignment is determined over the years by how we move (or don't), and much happens over time. Stress is a major player in loss of physical ease and balance. When we are afraid of or actually sustain any sort of harm or hurt, including psychological trauma, our muscles automatically contract in preparation for flight or defense. Sustained contraction leads to shortening of the muscles, breathing constriction, and decreased blood flow to the organs. The mental state associated with this physical reaction generally involves some combination of anxiety, anger, and emotional defensiveness. Emotional and physical stress reinforce each other and can quickly become indistinguishable.

Chronic tightness and shortening of tissues makes muscles susceptible to injuries that have their own possible consequences. When a large muscle is injured, for example, smaller muscles try to take up the slack, and movement is distorted. If you injure your quadriceps, you'll naturally shorten your stride as you try to protect the injured part. But the alteration of your stride challenges smaller muscles in the hip and leg, which can become strained as they work in ways for which they were not intended. This further impedes your ability to walk normally, rendering your gait that much stiffer. Without correction, you may never walk easily again.

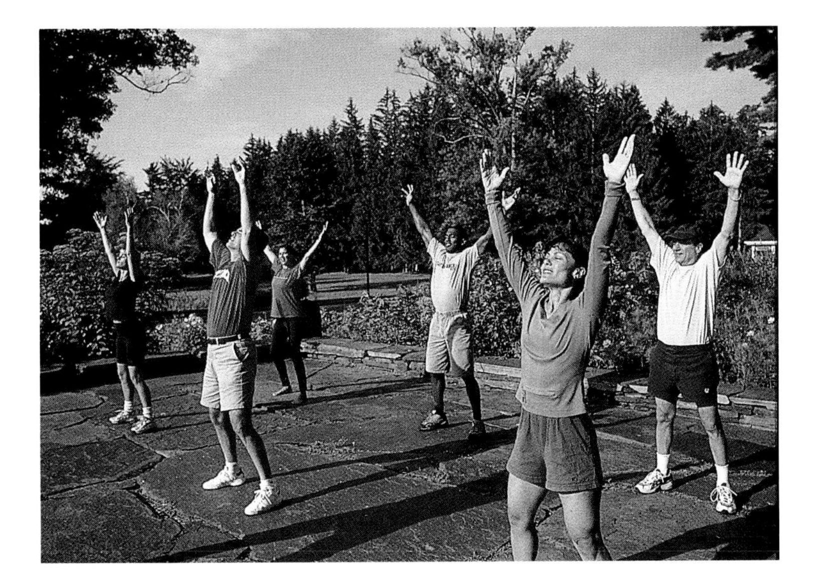

Similarly, a limp caused by a sprained ankle can cause your hip to tighten up. Left untreated, that tension can work its way up through the back, shoulders, and neck: our first warning that we're losing our sense of balance is often chronic pain, and the realization that we can't do what we used to. Maybe your neck hurts a little. Your shoulders don't move so readily. You probably ignore the early signs. Most of us have to feel real pain, caused by real damage, before we pay attention.

Movement therapists work on and through the body to change the physical patterns of trauma and stress to those of ease, comfort, and increased vitality. As the body regains its balance, mind, mood, and emotions relax and expand. Movement therapy and mind-body exercise are defined as *physical exercise executed with a non-judgmental, inwardly directed, meditative focus.*

Movement Therapy Basics

AS YOU MIGHT EXPECT, changing ingrained patterns of movement requires commitment and perseverance. However, various movement therapies—including Pilates, Feldenkrais, Trager, aqua therapy, and yoga—provide clear and structured paths to better movement.

All movement therapies address body change through the same basic avenues.

1. BREATHING EXERCISES

Breath literally defines life, from our first moment to our last. It's also our ground rhythm: the inflow and outflow of breath, coupled to the heartbeat, is the essential pulse of life. We are never without this rhythm. Breathing is one of the few autonomic systems that we can consciously override (to a point, of course). When we breathe deeply, whether in motion or at rest, we send nutrient-rich oxygenated

MARTIN CAME TO Canyon Ranch seeking help. He was in his sixties, big and burly, a prototypical example of the physically and intellectually imposing American business executive: hard-charging, confident, thriving. That wasn't the whole picture, however. As a young boy, Martin had contracted polio. He'd escaped paralysis, but had never been able to shake chronic pain in his lower back and legs. He had come to Canyon Ranch to see what he could do about it.

During a movement therapy session, the therapist tried to get him to stretch his hamstrings, but Martin told the therapist that he thought this movement would be so painful that he'd never really tried to do it before. He gave it a go, however, and it was then, as he moved into the stretch, that his whole body started to quiver and he suddenly experienced a flashback to his childhood. Martin's past returned to him, and he saw himself as a young boy again, in the same position, as his father pushed on his

blood to heal and revitalize our tissues. Deep, slow breathing is also a message to every system in the body that it's okay to relax.

2. RELEASING EXERCISES

Stretches and muscle-balancing and range-of-motion exercises lubricate the joints and facilitate blood flow to the tissues. By making the body more flexible and comfortable, these exercises help release stored tension throughout the musculoskeletal system. People who are in pain tend to tighten and, in tightening, constrict their muscles to shut off the feeling. This works for a while, but it inevitably creates more pain.

3. CORE STRENGTH EXERCISES

The heaviest bones in our body require the most muscular support. The pelvis and lower spine need firm abdominal and pelvic floor support, as well as support from the back muscles themselves. As the frame becomes better aligned and the suite of lower trunk muscles grows stronger and becomes better integrated, overworked individual muscles unclench, taking strain off distorted joints and pressure off irritated nerves.

4. STRENGTH/ENDURANCE EXERCISES

Muscular strength and endurance work helps maintain and increase bone density and enables us to perform daily activities with ease, thereby increasing our sense of physical competence and confidence and decreasing the risk of injury.

5. CARDIOVASCULAR EXERCISES

Cardio exercise promotes heart health, lowers cholesterol, stabilizes blood sugar levels, improves circulation, and burns fat at an increased rate.

back to help him stretch. He had forgotten, or tried to forget, about the difficult days of his slow recuperation from illness.

Martin was clearly on the brink of crying, though he struggled for control. Slowly, tension he'd been holding in his body for more than fifty years began to recede, and he experienced a huge physical and emotional release. Stretching became less difficult and his companion pain began to ease.

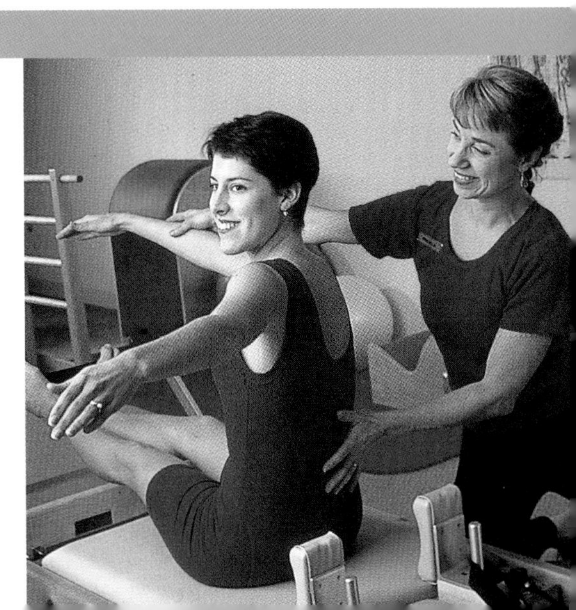

6. MEDITATION AND VISUALIZATION EXERCISES

These reduce stress, increase self-understanding, improve awareness of the body's signals, and lead to a greater sense of spiritual connection and well-being.

7. CREATIVE MOVEMENT/MINDFUL MOVEMENT

Creativity and play with no specific goal in mind encourages "being in the moment." In play, the emphasis shifts from who we *think* we are, leaving room to explore who we actually are. Creative movement helps participants overcome self-consciousness and self-imposed limitations. Mindful movement helps people connect mind and body through a moving meditation that increases awareness of breathing patterns, movement habits, and physical sensations. By becoming more aware through movement exploration, a person can self-correct patterns of pain, tension, and discomfort and learn how to move with fluidity and joy.

Movement therapy techniques improve strength, flexibility, coordination, and balance and teach individuals to correct their own bodies. The mental and emotional benefits—improved awareness, concentration, and empowerment—are often just as important.

Sports psychologists use mind-body techniques to improve focus and performance in athletes, and integrative medical practitioners incorporate movement therapies in their multidisciplinary approach to health and healing. Researchers are investigating the impact of movement therapy and mind-body exercise for chronic disease management, potential stress reduction, and containment of health-care costs. As the field of integrative medicine continues to grow, movement therapy techniques are becoming an increasingly valued part of health care.

The Therapies

ALEXANDER TECHNIQUE AND SOMATIC EDUCATION

These two therapies are intellectually joined because both focus on postural integrity, movement patterns, and gait. Changing patterns of habitual movement can release stress, improve alignment and body image, and decrease pain and tension. These therapies are particularly helpful to people who contend with repetitive stress at work or experience pain in movement.

AQUA THERAPY

"Bathing" in healing waters, an ancient and widespread therapy, is enjoying a current surge of popularity, as several movement and treatment systems have moved into the pools. For people with joint problems, back pain, arthritis, or other limitations that make movement difficult, passive therapies like Watsu (for *water* plus shiat*su*), a deeply relaxing combination of shiatsu massage and dance done in a warm pool, and exercise systems like ai chi—an aquatic form of tai chi—can be a godsend. Of course, they're also terrific for people with no limitations at all. Ongoing research shows that immersion, in and of itself, has a tonic effect on the whole body and particularly benefits the circulatory and lymphatic systems and kidney function.

CHI GONG

This slow, flowing meditation-in-motion focuses on mastery of the breath—the Chinese word *chi* (or qi) means "breath of life" or "energy," and *gong* denotes "cultivation" or "control." It is a gentle, calming discipline that promotes full integration of mind, spirit, and body. Chi gong is extremely useful for stress reduction. In China, millions of people practice chi gong and its offshoots to promote self-healing and maintain wellness. See page 22 for a simple chi gong exercise.

FELDENKRAIS

The aim of Feldenkrais is to improve quality of life by enhancing communication between the brain and body, improving the body's capacity to function in a variety of ways. The therapy emphasizes gentle, precise touch on a massage table, as well as classes designed to reprogram neuromuscular pathways.

This subtle yet powerful approach is based on the process of sensorimotor exploration that children go through while learning to move through the world. Feldenkrais has proven to be especially helpful to seniors and to people with limitations due to pain, stress, injury, or illness.

TRAGER

Trager stimulates good health through gentle bodywork designed to access and influence deep-seated psychophysical patterns. The process is described as sensitive feeling work: the therapist uses rhythmic touch to lull the client into safety and surrender. Working within this state of openness and diminished resistance, the therapist or practitioner can address the subconscious directly and speed the reprogramming at the most fundamental level. Once this meditative state has been achieved, every movement is initiated as gently as possible, with gravity completing the actions. Release is the key.

Below you'll find beginning programs in Pilates and yoga. We've chosen to include specific instructions for them because they're two of the most popular and accessible systems.

Pilates

PILATES IS AN EXERCISE system designed to develop the body uniformly by promoting strength, flexibility, ease of movement, balance, posture, and overall health. It has been used since 1926 in this country, where it was originally embraced by dancers and more recently by physical therapists and the fitness industry. The system's inventor, Joseph Pilates, adapted movements and postures derived from Asian and Western movement systems and refined them to build power, muscle integration, and flexibility, with special emphasis on the "powerhouse" muscles of the abdomen, pelvic floor, lower back, inner thighs, and buttocks. By working through a carefully controlled series of graceful movements with proper form—ideally with a certified instructor and using the specialized equipment Pilates invented—you can improve circulation, range of motion, coordination, flexibility, strength, and posture. Pilates exercises can also be done on the floor, without any equipment other than a mat. A basic mat routine you can do at home follows.

Joseph Pilates felt that certain aspects of traditional physical training needed correction. He saw that people tend to work obvious surface muscles, while neglecting weaker, smaller muscles that are just as important. A chain is only as strong as its weakest link, and most training systems promote a physique with many weak links.

Pilates works the whole body, strengthening and stretching key muscle groups simultaneously. This totality of action, engaging all the muscles at once but continually switching movements, is designed to build stamina without overloading any single group of muscles. Pilates is especially valuable for the way it works muscles deep inside the body, building a protective sheath for the vulnerable lower spine.

A GROWING LEGION of devotees can attest to Pilates' long list of benefits:

1. Conditioning of deep muscles
2. Strengthening of the abdomen and back
3. Restoration of natural posture
4. Development of overall strength, flexibility, and endurance
5. Muscle toning
6. Enhanced mobility and agility
7. Improved athletic performance
8. Decompression of the spine and joints; improved circulation
9. Alleviation of pain and tension

As you become proficient at the exercises, you will be able to flow from one movement to the next, and ideally your practice will become as natural as walking and running. The subconscious rhythm that regulates our ordinary movements provides the measure, the beat, for Pilates training.

Here are five principles of Pilates that you should bear in mind as you embark on this adventure in fitness:

1. Breath: Everything starts and ends with the breath. Inhale and exhale completely but without noise or exaggeration. Expel stale air from your lungs, and replenish your body with fresh air throughout your practice. Regular, deep breathing will help you control your exercise and movements and make them more efficient.

2. Concentration: To reap the maximum benefit from your training, focus on each movement as you perform it. The more intensely you concentrate, the better you will be able to perceive your body's response. The mind is an amazing instrument. Use it in your training.

3. Control: Muscle control determines the quality of each movement, and is key to making progress, as well as to avoiding injury. Injuries occur when control is relaxed and movement becomes awkward or erratic.

4. Precision: Since every movement serves a precise purpose, every movement should be done precisely. You can achieve your goals step by step, by defining those goals and working patiently toward them.

5. Fluidity: Never perform Pilates exercises in a jerky or mechanical way. Strive to make every movement flowing, dynamic, and graceful.

THE EXERCISES

The Hundred

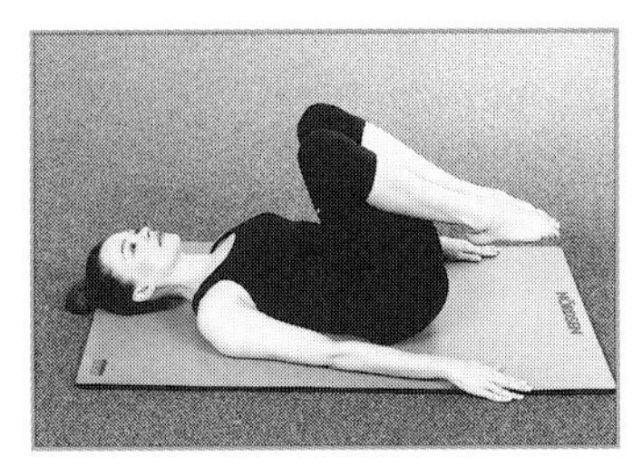

BEGIN lying on your back. Pull your knees to your chest.

YOUR breath is crucial. After inhaling as deeply as possible, exhale and try to press your chest and stomach through your back and into the ground.

TORSO flattened, raise your head and shoulders until you can see your midsection. Lift from your upper back and not your neck or head.

STRAIGHTEN your arms along the sides of your body, reaching long until the bottom of your shoulder blades are against the floor.

NOW lift the legs straight to the ceiling, so that they are perpendicular to your body. Press your legs tightly together.

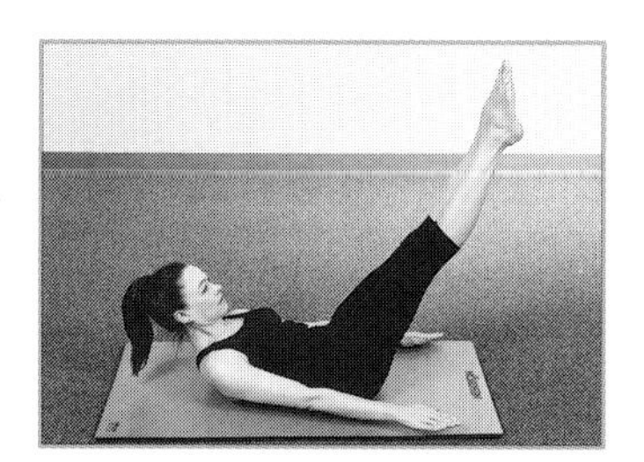

YOU'RE ready to start moving your arms, pumping them up and down in short, vigorous, controlled strokes. Keep the arms straight.

INHALE and exhale for five beats while continuing to pump the arms with control. (This is not a big motion.)

NOW shift the legs, lowering them halfway down, to a 45 degree angle. Holding this posture, belly still flattened against the lower spine, pump your arms up and down again no less than one hundred times.

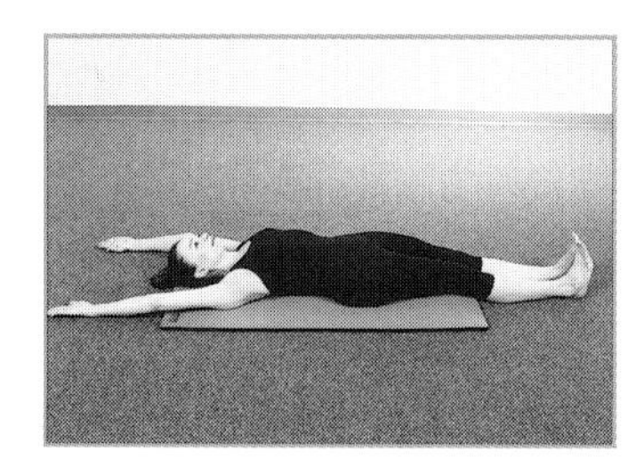

FINISH by lowering your head while you pull your knees toward your chest and rock gently from side to side for a moment.

EXTEND fully, arms stretched out above your head, in preparation for the next exercise.

The Roll-Up

TIGHTEN your buttocks, squeeze your thighs together, flex your feet, and raise your arms straight to the ceiling while lying on your back.

ONCE your arms are perpendicular to your trunk, inhale and begin to roll up and forward, starting with the head. (The lower body does not move.)

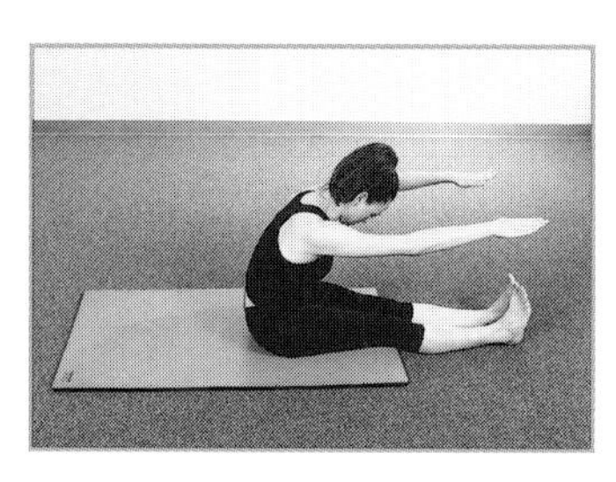

CONTINUE your forward roll, trying to peel one vertebra at a time off the mat as you come up. Your chin goes to your chest, your chest goes over your ribs, your ribs over your abs, your abs over your hips, and then reach out over your thighs, retaining the curve in your spine.

AS you reach your furthest point, exhale and try to reach further forward from your hips, all the while keeping your belly flattened.

YOU'VE made it up—now it's time to head back down. Inhale and tighten your buttocks again, press your midsection back, and tuck your tailbone beneath you.

EXHALE as you slowly curl back down, vertebra by vertebra, against the mat. When your shoulders make contact with the floor, bring your head down and return your arms to their original overhead position.

YOU'RE down, so start back up, with the goal of completing three to five reps.

Single-Leg Circles

PULL one knee to your chest and then raise the leg straight to the ceiling, holding your ankle or calf.

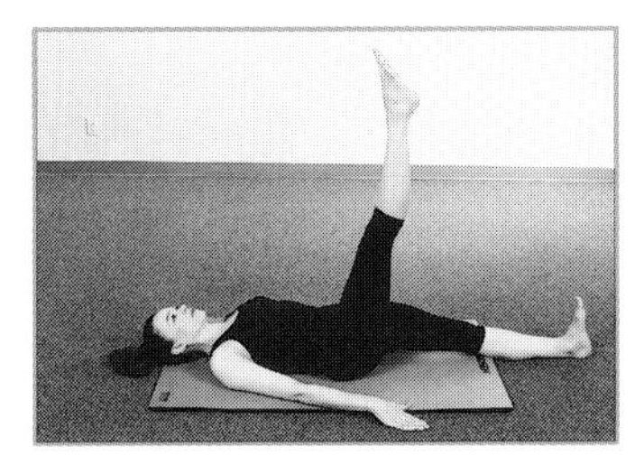

WITH your foot softly pointed, return the arms to your sides while keeping your other leg long, straight, and flat to the floor.

DRAW basketball-size circles in the air with your pointed toe, starting the circle by moving across your body, then heading down and progressing all the way around. Emphasize the movement across the body, and don't let the leg swing out too far as it moves away from the centerline.

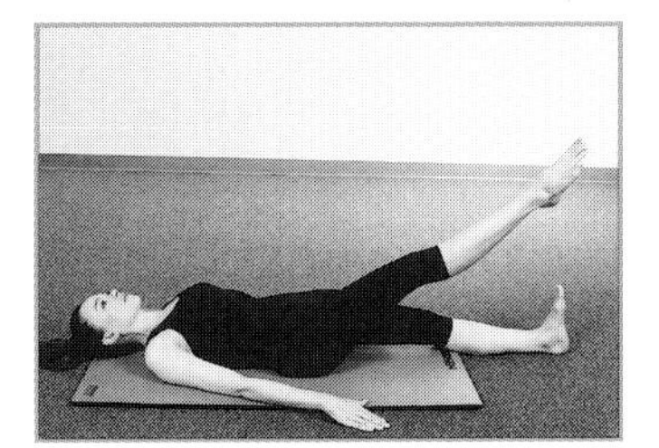

YOUR leg should move freely in the hip socket, but keep the hip in contact with the floor. Control the circles, consciously stabilizing the movement from the belly, and don't strain the hip joint.

WITH each repetition, complete one full breath—all the way in and all the way out. Do three to five reps.

STOP and complete a set of circles in the opposite direction, doing three to five more reps.

SWITCH to the other leg and repeat.

END by pulling both knees in and then rolling up to a sitting position.

NOW that you're sitting, pull your heels back toward the buttocks to prepare for the next exercise.

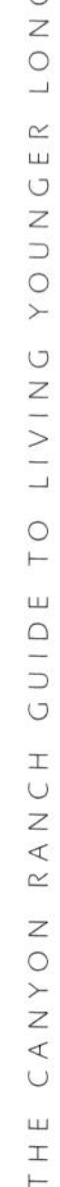

Rolling Like a Ball

TAKE hold of your ankles with your hands as you bend your knees into your chest. Your ankles should be aligned, and your elbows open out to the sides.

OPEN your knees just a bit as you raise your feet from the mat. You should feel that you're balancing on your sacrum.

TUCK your chin into your chest, look at your navel and pull your belly back toward your spine. Now you resemble a ball.

SINCE you're a ball, start rolling. Press your midsection even further into your spine to start the backward roll. Stay tucked, with the head forward.

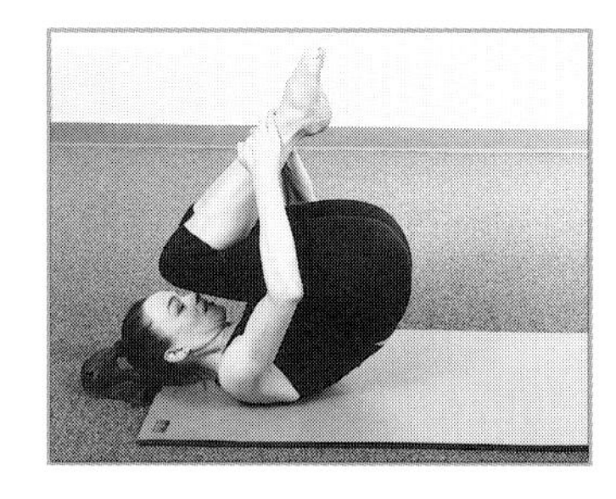

ROLL back to the tip of your shoulder blades as you inhale; exhale to reverse direction. Roll back up to your balance point.

BALANCE on your sacrum for just a second (put a foot down if you need to), then roll back again.

ROLL five to eight times.

END balanced on your sacrum, still tucked.

Single-Leg Stretch

TAKE hold of one ankle with your outside hand, and the knee with your inside hand, and pull the bent knee closer to your chest.

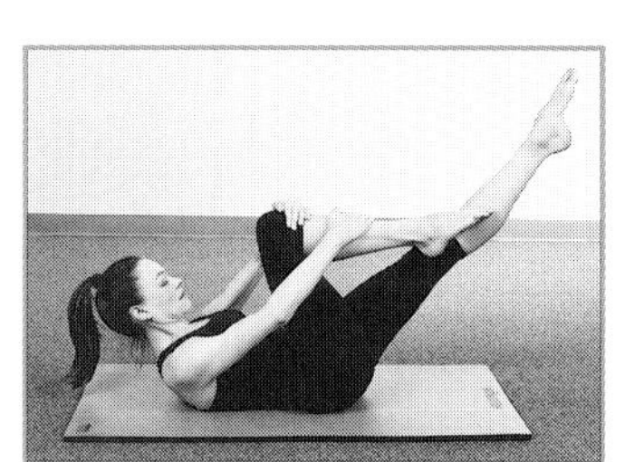

ROLL back down to the floor while stretching the other leg out straight and long. This straight leg is extended in the air, at a height that makes it possible for you to keep your back flattened to the floor.

WITH elbows out and head and upper back curled forward, inhale deeply and feel your midsection press down against your spine.

EXHALE and switch legs, being careful to mirror the placement of your hands on the bent leg. Keep the extended leg very straight and strong, and both feet softly pointed.

COMPLETE five to ten reps.

PULL both knees to your chest to get ready for the next exercise.

Double-Leg Stretch

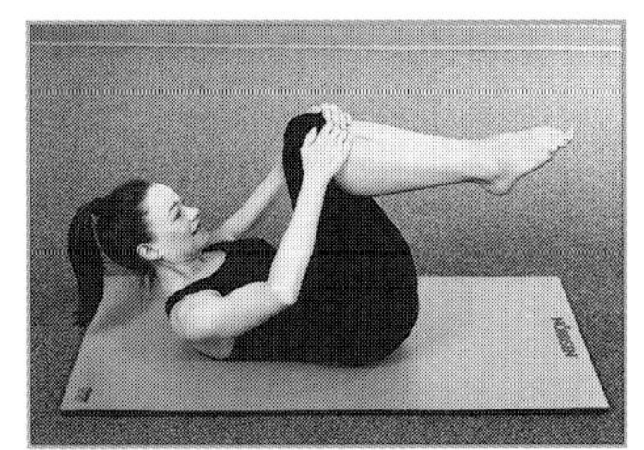

STILL on your back, knees to chest, elbows extended, head up, inhale deeply.

AS you inhale, stretch and open up, reaching up and back with your straight arms and out with your legs until your limbs are at 45 degree angles to the ground.

YOUR torso remains on the mat, midsection anchored to your spine, shoulders down and back (not hunched up around your ears).

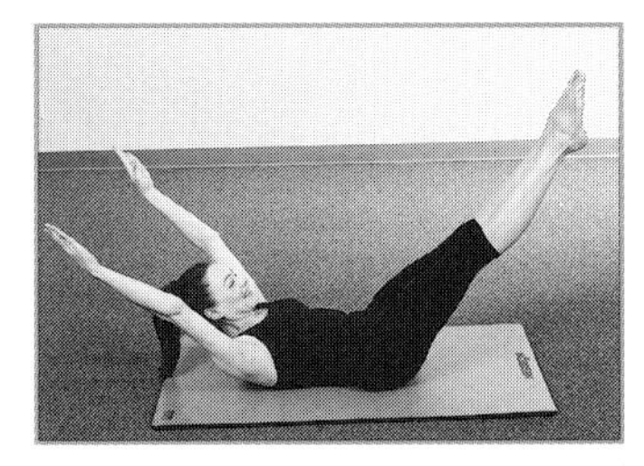

EXHALE and scoop everything back in, bringing your knees back to your chest and circling them with your arms.

PRESS even further into mat, making yourself a tighter package and exhaling the last drop of air.

REPEAT five to ten times.

YOU should end with both knees to your chest, hands on shins.

Spine Stretch Forward

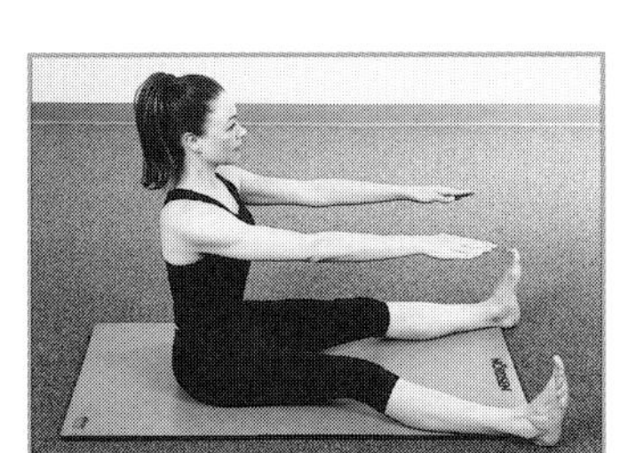

ROLL up into a sitting position, back straight, legs extended at an angle slightly wider than your hips, feet flexed. Shoulders are down and back, and the neck is long. Reach your arms straight out in front of you.

INHALE and try to sit up even taller, squeezing the glutes.

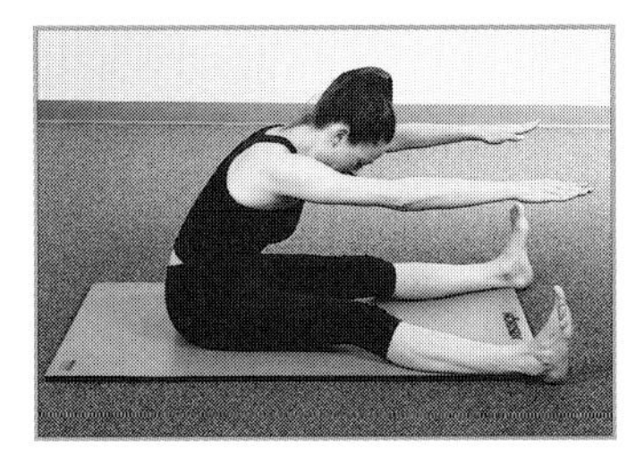

LOWER chin to your chest and round over toward your midsection, exhaling as you go and continuing to reach the arms long.

YOUR torso should resemble the letter C. Exhale as you stretch further, pulling the belly further back toward the spine.

INHALE and reverse the direction, rolling up vertebra by vertebra. Head comes up off the chest last.

RETURN to the starting position.

REPEAT three times, trying to curve and stretch the lower spine more each time.

END by sitting up tall, legs extended.

The Saw

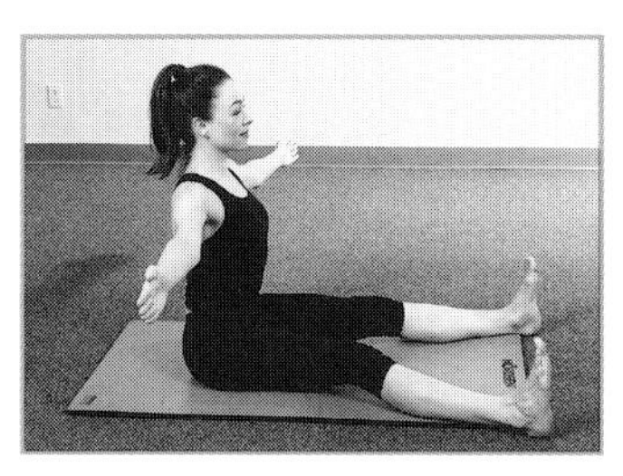

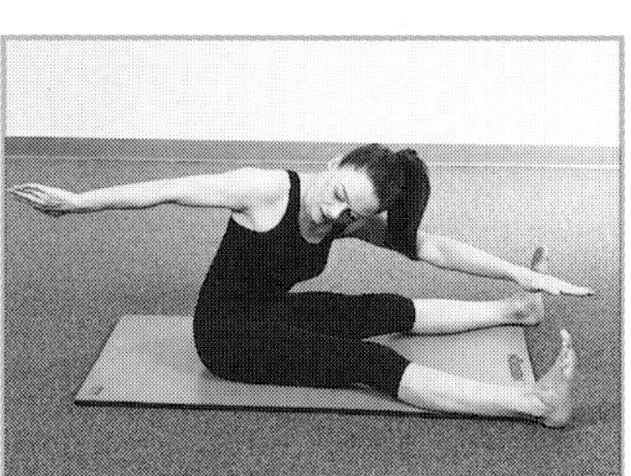

SIT tall and square on the hipbones, legs straight out and slightly wider than your hips, feet flexed, heels pressing into ground. Extend arms straight out to either side. Neck is long and shoulders are down and relaxed.

INHALE, tighten the glutes, and try to pull your midsection upward as you become as tall as possible.

AT the top of this movement, twist from your waist to one side, moving torso and arms as one unit, and leaving both hips flat on the floor. Remember, you are turning from your waist, and the opposite hip stays back and down. (Pressing your legs into the floor helps stabilize the hips.)

AS you exhale, reach for—ideally past—the little toe with the opposite hand, keeping the arms long and turning the head to look up at the arm that's behind you. Your pinkie finger should brush by your baby toe ("sawing" it), if possible.

DON'T stop stretching—feel your belly pull in as you reach your arms long and continue to exhale.

INHALE and come back up, initiating the movement from the waist.

RETURN to the starting position.

SWITCH sides and repeat. Complete four to six reps.

Side Kick—Front/Back

BEGIN on your side, head resting in your hand, with other hand solidly planted, palm down, in front of your midsection

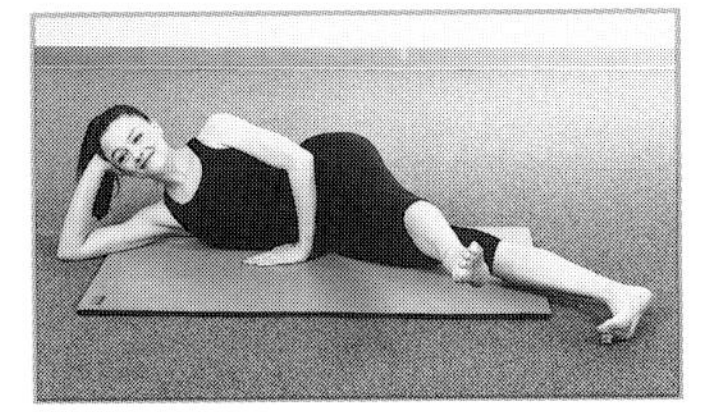

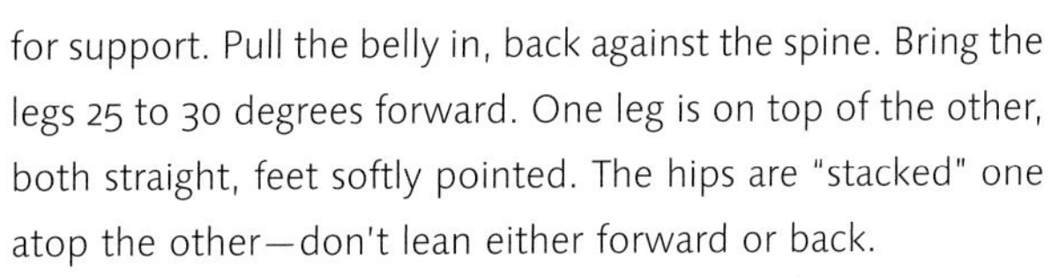

for support. Pull the belly in, back against the spine. Bring the legs 25 to 30 degrees forward. One leg is on top of the other, both straight, feet softly pointed. The hips are "stacked" one atop the other—don't lean either forward or back.

RAISE the top leg until the foot is at hip level. Turn the whole leg slightly out (up) from the hip. Inhale.

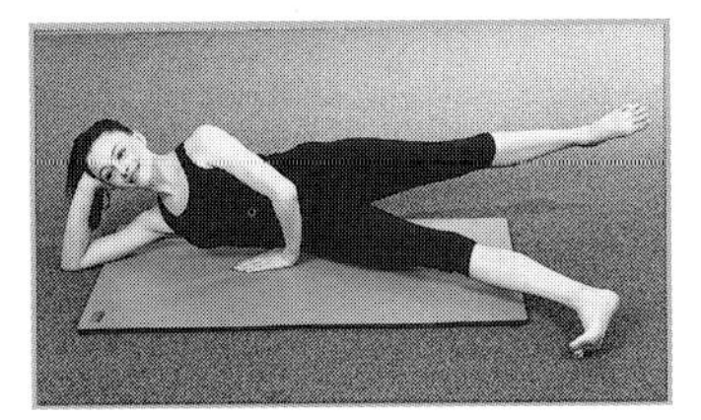

SWING the top leg forward, keeping it straight. Pulse twice, as far in front of you as you can, keeping the rest of the body still. Try to move only the leg.

EXHALE as you reach the leg back behind you, and pulse.

REPEAT six to ten times. Switch sides.

The Seal

NOW for the big finish—a wonderful rolling massage for your lower back.

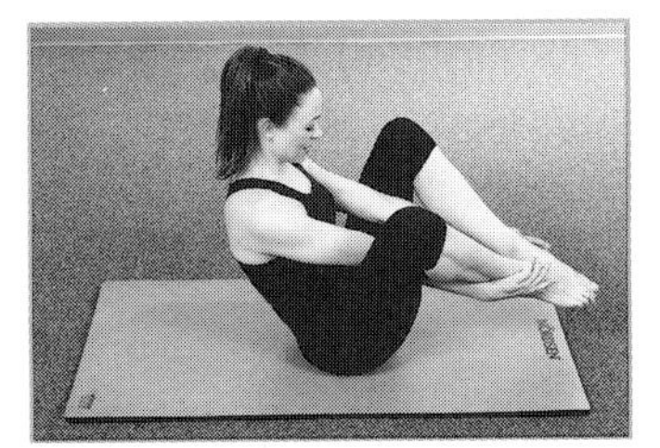

WITH knees bent to your chest, heels together, sit up tall. Open your knees to shoulder width, and take each ankle on the outside, coming inside the thigh and outside the calf with the arm. Pull your feet up so that you balance on the sacrum and the inside edges of your feet are together. Don't let the thighs get too wide apart, and start with the feet as close to the floor as you can get them and still balance. (This all sounds more complicated than it is. Check the photo.)

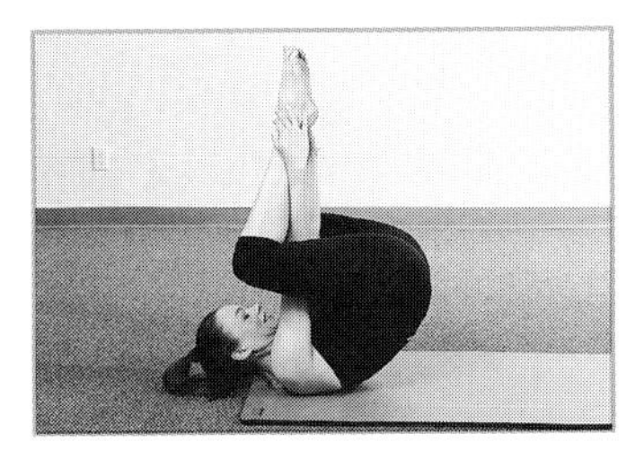

INHALE and roll back, pulling your belly in and rounding your lower back out so it rolls smoothly along the floor. Roll back to your shoulders—*not* onto your neck—and pause.

RIGHT there, clap your heels together. (At this instant, you can, if you wish, imagine that you're a seal.)

EXHALE on your forward roll, tucking the chin into your chest and keeping your belly pulled in.

BALANCE again on the sacrum and clap your heels. You can eventually work up to three quick claps.

REPEAT six to eight times.

And now you're done.

Advanced Pilates classes add more exercises, and even for this basic selection there are dozens of variations that are harder or easier. Several hundred other Pilates moves await you, the overwhelming majority of which are performed on Joseph Pilates' imposing machines under the supervision of an instructor. Nonetheless, this is a good start. Master these, or at least give them a shot, and if you want to pursue the method further, find a local studio or instructor and see how far you can go.

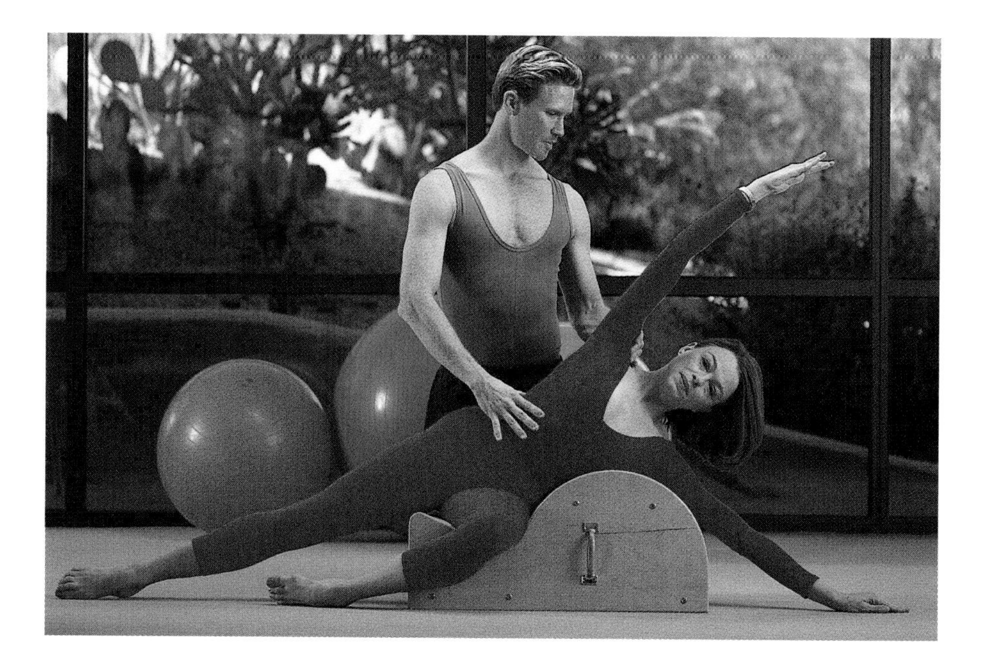

STYLES OF HATHA YOGA

IYENGAR, ASHTANGA, Kundalini, Kripalu, Sivananda, Bikram, and the many other "yogas" you may hear and read about—are all just styles of hatha yoga developed by various teachers.

Yoga is a house with many rooms. Some styles are vigorous and fast, others are more meditative and flowing; some are strict and rather formal, some are freely expressive. All are yoga. By all means, try various styles if you're interested, but don't be intimidated by the loyalties or preferences of others. The "best" style is the one that suits you.

Yoga

YOGA IS THE MOST ancient method of personal development known. It's a discipline with the power to profoundly affect both mind and body. The first evidence of yoga—postures etched on stone tablets—dates from 3000 B.C. Students and teachers have spent generations shaping its practices and understanding its powers.

Modern knowledge of yoga can be traced back to the sage Patanjali, who lived around 200 B.C. Patanjali codified yoga, defining it as an eight-fold path in his work *Yoga Sutras.* In the simplest terms, the sutras are an instruction manual for leading a full and productive life.

The eight paths or limbs of yoga are equally important, and, properly understood, they form a seamless whole. *Yama* is a set of ethical standards for correct behavior. *Niyama* is self-discipline. *Asana*—the practice of postures that make up hatha yoga, which we tend to think of as yoga itself—maintains the healthy body necessary for equanimity of spirit. *Pranayama* is control of breath, while *pratyahara,* or sensory withdrawal, and *dharana,* or concentration, form the basis of *dhyana,* meditation. The end point of the eight-fold path is *samadhi,* or transcendence, the union of the soul with the divine Spirit.

Asana (the physical postures), *pranayama* (breathing practices), and *dyana* (meditation) are the paths most familiar to the Western yoga student. The practice of the physical form of yoga (*asana*) eventually involves all the branches of which Patanjali speaks in the sutras. When we practice *asana,* we develop concentration and self-discipline. Breathing exercises give movement and life to our postures and help us develop meditative skills. All aspects of yoga are subtly interrelated, and benefits gradually reveal themselves through continued practice. Yoga also has the virtue of

HINTS FOR AN ENJOYABLE PRACTICE

Practice daily.

Don't practice on a full stomach.

Wear comfortable clothing you can move in.

Never force your body beyond its limits.

Never hold a pose longer than is comfortable.

Never hold your breath.

Listen to your body.

Think of the postures as a mindful dance of breath and body.

Take time to feel and reflect in each posture.

Increase the time you spend in each posture as your strength and agility improve.

Most important, enjoy!

being almost endless. There's always something more to learn and do in yoga, which means that it need never become boring.

On a physical level, continued *asana* practice, hatha yoga, gives strength and flexibility to the muscular, skeletal, and nervous systems. In addition, it fosters a supple, healthy spine; massages and improves blood supply to internal organs; and improves circulation and respiration. Over time, people who do yoga for its purely physical benefits often begin to feel more insight into their own natures and enjoy a calmer, clearer state of mind. Regular yoga practice creates a better quality of life on many different levels.

While it's possible to do some beginning yoga practice with just a book or videotape for guidance, as you become more interested you'll want to take classes with a qualified teacher. Alignment and proper technique are crucial if you are to enjoy all the many benefits of yoga, and it's easy to slip into subtly incorrect postures when you practice entirely by yourself.

Because of yoga's burgeoning popularity, many choices of styles and teachers are available at gyms, health clubs, and the growing number of facilities wholly devoted to yoga. You have so many choices that you may want to sit in on several different classes before signing up. Choose a teacher and a class that best suits your needs, and remember that the intent of yoga is to "honor your body." Never push past your comfort zone.

THE WORD *yoga* is derived from the Sanskrit word *yuj*, which means "to yoke" or "join." The goal of yoga is the union of all opposites in a balanced, seamless whole.

The following postures come from our begining yoga class at Canyon Ranch. To do them, you'll need comfortable clothes, a yoga mat, a strap or soft belt, and a towel. The yoga mat should be a "sticky mat," which provides a nonslip surface for your postures. (Always do yoga with bare feet.) These items can be purchased from almost any yoga studio or ordered through a yoga supply house—there are many on the Internet.

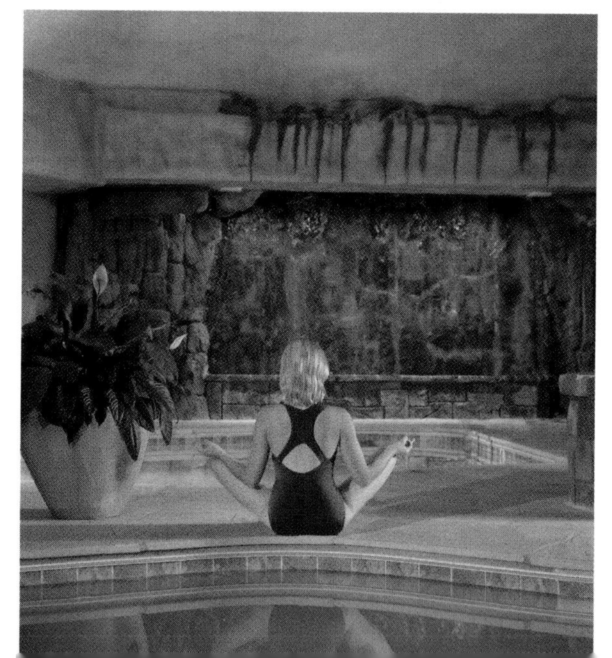

THE POSTURES

Note: When lying on the floor, support your neck or head with a folded blanket if it's more comfortable.

Tadasana—Mountain Pose

Benefits: **Develops proper posture and skeletal alignment. Balances the mind-body system.**

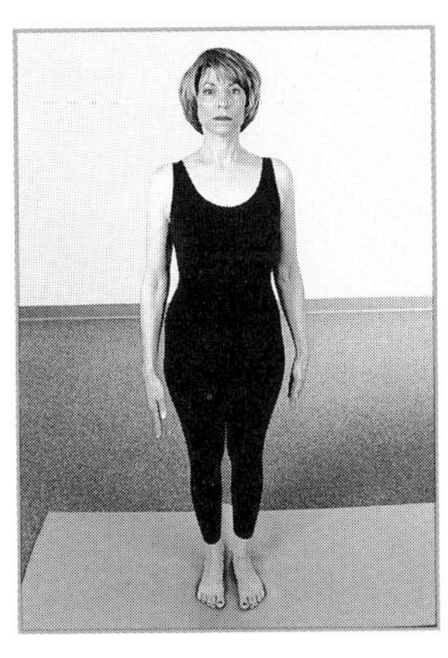

STAND with your feet slightly apart and parallel. Keep your weight balanced evenly on the balls and heels of your feet.

Firmly press your feet into your mat, tighten your thigh muscles (think of pulling the kneecaps up), and relax your shoulders back and down. Arms and hands stay active but relaxed at your sides, palms facing your hips.

IMAGINE a line of energy running from the base of the spine to the top of your head.

LENGTHEN your spine on an inhale. Keep this length as you exhale.

BREATHE gently and evenly, keeping your eyes soft and your jaw relaxed. Take a few moments for self-reflection.

VARIATION:

STANDING tall, on an exhale reach your arms up, palms facing one another.

KEEP your shoulders and neck muscles relaxed. Continue to stretch the body upward as you breathe full, easy breaths. Hold for 30 seconds.

Utthita Trikonasana—Triangle Pose

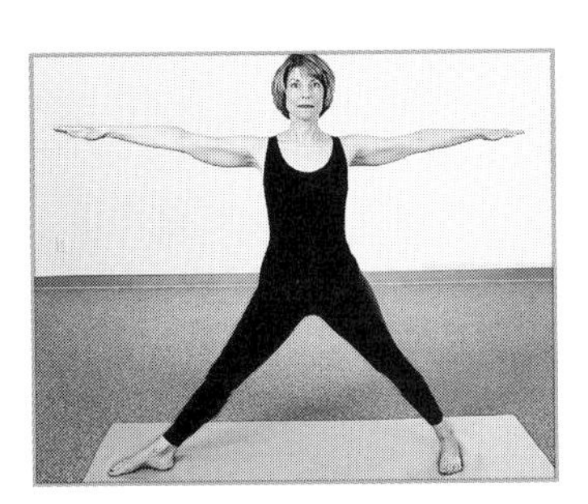

Benefits: **Tones the leg muscles, brings flexibility to hips, knees, neck, and shoulders. Like all the standing postures, it improves circulation and breathing.**

STAND with your feet 3 to 3 1/2 feet apart.

TURN your right foot out about 90 degrees, turn your left foot in slightly, to about 15 degrees. Adjust the feet so that the right foot is in alignment with the left arch.

PRESS the soles of your feet firmly into your mat. At the same time, tighten your thigh muscles. Raise your arms to shoulder height, palms facing down.

INHALE and lengthen your spine up. Be mindful of the expansion in your body; exhale as you need to.

INHALE again, and on an exhalation shift your trunk sideways to the right, keeping your spine long. Bend and stretch from your right hip joint and arch over to the right, moving your arms, shoulders and trunk as a unit. Place your right hand lightly on your leg or ankle as your left arm reaches up, palm facing forward.

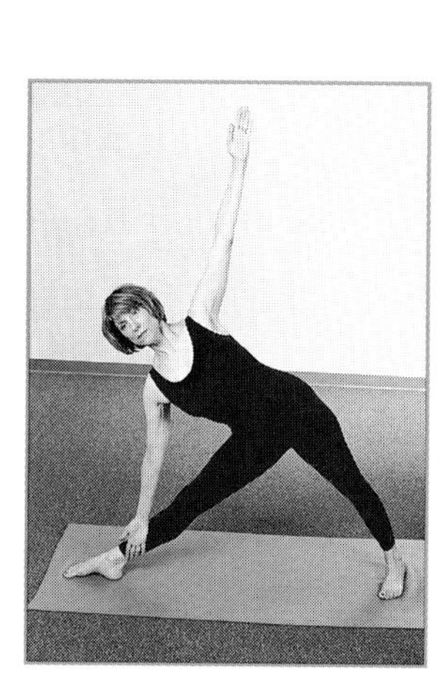

Your left arm should be in line with your right arm. Keep your head in line with your spine and facing forward. Keep the legs active, muscles working, shoulders and neck strong but not tense.

REMEMBER to keep the breath flowing gently and easily while you are in the pose.

HOLD the posture for 20–30 seconds.

On your last inhale come back to center.

TAKE a few breaths and repeat to the left side.

When you finish the posture, give yourself time to feel its effects.

Virabhadrasana II—Warrior Pose

***Benefits:* Creates strength and suppleness in the leg and back muscles, tones the abdominal organs, and instills a feeling of confidence.**

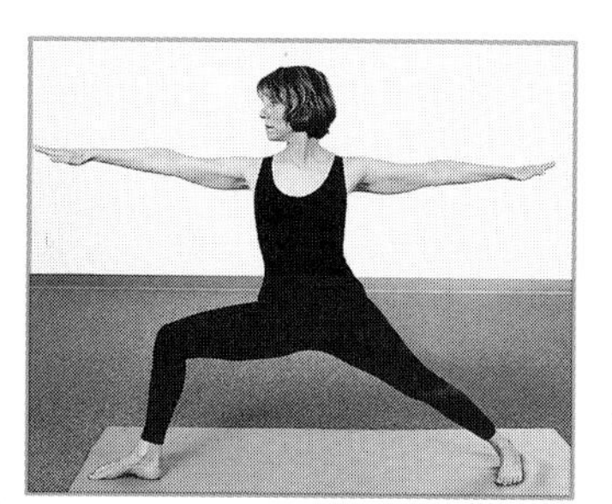

STAND with your feet 4 to 4 1/2 feet apart.

FIND your balance and turn your right foot out to 90 degrees and your left foot in, to 15 degrees. Align the right foot with the arch of the left.

NOTICE the contact of the balls and heels of the feet with the mat. Inhale and lift your arms to shoulder level, palms facing down.

KEEP the breath continually moving through your body. Inhale and lengthen your spine.

EXHALE and bend the right leg to a right angle. Be sure to keep the right knee directly above the right ankle.

CENTER your weight between the two asymmetrical legs by pressing strongly into the left foot. When you feel centered, slowly turn your head and look at the fingers of the right hand.

STAY in the pose for 20–30 seconds, breathing normally.

INHALE and come up by pressing the ball of the right foot and the outer edge of the left foot into your mat.

TAKE time to reflect, then repeat on the left side.

Vrksasana—Tree Pose

***Benefits:* Strengthens the legs and feet; improves balance and concentration, circulation, and breathing.**

STAND with your feet apart (no wider than hip width), feet and knees facing forward.

BRING awareness to the soles of your feet, firm the muscles of your legs, and lengthen your spine.

FOCUS on a point in front of you, soften your eyes and face, and breathe naturally. When you feel centered, shift your weight to the right leg.

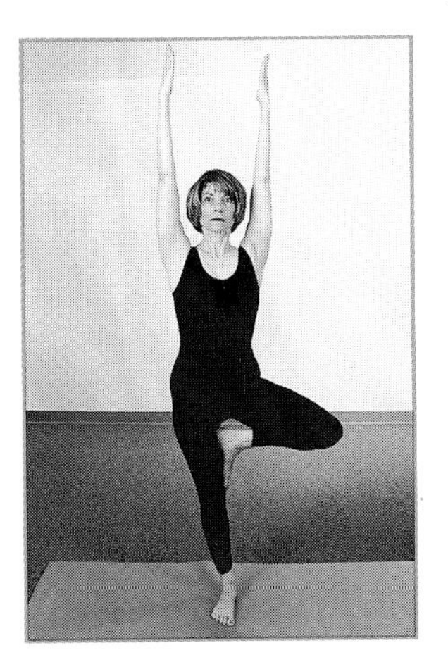

BEND the left knee to the side and place the sole of your left foot on the right inner calf or thigh, toes toward the floor. Use your hand, if necessary.

KEEP the muscles of the standing leg firm and your spine long. Place your hands in prayer position. Press the foot into the thigh and the thigh into the foot to stabilize your balance.

If you feel ready, extend your arms overhead, palms facing one another.

KEEP your breath relaxed and easy. Hold the posture for 10–30 seconds.

***NOTE:* IT'S especially important to practice balance postures regularly since balance can deteriorate with age. Until you find your balance in the pose, practice holding on to a chair or touching a wall.**

PLACE your left foot to the floor.

REPEAT the posture on the left leg when you are ready.

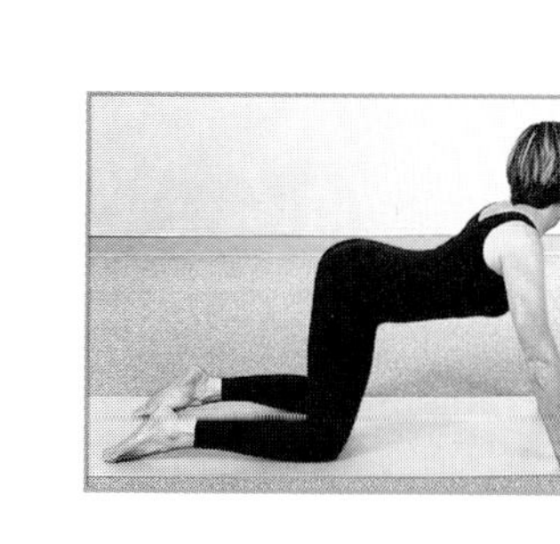

Cakravakasana—Cat Pose

Benefits: Stretches and balances the spinal column, relieves lower back tension, brings nutrients to the abdominal organs, and improves respiration.

BEGIN on your hands and knees. Your shoulders should be vertically above your wrists and your hips above your knees.

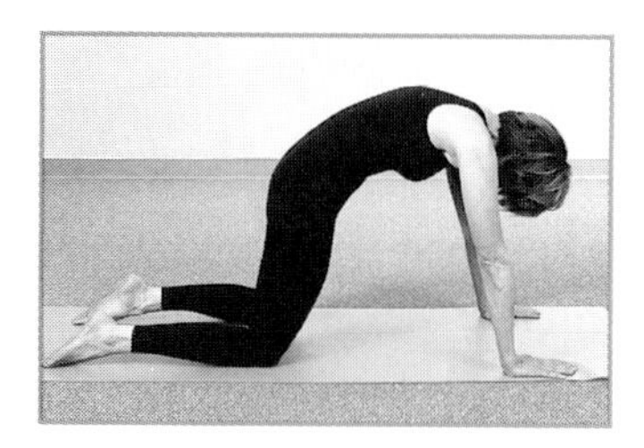

INHALE and tilt your buttocks toward the ceiling, gently arching your lower back and letting your chest drop toward the floor. Look up slightly.

EXHALE and pull the abdomen toward your spine. Round your back.

REPEAT several times, coordinating your breath with the movement. Move slowly and mindfully.

Balasana—Child Pose

Benefits: Relaxes and lengthens the spinal muscles; nourishes the disks between the vertebrae by creating space between them, thus relieving compression.

Note: The Child Pose and the Cat Pose work well in conjunction.

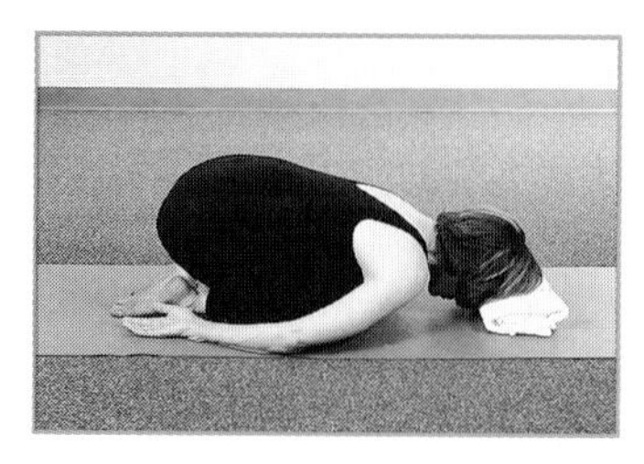

BEGIN on your hands and knees. Hands are below the shoulders, knees below the hips.

EXHALE and move your buttocks toward your heels, placing your forehead on the floor.

REST your hands palms up at your sides as you continue to watch your breath. If your buttocks do not reach your heels, place a folded towel or a pillow on your calves and rest on that.

If your head does not reach the floor, place a folded towel under your forehead.

NOTICE how the posture passively lengthens your spine as you keep your attention focused on your breath. Let the muscles of the back relax—imagine them as a heavy blanket. Stay in the pose as long as you're comfortable.

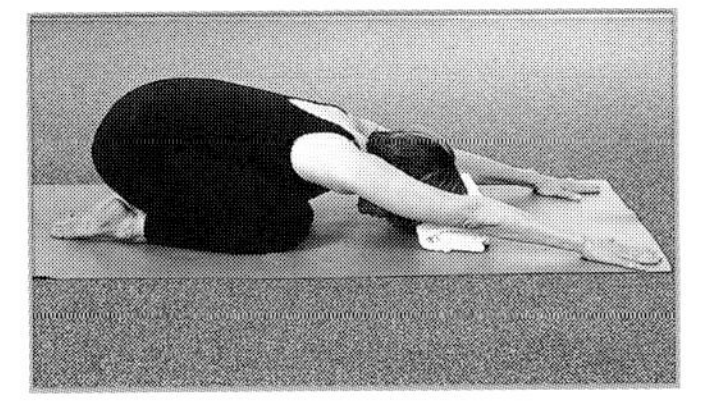

VARIATION:

After you are in the pose for a few breaths, extend your arms in front of you on the floor.

LET the shoulders relax as you increase the stretch in the chest, waist, and arms.

Adho Mukha Svanasana—Downward Facing Dog Pose

Benefits: **Helps relieve fatigue; brings flexibility and strength to arms, shoulders, legs, and feet.**

BEGIN on your hands and knees. Place your hands shoulder width apart. Keep your shoulders above your wrists.

KEEP your knees hip width apart and slightly behind your hips.

PRESS your fingers and palms into the mat as you firm the arm muscles.

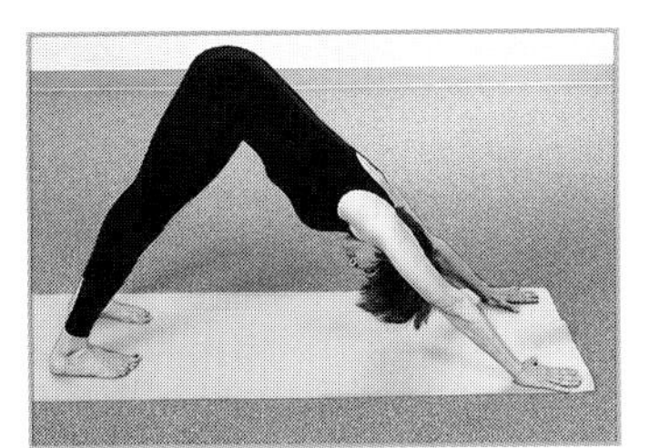

TURN your toes under and on an exhale lift your buttocks toward the ceiling.

KEEP your heels raised as you lift the hips and buttocks higher. Relax your head and neck muscles. Keep your breath easy and unrestrained.

HOLD the posture for a few breaths and return to your hands and knees.

As you become stronger, try lowering your heels to the floor, remembering to keep the thigh muscles firm and pulled up.

EASIER VARIATION:

STAND facing a wall. Walk to the wall and place your fingers on the wall at hip level.

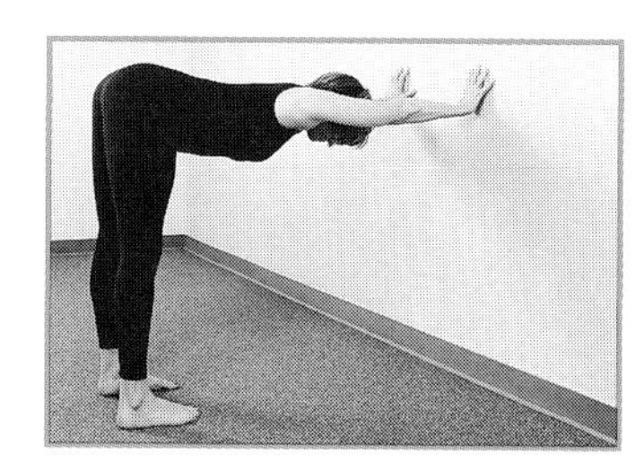

SEPARATE your feet as wide as your hips.

STEP back from the wall, pressing fingertips into it while straightening your arms.

CONTINUE to lengthen your spine, keeping your neck in line with your spine.

HOLD for a few breaths, enjoying the stretch. When ready, walk toward the wall to come up.

Bhujangasana—Cobra Pose

Benefits: **This posture strengthens the back muscles and keeps the spine supple, thus improving posture. It also massages the abdominal organs.**

LIE on your stomach with your legs hip width apart.

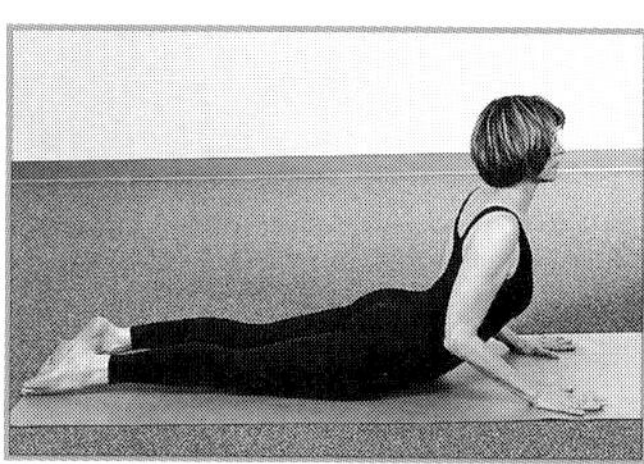

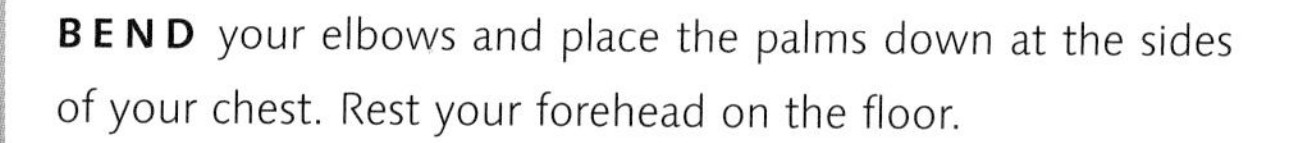

BEND your elbows and place the palms down at the sides of your chest. Rest your forehead on the floor.

PRESS the palms into the mat.

INHALE, raise the forehead, chin, and chest from the floor and look straight ahead.

KEEP your pelvis in contact with the floor or mat, and keep buttocks firm.

REMEMBER to use your back muscles to curl the spine up. Use your arms and hands for balance and support.

DO NOT strain or force the posture. Come up only as far as you are comfortable.

HOLD the posture for 10–20 seconds, breathing naturally.

COME down slowly, uncurling the spine and bringing the chest, chin, and then forehead back to the mat.

TURN your head to one side, place it on the mat, and feel the effects of the pose.

Supta Padangusthasana—Lying Down Big Toe Pose

***Benefits:* This posture lengthens the leg muscles and relieves tightness in the legs and hips.**

Note: The classical form of this asana is done holding the big toe. We use a strap, making it easier to stretch tight leg muscles without placing a strain on the back.

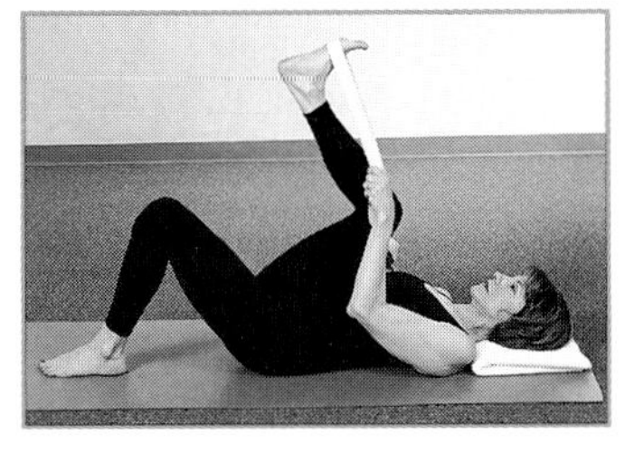

LIE on your back with knees bent, feet flat on the floor. If needed, support your head or neck with a folded blanket.

ALLOW your lower back to sink toward the floor. Bend your right knee toward your chest.

PLACE your yoga strap or a soft belt around the ball of your right foot.

HOLD the strap in your right hand. Place your left arm down at your side or in line with your left shoulder on the floor.

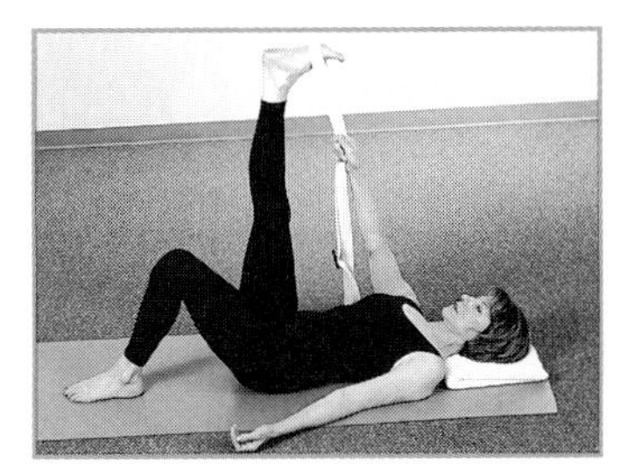

STRAIGHTEN your right leg gently and slowly.

KEEP your lower back on the floor; do not arch as you deepen your leg stretch.

BREATHE naturally and continue to move your leg closer to your face—but do not force the stretch. Be mindful of your "edge."

MAKE this pose more challenging by practicing it with your bottom (left) leg straight. Be sure to keep the muscles of that leg firm.

HOLD for about 30 seconds, making sure that you don't tense head, neck, or shoulders.

RELEASE by bending your right leg, then extend both legs on the floor. Take a moment to notice the feeling in your "newly stretched" leg.

STRETCH the opposite leg when you're ready.

Variation of Jathara Parivartanasana—Lying Down Bent Knee Twist

Benefits: **This posture tones the abdominal area and helps relieve tension in the lower back.**

LIE down with your arms stretched out to the sides, palms facing up.

BEND your knees and bring them toward your chest, then slowly move your knees to the right, keeping both shoulders and arms on the floor.

If they do not touch the floor, you can support them by placing a pillow under the knee.

STAY in the pose for a few breaths, allowing the lower back and spinal muscles to relax.

BRING your knees to center and move them to the left.

REPEAT this pose a few times to each side. Remember to contract your abdominal muscles when you bring your knees back up to the centerline of your body. Enjoy the release in your lower back.

Savasana—Corpselike Pose

Benefits: **This pose allows the body to renew and restore its own energy by releasing fatigue and quieting the mind. In essence, it is a pose of relaxation.**

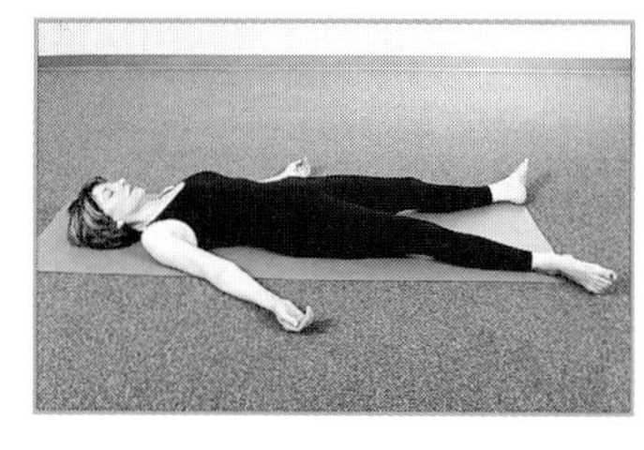

LIE on your back. Place your legs a comfortable distance apart.

RELAX your toes, feet, and legs.

TURN your upper arms out, turn palms up, and relax your arms.

KEEP your arms slightly away from your body.

TAKE a moment to observe your body; this position should produce a sense of ease. If need be, adjust your body so that it rests in a state of complete comfort.

CLOSE your eyes and release any tension in the eyelids; allow them to be "soft."

RELAX your facial muscles, jaw, mouth, lips, and throat. Release any tightness in your neck and shoulders.

ALLOW your body to melt into the floor.

CONTINUE to breathe normally, observing the gentle flow of your breath.

ALLOW the mind to quiet and the body to let go even further. Rest in the pose as long as you wish.

COME out of the pose by deepening your breath and bring gentle movement to fingertips and toes; slowly open your eyes.

BEND your knees, roll to one side, stay in a fetal position for a few breaths. Then get up.

Balance, Movement, and You

BALANCE COMES TO US as whole beings. We intuitively understand why this should be: when we feel good emotionally, we're at ease physically. We move more briskly, lightly, and with more confidence, and, as we enjoy our free and comfortable movement through space, our mood improves further. A comfortable, strong body and a mind at peace reinforce each other.

As scientists identify more precisely the intricate linkages between body and brain, we understand better than ever before why reprogramming one can be so beneficial to the other. Healthy movement eventually leads to a new sense of ease and self-possession.

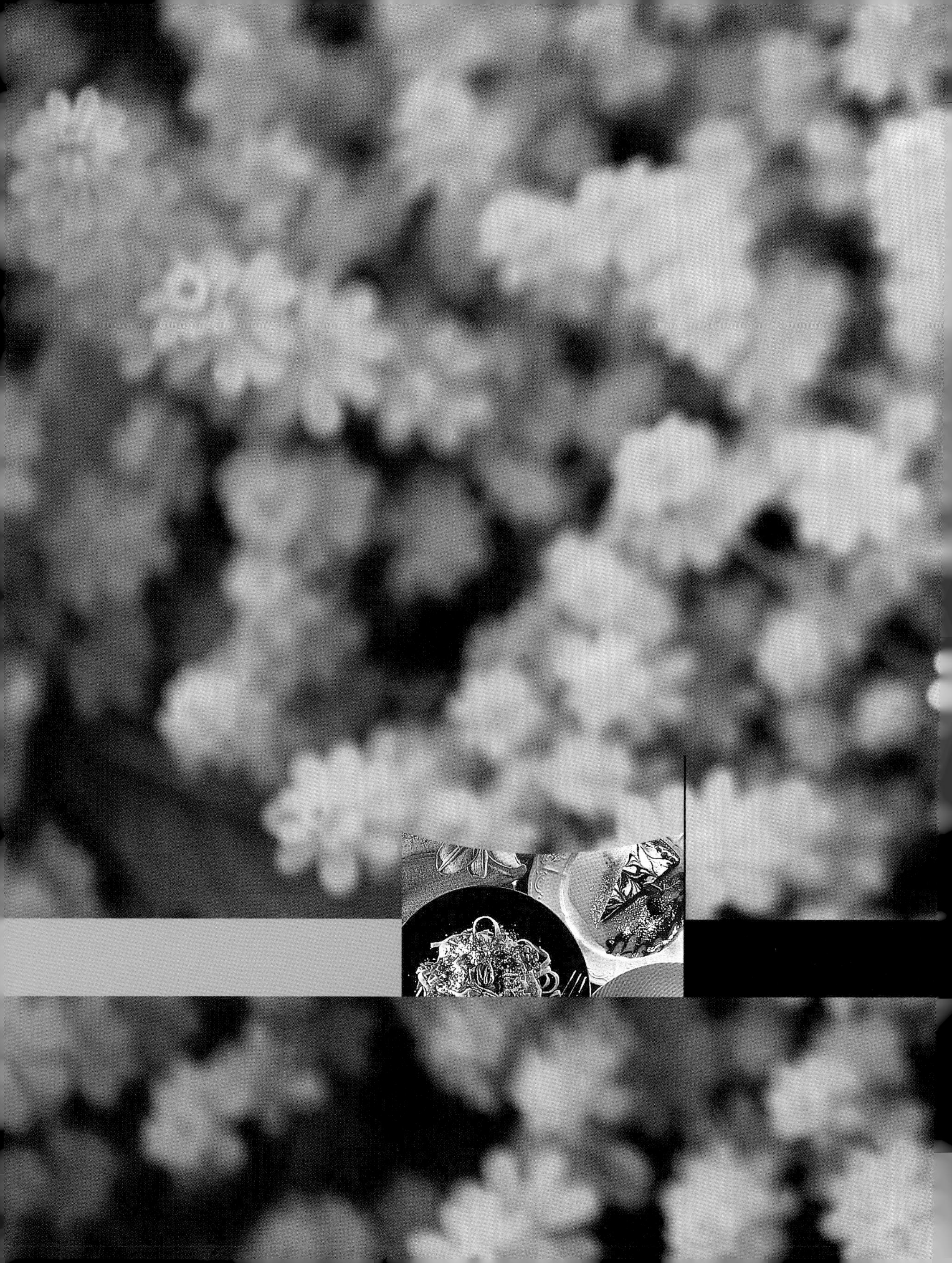

6

THE HEALTHY WEIGHT PHILOSOPHY:

The Dangers of Dieting

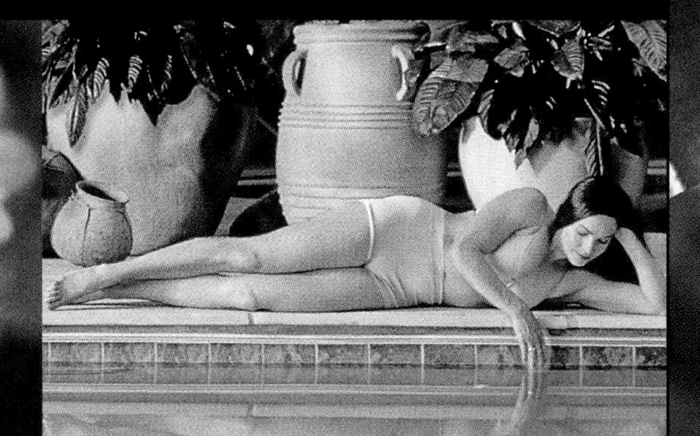

When Canyon Ranch started more than two decades ago, people came here to lose weight fast. And they did. It wasn't unusual for a guest to lose ten or twelve pounds during a ten-day stay. A strenuous walk first thing in the morning and five, six, or seven hour-long fitness classes a day, all on 800 calories, did the trick. Our guests weighed in before they checked in and weighed out just before they got on the van for the airport, so we knew just how dramatic those losses were.

We did great return business, too. (We still do, actually, but for more satisfying reasons.) As soon as our guests stepped off the property, most of them began putting the weight back on. Who's got seven hours a day to exercise in the real world? Never mind the impossibility of sticking to a starvation diet.

By the early nineties, we had become very uneasy about this pattern—lose it at the ranch, pack it back on, come back for another fat-melting stay. So uneasy that key members of our medical, exercise physiology, and nutrition staffs sat down and reviewed the program of weight loss we recommended to our guests. We were concerned about what we'd seen ourselves, and startled by a 1991 finding by the National Institutes of Health: 95 to 98 percent of all people who lose weight by going on a diet regain it within five years. We'd also seen research that suggested that a stable, heavier weight might be healthier, in the long run, than yo-yo dieting.

Our first question was whether we believed that long-term, permanent weight loss *is even possible.* Yes, was the answer, under certain conditions and with qualifications. We then went back through fifty years of research, looking for clues as to why losing and keeping weight off is so hard—and for leads to what might actually work.

The result is the Canyon Ranch Healthy Weight Philosophy—the least specific "diet plan" you'll ever see. It's also the most enlightening, realistic, and potentially empowering approach to body-weight issues you've ever encountered. It's what we tell our guests at Canyon Ranch, and it's our best advice.

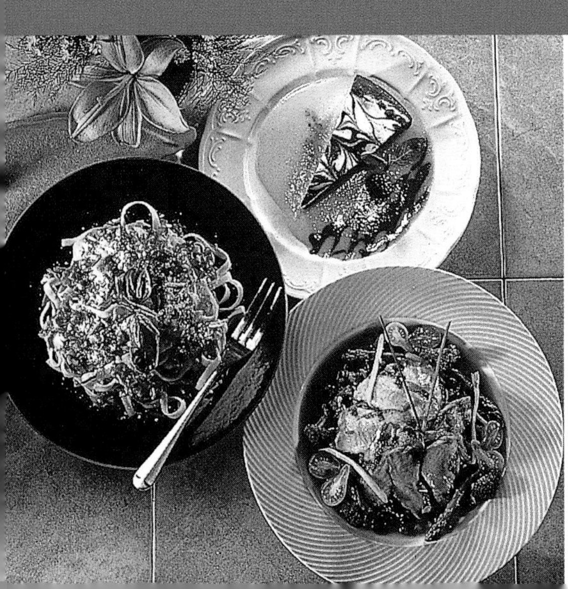

IN THE EARLY NINETIES, researchers involved sedentary nursing home residents in a consistent program of weight training. The last group studied were men and women between the ages of eighty-six and ninety-six. In the course of ten to twelve weeks, the strength of the muscles trained doubled, greatly increasing the mobility and quality of life of the near-centenarian participants. The capacity of the human body to adapt when challenged—even in extreme old age—is astounding.

Your Perfect Body

YOUR BODY, AS IT is at this moment, is perfect.

We're not kidding, and here's what we mean: your body is perfectly adapted to the way you live, and it reflects, perfectly, what you do every day, given your genetic inheritance.

What you have is what you get when you eat the way you've been eating and exercise the way you've been exercising. Period. You might as well just stop stewing about what Kate Moss, Jennifer Lopez, or your skinny, potato-chip-munching sister-in-law looks like, because it's irrelevant to *you,* to your physiology.

So are we saying that you're stuck with what you have right now? No: the evidence is overwhelming that the human body adapts beautifully to whatever we ask of it. What follows from this? One simple rule: change your life, and your body, given time, *will* change. It will never be exactly the supermodel body that our culture keeps insisting you must have to be happy, but your body will change within the parameters of your genetic inheritance, and those changes will faithfully reflect your efforts. But whatever you do to lose weight, you must keep doing, or your ever-adaptable body will readapt.

Why the Accounting Approach Doesn't Work

WE ALL LONG FOR CERTAINTIES, for hard edges and promises and definite numbers. We love height-and-weight charts, even though most of us, once we've found the place where our height and weight converge, instantly decide that we must be big-boned. We like the Body Mass Index, which divides height in meters (squared) into weight in kilograms, even though all those conversions and calculations don't take body composition into account and consequently indicate that some heavily muscled athletes are overweight. These charts work well for characterizing populations, but they're often misused. They don't allow for the enormous variability of the human body and consequently have limited relevance to individuals.

The numeric, or accounting, approach is also limited when it comes to calorie counting. You want numbers? Here's numbers:

- The average American gains about one pound a year, or ten pounds a decade, between the ages of thirty and sixty.
- Take that ten pounds, multiply by 3,500 excess calories per pound, then divide by ten years times 365 days, and you arrive at an excess consumption of 9.5 calories a day. That's nothing. It's six Tic-Tacs. It's less than the variation between one serving

A GUEST TOLD us that at the end of a long transit strike in Paris a few years back, a French newspaper reported that the average Parisian, who was forced to walk everywhere, had lost five pounds. Six months later, the average Parisian, back riding the bus, subway, and train every day, had regained the weight.

and the next of fruit-juice-sweetened chocolate sauce on the ice cream sundaes we serve at Canyon Ranch—and our cooks are extremely careful about portion size. Nine and a half calories a day is less than you can conceivably keep track of.

Does this mean that there's no point in trying to control your weight? Just the opposite, but it does mean that we need to look at weight control in a new light. What we need to do to be thinner is to eliminate three key saboteurs of healthy weight.

I. THE FIRST SABOTEUR: INACTIVITY

Our bodies are, as we've said, tremendously adaptable. They can even adapt to no exercise at all. One of the results of this particular adaptation, however, is an almost total loss of natural weight regulation.

This, too, can be explained in terms of adaptation to functional demand. Take a day in the life of Liz. Liz gets up in the morning, eats, showers, dresses, walks to her garage, unlocks her car with a remote, opens the garage door with another remote, drives to work, parks in an executive parking place—right by the front door—takes an elevator to her office, and proceeds to put in a twelve-hour day, never leaving her desk. She doesn't have time to go out for lunch, so she orders in. She doesn't have time to walk down the hall to talk to co-workers, so she calls them. At the end of the day, exhausted (and who wouldn't be?), she repeats the going-to-work sequence in reverse, microwaves dinner, and either flops on the couch to read or watch TV, or, more likely, sits down at her home computer to do a few more hours of work before falling into bed, totally wiped.

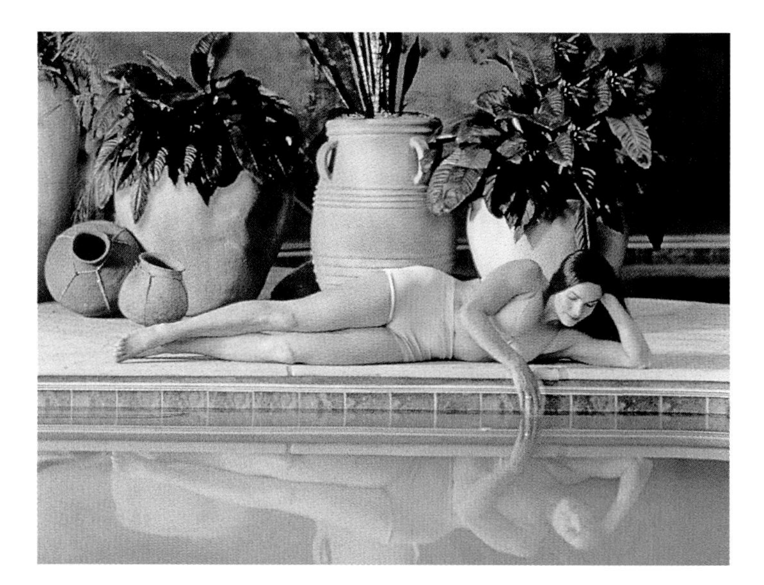

Liz works hard, but there is nothing about her physical existence, no demand whatsoever, that would make it biologically disadvantageous for her to weigh 250, or even 350 pounds, and to have no cardiovascular endurance beyond that required for prolonged sitting, talking, typing, and walking distances of less than a block. It doesn't take long for a body to adapt completely to a sedentary way of life. This is happening today to millions of Americans, and if you don't believe it, go the nearest mall and look around. Our bodies are changing to reflect precisely the physical challenges presented by the world in which we live.

How surprising is it that we're in the midst of an epidemic of obesity in this country? Four generations isn't enough time for any organism to change significantly, but look at how life has changed for the average American. Consider what your great-grandmother probably did in a typical day: an hour or more of heavy labor (washing clothes by hand, chopping wood), and several more hours, at least, of light to moderate physical activity (cleaning, gardening, cooking, tending to animals and children). When she sat down to eat, she refueled her body, very largely, with the fruits of her own labor.

You and I, by contrast, can flip open a cell phone and order a pizza (roughly 2,500 calories) delivered, expending maybe 5 calories in the process. And we will not have worked very hard physically or mentally to pay for this gigantic feast: food in this country is not only abundant but unbelievably cheap.

How do you avoid becoming a miserably overweight victim of the good life? You know the answer already: move your body. Huge amounts of exercise aren't needed for the body to balance appetite and energy expenditure, but *some* regular physical activity is. A recent study recorded in the National Weight Control Registry, for example, suggests that frequency of exercise is more important for weight control than other factors, such as intensity. If you're doing nothing now, just walking for twenty minutes every day will make a measurable difference in your body's ability to self-regulate.

II. THE SECOND SABOTEUR: DIETING

The second saboteur of our perfect body's perfect self-regulation is dieting itself.

Dieting is starvation, as far as your body is concerned. The body has very effective defensive responses to starvation, which include shedding of lean muscle mass, conservation of fat, and slowing of metabolism. What you get when you starve is a starved body. It is not the body you want.

The classic, irreplaceable study on dieting is, surprisingly, more than fifty years old, and the point of it was not to study dieting but to learn how to best feed people who'd been starved.

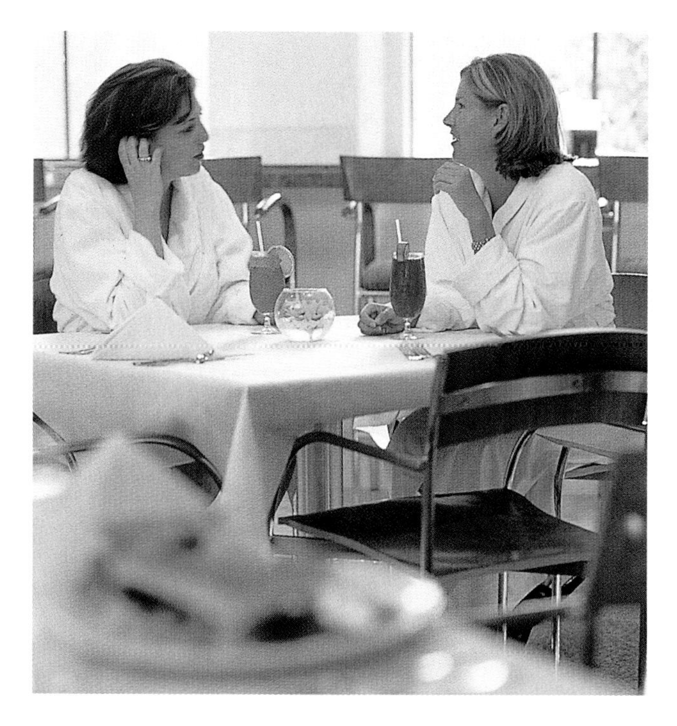

Toward the end of World War II, scientists at the University of Minnesota started working on how best to nourish and return to health the severely emaciated survivors of concentration and prisoner-of-war camps. To do their experiments, however, they needed people who were starving—and, obviously, not the victims they wanted to help. So they got a group of conscientious objectors, young pacifist men who volunteered to participate as an alternative to war service. The researchers then starved them for about four months—on a 1,500-calorie-a-day diet.

That is not a misprint. The study subjects were, of course, young men, but their calorie intake over that period was roughly equivalent to a 1,000- to 1,200-calorie-a-day diet for the average woman. And this did, in fact, constitute starvation—after three to four months, the young men had lost 25 percent of their initial body weight, which was the goal the researchers set as a marker of starvation.

What makes the Minnesota study so valuable for us is the inquisitive alertness of the researchers, who carefully recorded the extraordinary things they saw happening to their subjects.

The hungry young men in the dormitories at the University of Minnesota

- Lost significant lean muscle mass (current studies show that between one third and one half of total pounds lost on a diet are muscle)
- Began guarding and hoarding food and changed the way they ate their meals—some developed long, drawn-out eating rituals, while others bolted their food

- After about two weeks, took down their pinups and pictures of girlfriends and replaced them with pictures of food
- Talked exclusively about food
- Began to experience irritability, difficulty concentrating, and sleeplessness
- After they had returned to their normal weight, experienced unprecedented episodes of binging

One of the fascinating conclusions nutritionists have drawn from the Minnesota study is that the behavioral effects of starvation (dieting) are rooted in biology, in the unchangeable history of the species.

Since dieting feels just like famine to our bodies, when we try to go down a dress size on, say, the cabbage-soup diet, a biological emergency system kicks in, causing changes that optimize our chances for survival until the next big kill or good harvest.

And if you still don't think that undereating is a bad way to lose weight, consider the practices of research labs that fatten rats to the point of obesity for experimental trials. They use a strain of rat that tends to get fat easily, and you'd think they'd just put them in tiny cages and overfeed them. What lab workers have found, though, is that the fat rats get fatter quicker if they're deprived of food for a day or so, then overfed again. It's true: dieting makes people, and rats, fat.

Calories, Diets, and All That

Canyon Ranch nutritionists would really rather not talk about calories: they've learned the hard way that guests tend to make a graven-in-stone goal of whatever number they hear at the ranch. The nutritionists do, however, sometimes use the

Effect of Dieting	Biological Reason
Loss of lean muscle	Muscle burns more precious calories than fat, and vital organs must be protected. Muscle is expendable for now.
Loss of sex drive	A famine is a disastrous time to be pregnant.
Obsession with food	The individual who's looking for food all the time is more likely to find what there is, and to survive the famine, than someone who's casual or indifferent.
Poststarvation binging	It could happen again. The individual with a big fat reserve will weather the next famine better.

following formula as a guideline. Someone who wants to lose weight can go this low without jeopardizing his health: calories per day = weight (in pounds) times 10. This is based on a rough estimate of resting metabolic rate—the rate at which the average person burns calories when doing absolutely nothing (not even digesting food). In other words, if you weigh 160 pounds, you need *no fewer* than 1,600 calories a day for energy and to keep your body healthy and functioning.

We repeat: this formula gives you the *bottom* limit. Ranch nutritionists actually recommend a weight-loss diet 25 to 30 percent higher than this figure for moderate weight loss. That comes out to 2,000 to 2,080 calories a day for our 160-pound dieter. If that seems much too high, read on.

Canyon Ranch strongly recommends that people who want to lose weight achieve most of the necessary calorie deficit by stepping up their physical activity, with a moderate cut-back in food contributing only a modest fraction of the deficit. In other words, eat a little less and get a *lot* more exercise.

Nutrition professionals are critical of most of the popular diets out there for a variety of reasons. Their overarching concern is that fad diets are necessarily one-size-fits all: Most do not address the wide variation in needs and preferences among individuals. In addition, most popular weight-loss diets

- Are calorically inadequate for health or energy
- Eliminate whole categories of food necessary for balanced nutrition
- Are hard to plan for and follow, since they require people to change their way of eating overnight
- Encourage dieters to give control to "the diet" instead of developing internal awareness and choice

To lose weight, eat sensible portions and cut out junk food, get enough sleep, drink lots of water, and get plenty of exercise.

Calories are never the whole story.

Dieting: What Works

At Canyon Ranch, when we talk about a diet working, we mean that the weight comes off and stays off for a long time—at least three years. Fascinating clues to sustainable weight loss come from the more than two thousand weight-loss heroes of the National Weight Control Registry. (www.uchsc.edu/nutrition/nwer.htm).

The registry is a database of successful dieters: their average weight loss is sixty pounds, and they've kept it off for an average of seven years. They are to dieting what centenarians are to aging.

Here are some of the facts gleaned from their experience:

- Virtually everyone in the registry exercises seven days a week. Ninety minutes of walking is the average length of exercise. (Remember, these are people who have lost and maintained an average loss of sixty pounds.)
- They eat regular meals—very few skip breakfast.
- They regularly monitor their weight.
- They tend to target something in their diet that they carefully watch. These "targeted" foods vary from individual to individual: some people limit fats, some watch carbohydrates, some stay away from sweets, some consciously limit alcohol consumption. People who keep weight off seem to come to an understanding of what they, as individuals, need to limit. Denying themselves everything isn't how they've succeeded. This, by the way, is reflected in one of Canyon Ranch's recommendations for permanent, sustainable weight loss: make consistent, measurable changes you can live with.

Moderate, reasonable eating is the key. This is something you are going to have to work at because you're surrounded by the third thing that conspires to keep your body off-kilter.

III. THE THIRD SABOTEUR: GIANT-SIZE FOOD

Bottom line from the nutritionists at Canyon Ranch: eat less. Don't diet; just eat less, because if you're an American at the beginning of the new millennium, it's a safe bet that you're overeating. The FDA recently estimated that our food industry is now producing 3,600 calories a day for every man, woman, and child in this country. That's too much.

We live in a world in which eating is a major form of entertainment, and possibly *the* most popular leisure-time activity in the United States. Food and advertisements for food are everywhere, all the time. America is now the land of super-size, over-size food: stuffed-crust super-giant pizzas, 72-ounce soft drinks, and 800-calorie bran muffins the size of softballs. As with everything else, we want our money's worth—we want a deal. (And you'll notice that the food that's advertised most is the food that's least nutritious. When did you last see an ad for fruit?)

The trouble is that when it comes to food, this is crazy. As a culture, we eat not in response to hunger, but in response to everything and as if we were all terrified of going hungry. Our children have newly discovered eating disorders while we've become the fattest nation in the history of the world. It's so bad that one nutritionist simply declared the United States "a toxic food environment."

If you want to be healthy, you must swim against the tide and fight the subliminal message that enough is never, ever enough. You need to pay attention to how much you eat. Portion size counts.

Paring Down Portions

- Use the palm of your hand as the right size for a portion of lean meat, chicken, or fish.
- Keep cheese portions to the size of a one-inch cube.
- The size of a D-cell battery is right for a serving of dried fruit or salad dressing.
- Use a tennis ball as the right size for a serving of rice or potatoes.
- A large marshmallow is the size of a reasonable portion of salad dressing.
- Use a Ping-Pong ball as a reference for a serving of nuts or nut butter.

Restaurant Strategies

Even dietitians have a terrible time guessing the calories in a restaurant meal—they almost invariably underestimate radically. Does this mean you never get to eat out again? Of course not, and an occasional splurge is no big deal. (What you do once in a while is irrelevant; it's what you do all the time that matters.)

- Stop to notice how hungry you really are and order accordingly. *Of course* they want you to go for a three-course meal, but that doesn't mean you really need one.
- Have a salad (dressing on the side) or a cup of (noncreamy) soup first, or maybe just stop right there.
- Leave that bread or chip basket alone—it's easier not to start.
- Drink lots of water or tea; see if they'll leave the pitcher on your table.
- Split entrées and share, or have your server box up half your plate *at the beginning of the meal* to outwit that clean-your-plate training.
- If waste doesn't bother you, make it a rule to eat half of what you're served on all occasions. Setting up your own inflexible rule counter to "Clean your plate" can help you control your eating without having to think too much about it.
- If you're full, don't even *look* at the dessert menu. Have a decaf cappuccino or concentrate on the single Peanut Butter Cup you'll buy yourself later as a reward.
- Remember: life is long. This is not your only chance ever to eat good things.

Your Ideal Weight

Finally, we get to Canyon Ranch's best and final word about your ideal weight. Ready?

Your ideal weight is your weight after a period of time in which you 1) eat as well as you can reasonably eat, and 2) exercise as much as you can reasonably exercise.

That's it. That's all. (There's typically an audible, roomwide "Oh" of disappointment when presenters give this program at the ranch.)

But think back over everything we've covered so far in this chapter. This is actually a subtle and liberating formula. Folded into it are the following assumptions:

1. Your body and your life are unique.
2. If you eat properly and exercise consistently over a period of time, you *will* have a leaner, stronger, healthier body. That's guaranteed. The person who starts from ground zero—complete inactivity—will see more dramatic changes than someone in decent shape who gets into better shape, but everyone will see and feel improvement as the small, cumulative changes add up.
3. You cannot do more than is reasonable, for you, over time, and any effort you can't sustain is counterproductive. The body you get when you make a reasonable effort is ideal.

But what if your ideal body just isn't good enough?

Then you have three choices. The first involves surgery, and we generally do not recommend it.

The second is to do more. Say you've worked up some steam and you're ready to improve your diet even more and add maybe another ten minutes to your walking routine, or start some weight training, or add a weekly yoga class. If more has come to seem reasonable, then that's great, and you'll see and feel more change after a reasonable length of time.

But if you're doing all you reasonably can and you're still not happy with the body you have, then our advice is to start practicing some self-acceptance.

Who *said* you had to look like a movie star? And even if you could somehow achieve someone's ideal of physical perfection, what good would it do you, really? Judging from their rate of admission to rehab, the most beautiful people in the world don't seem to be the happiest.

Stop beating yourself up.

And now go on out there and be reasonable.

Mindful Eating

At the core of a balanced life is mindfulness: living in the moment, being conscious of all that you do and feel. It can turn ordinary activities into meditations. Mindfulness naturally extends to eating—being aware of eating, experiencing tastes and textures, remembering why we eat, being in touch with appetite and hunger. It is one of the best innate tools we have to control appetite and bring a sense of enjoyment and satisfaction back to eating.

Some of the tools we recommend in mindful eating are:

- Say grace or a personal affirmation before meals. This practice has been lost in many households. Whether religious or secular, it's a lovely ritual and an opportunity to use words as an acknowledgment that you are choosing the foods that are best for you.
- Clear and quiet your mind before a meal. Take one or two deep, cleansing breaths before you begin to eat. This allows you to focus your thoughts on the meal before you.
- Visualize the process of food arriving at your table. From orchard or field to table, the process food goes through to get to you involves many transformations and the work of many people. This visualization can help you understand the connectedness of all living things—essential for fully appreciating what it takes to nourish you.

- Eat slowly. Rapid eating is usually unconscious eating. Slowing the pace of your eating allows you to become more aware of the sensory pleasures of food. You're also better able to match your food intake with your actual hunger. It takes a while for your hunger control mechanisms to recognize that your hunger is being satisfied. Relax, slow down, and give eating the respect it deserves.
- Become aware of your physical hunger. After saying grace or taking your cleansing breaths, and before you begin eating, check out your hunger. Rate your hunger on a scale of 0 (for ravenous) to 10 (Thanksgiving full).

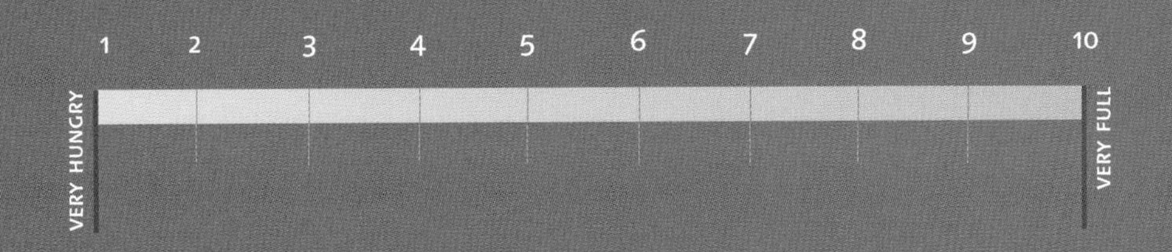

About halfway through your meal, ask yourself the critical question, "Am I full?" If the answer is no, keep eating. If the answer is yes, ask yourself if you want to continue eating. Even if your food is so enjoyable that you choose to eat more, you are now doing so consciously.

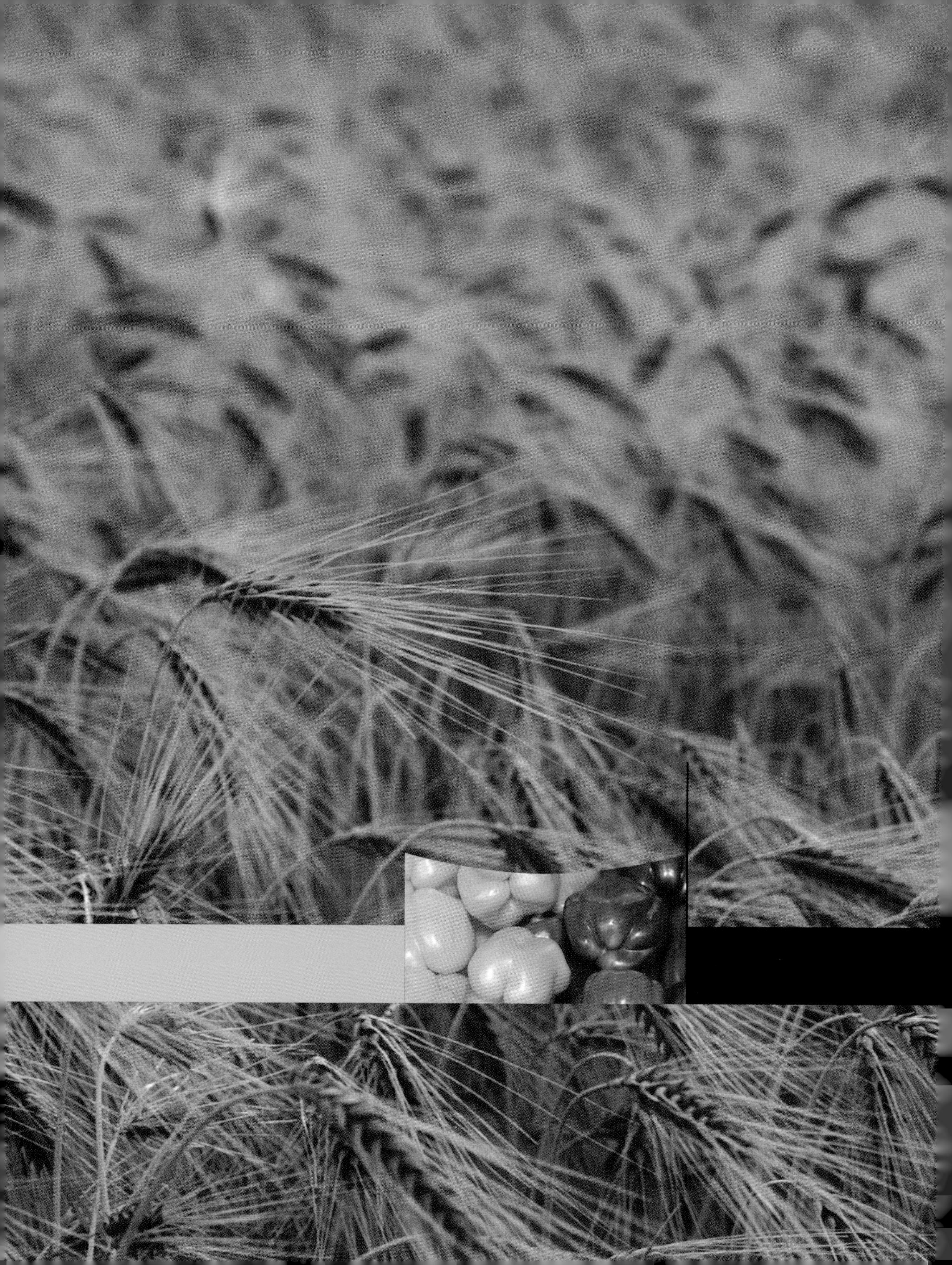

7 NUTRITIONAL INTELLIGENCE: *The Five Principles of Healthy Eating*

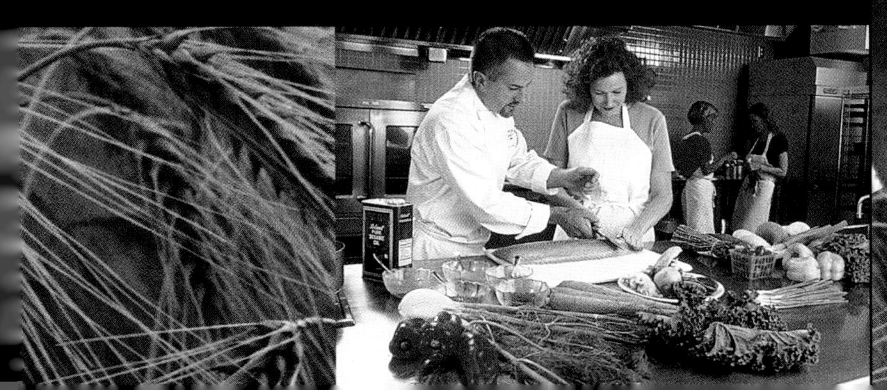

As Canyon Ranch begins its third decade, our approach to nutrition has come a long way. The food here has always been beautifully prepared, delicious, pure, and fresh—we're the folks who invented spa cuisine—but when we started out we were a little, well, stingy with it. People came to us primarily to lose weight, and we fed them just 800 low-fat calories a day, served nothing containing caffeine, and absolutely no chocolate. We were very, very strict.

Not surprisingly, in those days there were a lot of quiet trips "off property" to local restaurants, and the housekeeping staff was kept amused by the candy wrappers that turned up in wastebaskets. (For our first year or two, we often had only a dozen guests at a time, so gossip got around fast.)

We've learned, though, as have our guests. Looking back, all that hunger and cheating seems pretty silly. We've moved away from deprivation and toward moderation: a diet you can't live with is a diet that won't do you a bit of good in the long run. The key to a healthy relationship with food, we now know, is balance, mindfulness, and plenty of knowledge.

In this chapter, we'll hand you all the tools we give our guests: the five guiding principles of Canyon Ranch Nutritional Intelligence, plus ten simple rules to help you implement them in your life—not to mention recipes from our kitchens.

Guiding Principles of Nutritional Intelligence

1. HONOR YOUR INDIVIDUALITY

Your nutritional needs may be different from someone else's. Many factors influence your nutrient requirements: genetics, health and medical history, eating preferences,

CLEAN EATING GUIDELINES

PRODUCE: Buy a variety of seasonally fresh, locally grown, and certified organic produce. The following is a priority list for purchasing organic produce: strawberries, grapes, cherries, apricots, peaches, apples, pears, and spinach. You can also reduce your exposure to pesticides and bacteria by following these smart washing and peeling techniques:

- Prepare a vegetable wash solution using one teaspoon mild soap in one gallon of water or purchase a prepared vegetable wash solution such as VegiWash (800-282-WASH) or Fit Fruit and Vegetable Rinse (800-434-8348) to wash all produce.
- Use a vegetable brush on potatoes, sweet potatoes, carrots, and other hard produce whose skin you plan to eat.
- Wash and peel nonorganic fruit and vegetables that have obvious wax coatings. Likely candidates are cucumbers, apples, peppers, and eggplants. This will remove pesticides that are often sealed in by the waxes.

lifestyle, and more. Your eating experiences should allow you to discover your natural ability to make food choices that reflect your uniqueness.

2. ENJOY THE SENSUAL AND SOCIAL ASPECTS OF EATING

Indulge your preferences for flavors and textures, ritual and conversation. Eating should be a joyful experience, one in which we participate with all our physical and emotional senses.

3. CONSIDER THE BALANCE OF YOUR MEALS

Choose a variety of foods, including generous amounts of vegetables and fruits, moderate amounts of protein-rich foods and whole grains, and small amounts of healthy fats and oils. A balanced approach to eating energizes the body, stimulates the mind, and enriches the spirit.

4. EAT TO GENTLY SATISFY YOUR APPETITE

Establish a pattern of eating regularly throughout the day to prevent extremes in hunger that can lead to fatigue and overeating. Learn to moderate your portions by eating with awareness and attention to your physical hunger.

5. FOCUS ON CLEAN AND WHOLESOME FOOD

Choose fresh, seasonal vegetables and fruits, and foods free from preservatives, additives, hormones, antibiotics, and other unnecessary chemicals. Explore the pleasures of natural-food shopping and enjoy the discovery of great tastes and the rewards of supporting a cleaner and safer environment.

- Discard the outer leaves of cabbage and head lettuce.

PROTEIN AND PACKAGED FOODS: Buy a variety of minimally processed foods. Choose antibiotic- and hormone-free animal poultry and meats. Avoid foods with additives such as artificial colorings, flavorings, and sweeteners and preservatives. A great source of information on this issue is "Food Additives to Avoid," a readable summary by the Center for Science in the Public Interest. It's available online at www.cspinet.org/reports/food.htm.

FATS: Choose foods without *hydrogenated* or *partially hydrogenated* oils or synthetic, "fake" fats like Olestra.

WATER: If you have concerns about your drinking water, consider a water-purifying system for your home. Distillers are more expensive; reverse osmosis systems are good and less expensive. Buying bottled water is another alternative—choose glass or hard plastic containers.

How to Make These Principles Part of Your Life

I. BEGIN BY ASSESSING YOUR PERSONAL NEEDS OR GOALS

You are the ultimate expert on you. Explore what you need to know about yourself to improve your diet:

- Your family health history
- Your body type
- Your personal health issues
- Your likes and dislikes
- Your eating style
- Your daily routine
- Your lifetime experience with food

It can be very helpful, if you have the opportunity, to talk with a nutritionist about your unique nutritional needs. A nutritionist can tell you if a lower fat or lower carbohydrate diet is best for you, can derive nutritional meaning from lab tests, and can evaluate what types and amounts of supplements may be important for you. A good nutrition counselor understands the role food plays in your life and can work with you to develop a healthier relationship with food.

II. ESTABLISH A PATTERN OF EATING REGULARLY

Nourishing your body by eating regularly throughout the day can prevent the extremes of hunger that lead to overeating and fatigue. Try to eat every three to five hours, and work toward a pattern of breakfast, lunch, and dinner—and an afternoon snack, if necessary. It's easy to overlook eating in a busy day, but this strategy can help you cope better with a demanding schedule.

Know yourself. Learn what it takes to maximize your energy and minimize your hunger.

- Honor your body's rhythms and individual needs.
- Notice your energy, appetite, and mood after a balanced meal.
- How long do you feel comfortable after a meal? Does it depend on the size of the meal or what you ate?
- Learn to recognize the symptoms of low blood sugar as signals that your body needs food. Symptoms include shakiness, fatigue, headache, inability to concentrate, and irritability.

Almond Butter Delight

Try this low-fat spread on toast, crackers, or fresh apple slices.

1 cup nonfat ricotta cheese
2 teaspoons vanilla extract
½ teaspoon ground cinnamon
1½ tablespoons honey
¼ cup almond butter (without added salt)

Combine all ingredients in a blender container and puree until smooth. Chill in refrigerator until ready to use.

MAKES 10 (2 TABLESPOON) SERVINGS, EACH CONTAINING APPROXIMATELY:
65 calories, 4 gm fat, 5 gm protein, 5 gm carbohydrate, 2 mg cholesterol, 12 mg sodium, Trace fiber

III. BE MINDFUL OF PORTION SIZES

Learn to moderate the amount you eat to gently satisfy your hunger. Further, learn to distinguish between physical hunger and hunger associated with stress, anxiety, or sadness. Choose moderate portions of protein-rich food, side dishes, and fruit; enjoy generous servings of vegetables. Share entrées in restaurants, or order a salad and an appetizer instead of an entrée. (See Chapter 6 for more information on portion control.) And remember, you'll be much more likely to actually use these strategies if you don't wait to eat until you're ravenous.

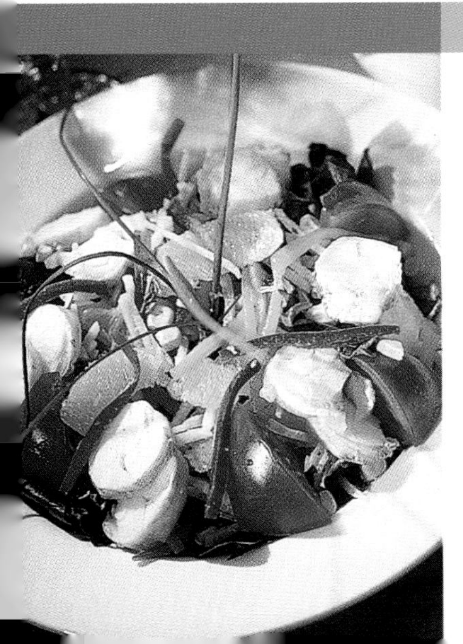

DON'T KID YOURSELF ABOUT CARBS

A SLICE OF SANDWICH bread is 70–100 calories, about the same as

- 1 corn tortilla
- *Half* an English muffin
- *Half* a small dinner roll
- *Half* a hamburger bun
- *Half* a medium (10 inch) flour tortilla
- A *quarter* of an average bagel
- A *quarter* of a sub roll
- A *quarter* of an average muffin
- A *sixth* of an average restaurant portion of pasta

Fennel-Crusted Lamb with Olive Relish

16 ounces lamb chops, trimmed of all fat
1 ½ teaspoons fennel seed
½ teaspoon peppercorns
½ teaspoon salt

OLIVE RELISH:

¼ cup minced red onion
¼ cup minced red bell pepper
2 teaspoons lemon peel
1 ½ tablespoons lemon juice
¾ cup chopped kalamata olives
2 tablespoons fresh basil, julienned
2 teaspoons fresh chopped mint
Pinch black pepper

Preheat broiler or prepare hot coals for grill.

Grind fennel seed, peppercorns, and salt together in a spice grinder. Dust lamb chops on each side with fennel mixture. Broil or grill until cooked through, about 3 to 5 minutes on each side.

Combine remaining ingredients in a medium bowl and mix well.

Serve ¼ cup relish with 3 ounces cooked lamb chop.

MAKES 4 SERVINGS, EACH CONTAINING APPROXIMATELY:
155 calories, 5 gm carbohydrate, 8 gm fat, 207 mg cholesterol, 17 gm protein, 351 mg sodium, 2 gm fiber

IV. EAT 8–10 SERVINGS OF VEGETABLES AND FRUIT EACH DAY

This is the category of food with the most power to prevent disease. You can make a major improvement in your diet simply by thinking of at least three new ways to conveniently add vegetables or fruit to your daily routine: have fruit—or fruit juice—at breakfast, enjoy a medium to large salad once a day, be sure that each of your meals includes vegetables or fruit, and always include fruit in your afternoon snack. Finally, buy organic whenever possible.

Everything You Need to Know About Phytochemicals

One of the hottest nutrition research topics in recent years is phytochemicals. The Greek word *phyto* means "plant"—phytochemicals are plant chemicals. They're not vitamins or minerals but biologically active substances that protect plants from too much sunlight, blight, and pollution.

What's exciting is that we are discovering that phytochemicals also enhance and protect human health: they're cancer and diabetes fighters, heart protectors, immune system boosters, and antiaging agents.

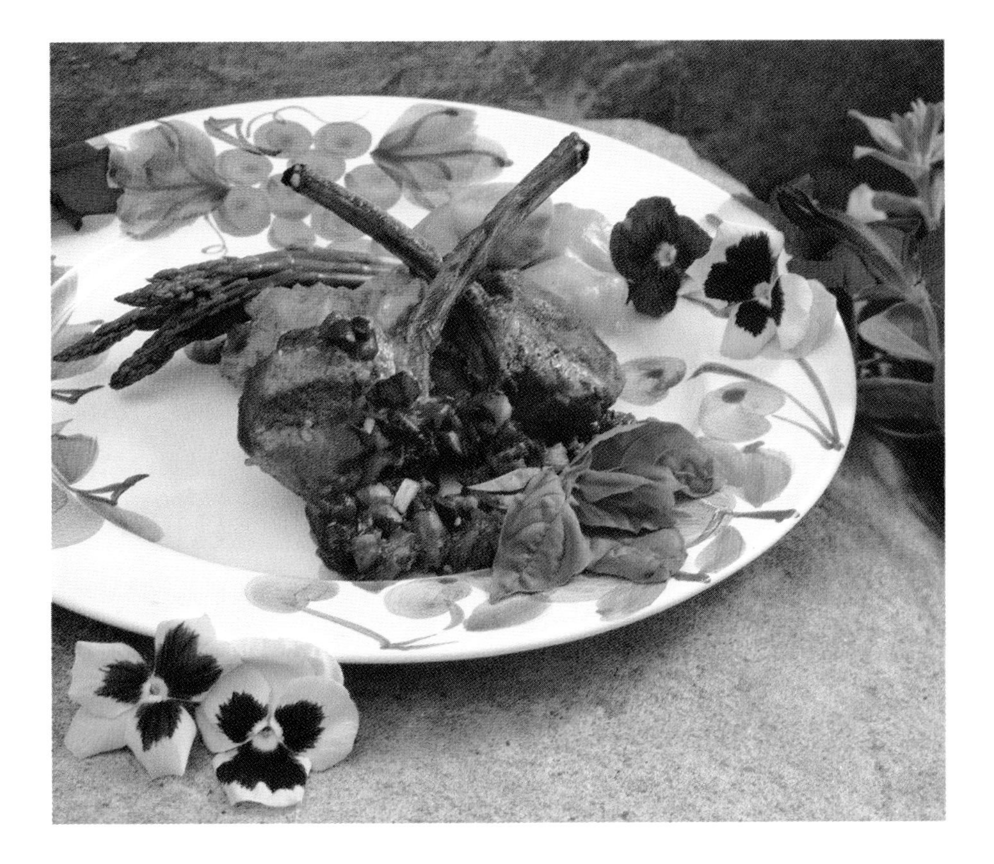

Phytochemicals

Food	Benefit
Red, yellow, and orange vegetables and fruits	Rich in antioxidants, such as the carotenoids lycopene and lutein, which neutralize free radicals and prevent degenerative diseases.
Dark green leafy vegetables	Rich in fiber for intestinal health, and in antioxidants such as carotenoids, specifically lutein, which neutralize free radicals.
Dark red, blue, and purple fruits and vegetables	Rich in antioxidants such as phenols, specifically anthocyanoside and ellargic acid, and in terpenes, which help boost the immune system and have anticarcinogenic properties.
Allium vegetables (onions, garlic, leeks, shallots)	Rich in organosulfur compounds, which produce enzymes that help rid the body of cancer-causing toxins. Also rich in phenols such as quercetin, which has antiviral and anti-inflammatory properties.
Cruciferous vegetables (cabbage, kale, cauliflower, brussels sprouts, broccoli)	Rich in indoles and isothiocyanates, phytochemicals that block cancer-causing agents from reaching cells.
Citrus fruits	Rich in limonene, from the terpene family, which helps prevent cancer and heart disease; carotenoids such as beta-carotene, lycopene, and lutein; the flavonoid hesperedin, particularly noted for fighting breast cancer; and perillyl alcohol, which helps boost the immune system.
Flaxseed	Rich in fiber, which promotes intestinal health, and in lignan, a phytoestrogen that helps promote beneficial intestinal bacteria and may help alleviate mild menopausal symptoms.
Legumes	Rich in fiber for intestinal health and in protease inhibitors, flavonoids, and saponins, phytochemicals that help prevent heart disease and cancer and enhance the immune system.
Soybeans and soy products	Rich in the phytoestrogens genistein and daidzein, and in the protease inhibitor BBI, which provides protection against cancer.
Tea (green and black)	Rich in flavonoids, antioxidants that help prevent cancer and heart disease.
Sea vegetables	Rich in carotenoids, which neutralize free radicals, and in elligic acid, a phenol noted for cancer prevention.

The basic rule for making sure that you get plenty of these miracle chemicals in your diet is simple: look for color. To get lots of different phytochemicals, eat plant foods across the color spectrum.

RED
Strawberries
Raspberries
Red grapes
Cherries
Red bell pepper
Watermelon
Rhubarb
Tomatoes
Chili peppers

ORANGE
Oranges
Orange bell pepper
Sweet potatoes
Carrots
Butternut squash
Apricots
Mangos
Papayas
Cantaloupe
Peaches

YELLOW
Corn
Lemons
Grapefruit
Crookneck squash
Yellow onions
Pineapple

GREEN
Kale
Spinach
Broccoli
Brussels sprouts
Asparagus
Romaine lettuce
Green leaf lettuce
Green onions
Sea vegetables
Kiwi
Lime
Arugula
Mustard and turnip greens
Swiss chard

BLUE AND PURPLE
Blueberries
Blackberries
Plums
Beets
Eggplant
Red onions
Purple grapes
Red cabbage
Radicchio

WHITE
Jicama
Cauliflower
White onions
Garlic
Shallots
Leeks

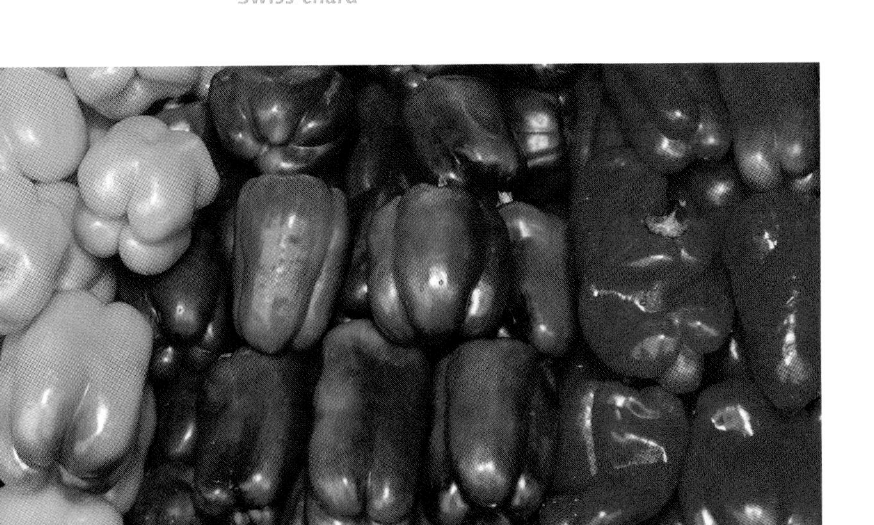

Roasted Butternut Squash Soup

1 medium butternut squash, cut in half and seeded
½ cup diced onions
2 tablespoons diced carrots
2 tablespoons diced celery
1 teaspoon olive oil
Pinch ground cloves
Pinch ground nutmeg
Pinch cinnamon
Pinch ground ginger
1 teaspoon curry powder
1 whole bay leaf
2 tablespoons white wine
5 cups vegetable stock
¼ cup apple juice
2 tablespoons honey
1 teaspoon lemon juice
½ teaspoon Worcestershire sauce
¼ teaspoon black pepper
½ teaspoon salt (optional)
1 tablespoon cornstarch (optional)

Preheat oven to 350 degrees. Fill a shallow baking pan with ½ inch water. Place squash halves skin side up in pan and bake for 1 hour. When cool, scoop out pulp and measure 1 to 1 ¼ cups.

In a large saucepan, sauté onions, carrots, and celery in olive oil until onions are translucent. Add dry spices and squash. Add white wine and simmer for 5 minutes over medium heat.

Add vegetable stock, apple juice, honey, lemon juice, and Worcestershire sauce. Simmer 30 minutes. Season with salt and pepper. Cool, remove bay leaf, and puree in a blender until smooth. If soup is not thick enough, mix cornstarch with an equal amount of water, return to saucepan, and simmer for 2 more minutes, or until soup is thickened.

MAKES 8 (3/4 CUP) SERVINGS, EACH CONTAINING APPROXIMATELY:
65 calories, 13 gm carbohydrate, Trace fat, 0 mg cholesterol, 1 gm protein, 151 mg sodium, 1 gm fiber

Poached Anjou Pear

2 cups white grape juice
1 cup water
1 star anise
1 cinnamon stick
½ vanilla bean
1½ teaspoons orange peel
2 large red Anjou pears, peeled and sliced in half

Bring grape juice, water, spices, and orange peel to a boil in a large saucepan. Reduce heat to low, add pears, and simmer until tender, about 45 minutes.

Remove saucepan from heat and place in an ice bath to cool. Remove pears and reserve liquid.

Remove spices from liquid, reserve 1 cup, and bring it to a boil. Simmer until liquid has reduced by ½, about 20 minutes.

Serve ½ pear with 2 tablespoons of sauce.

MAKES 4 SERVINGS, EACH CONTAINING APPROXIMATELY:
60 calories, 17 gm carbohydrate, Trace fat, 0 mg cholesterol, Trace protein, 1 mg sodium, 2 gm fiber

V. EMPHASIZE WHOLE GRAINS

Whole grains provide fiber, vitamins, and minerals and help keep blood sugar levels stable for several hours after eating. Other great sources of carbohydrates include beans, sweet potatoes, barley, and pasta cooked al dente. Experiment with delicious grains you perhaps haven't tried, such as quinoa, brown rice, and wild rice.

Personal Fiber Intake Assessment

Most of us don't get enough fiber. Take this quiz to see how your diet measures up. How many servings of the following foods do you eat every day?

	number of servings			fiber in grams
Beans and peas (serving is ½ cup)	_____	x 8	=	_____
Bran cereal (serving is ½ c.)	_____	x 8	=	_____
Whole grain cereals (serving is ½ c.)	_____	x 3	=	_____
Nuts/seeds (serving is 1 oz.)	_____	x 3	=	_____
Peanut butter (serving is 2 tbs.)	_____	x 3	=	_____
Starchy vegetable (such as potato)	_____	x 3	=	_____
Bread (1 slice) or crackers (5)	_____	x 2	=	_____
Vegetables (serving is ½ c.)	_____	x 2	=	_____
Fruit (1 piece or ½ c.)	_____	x 2	=	_____
Milk (1 c.)	_____	x 0	=	_____
Meat, fish, poultry (3 oz.)	_____	x 0	=	_____
		Total		_____

The recommended daily fiber intake is 25–40 grams. How did you do?

WITH FOOD CHOICES, you can moderate your blood sugar level to help control appetite, fat storage, and swings of low blood sugar, known as hypoglycemia.

Blood sugar levels are affected by the amount and type of carbohydrate-rich foods you eat. Eating less of such foods help maintain lower blood sugar levels—but restricting them too much may leave you without enough fuel. You can also control blood sugar levels by your choices among foods you may not think of as being high in carbohydrates. Different foods are digested and absorbed at different rates and raise blood sugar accordingly.

To make informed food choices, it helps to know how different foods affect your blood sugar. The glycemic index measures how high your blood sugar rises after a particular food is eaten alone. Each food is

GLYCEMIC INDEX OF COMMON FOODS

100 PERCENT

- glucose

80 TO 90 PERCENT

- cornflakes
- pretzels
- baked potato
- rice cakes
- jelly beans

70 TO 80 PERCENT

- waffles
- french fries
- soda crackers
- bran flakes
- bagel
- corn chips
- watermelon
- white bread

60 TO 70 PERCENT

- whole-wheat bread
- angel food cake
- GrapeNuts
- pineapple
- cantaloupe
- couscous
- table sugar
- raisins
- cola
- granola bars
- pizza

50 TO 60 PERCENT

- PowerBar
- papaya
- white rice
- brown rice
- mango
- banana
- sweet corn
- popcorn
- sweet potato
- stoneground wheat bread
- kiwi fruit
- sourdough bread
- pumpernickel bread

40 TO 50 PERCENT

- oatmeal
- chocolate bar
- green peas
- bulgur
- orange juice
- grapes
- pinto beans
- spaghetti
- orange
- garbanzo beans
- peach
- apple juice

30 TO 40 PERCENT

- tomato soup
- apple
- pear
- yogurt
- skim milk
- dried apricots
- lentils

LESS THAN 30 PERCENT

- kidney beans
- barley
- grapefruit
- fructose
- cherries
- soybeans
- peanuts

compared to glucose as the standard glycemic index of 100.

A high glycemic index means that the food causes blood sugar to rise in a way that demands a surge of insulin. To control blood sugar levels, we suggest:

- Choosing lower glycemic-index foods when possible.
- Eating higher index foods—some of which have great nutritional value—with lower index foods. The glycemic index of a meal is essentially the average of the individual foods.

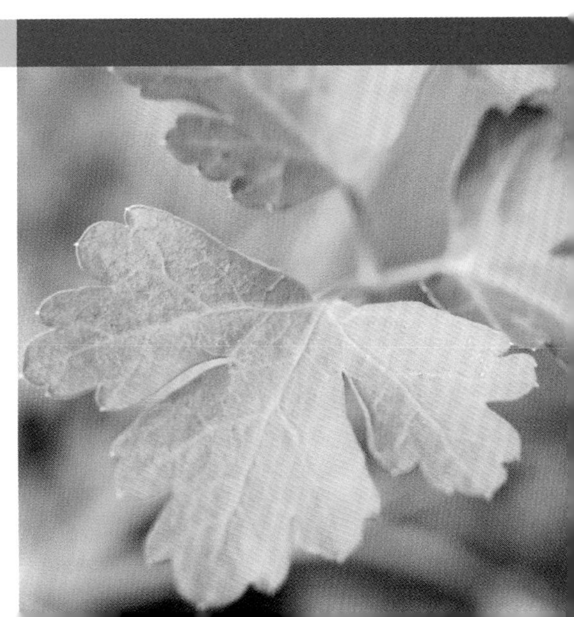

Whole-Wheat Buttermilk Pancakes with Fruit

This batter also works well for waffles. For successful waffles, spray the heated iron thoroughly with canola oil, and start with ¾ cup of batter.

¾ cup bread flour
¾ cup whole wheat flour
3 tablespoons sugar
¼ teaspoon salt
2 ½ teaspoons baking powder
1 teaspoon baking soda
1 tablespoon maple syrup
1 large egg
1 cup buttermilk
¾ cup 2 percent milk
2 ½ tablespoons canola oil
1 cup berries or chopped fruit

In a large bowl, combine all dry ingredients. In a medium bowl, combine remaining wet ingredients and mix well. Add wet ingredients to dry ingredients and mix until smooth.

Lightly coat a griddle or large skillet with canola oil. Place on burner over medium heat until hot. Portion approximately 3 tablespoons batter on griddle and sprinkle with 1 tablespoon berries. Cover berries with 1 additional tablespoon batter and cook until bubbles form. Flip and cook other side to golden brown.

MAKES 6 (3 PANCAKE) SERVINGS, EACH CONTAINING APPROXIMATELY:
335 calories, 59 gm carbohydrate, 8 gm fat, 48 mg cholesterol, 8 gm protein, 572 mg sodium, 4 gm fiber

Caramelized Vegetable and Tofu Stir-fry

10 ounces sliced tofu
2 tablespoons low-sodium soy sauce, preferably tamari
2 tablespoons brown sugar
Pinch chili flakes
2 teaspoons sesame tahini
1 ½ tablespoons olive oil
1 tablespoon minced garlic
1 tablespoon minced gingerroot
1 cup sliced scallions
1 cup sliced jicama
1 medium red bell pepper, cut into 1-inch cubes
2 cups broccoli florets, blanched
1 ½ cups sliced mushrooms
¼ cup vegetable stock
2 cups cooked chuka soba or buckwheat soba noodles

Heat a wok or large skillet and cook tofu until golden brown on each side. Remove from pan and cut into cubes.

In a small saucepan, combine soy sauce, brown sugar, chili flakes, and tahini. Simmer until sugar is melted and mixture becomes a syrup, about 5 minutes. Set aside.

Add oil to wok and, when hot, add garlic and ginger. Stir-fry briefly. Add remaining vegetables in order and stir-fry for about 30 seconds. Add tofu and continue to stir-fry until vegetables are tender but crisp. Add soy-sauce mixture and stir-fry until vegetables are coated.

Divide stir-fry into 4 equal portions and serve each portion over ½ cup cooked noodles.

MAKES 4 SERVINGS, EACH CONTAINING APPROXIMATELY:
325 calories, 44 gm carbohydrate, 12 gm fat, 0 mg cholesterol, 19 gm protein, 429 mg sodium, 7 gm fiber

VI. FOCUS ON HEALTHY FATS AND OILS

Fat is an essential part of your diet: for starters, adequate fat intake is critical if you want healthy hair, skin, and nails. We recommend a daily range of 20–30 percent of calories from fat for most people, with an emphasis on those fats that have a positive impact on health. In the last couple of decades we've learned a great deal about dietary fat, and many people have been frustrated and confused by seemingly conflicting messages in the media. Here at the ranch, we tell our guests that the *type* of fats in their diet may be as important to their well-being as the *amount*.

1. Emphasize the monounsaturated fats found in extra virgin olive oil, canola oil, avocados, olives, and nuts.

Dress your salads lightly with an olive oil vinaigrette, and experiment with a variety of delicious vinegars and citrus juices. Sauté vegetables in olive oil and garlic. Eat small amounts of nuts each day and add avocado slices to sandwiches and salads.

Rosemary Vinaigrette Salad Dressing

⅔ cup red wine vinegar
⅔ cup champagne vinegar
½ cup vegetable stock
1 tablespoon shallots
2 teaspoons black pepper
4 teaspoons white miso
1 tablespoon chopped fresh oregano
1 tablespoon chopped fresh rosemary

In a blender container, combine all ingredients except for oregano and rosemary. Add herbs and mix by hand.

Pour into storage container and refrigerate.

MAKES 16 (2 TABLESPOON) SERVINGS, EACH CONTAINING APPROXIMATELY:
10 calories, 2 gm carbohydrate, Trace fat, 0 mg cholesterol, Trace protein, 292 mg sodium, Trace fiber

2. Have a daily source of omega-3 fat in your diet.

Add freshly ground flaxseeds to breads and muffins you bake at home, or sprinkle over cereal or salads. Use fresh walnuts and pumpkin seeds in salads and sauces and eat them for snacks. Try eggs that contain higher omega-3 fat in the yolk. Several times a week, eat cold-water fish—salmon, albacore tuna, trout, arctic char, sardines, black cod (sablefish), mackerel, herring, pompano, smelt.

Flaxseed Apple Batter French Toast with Fruit Compote

FRUIT COMPOTE:

¼ cup orange juice
¼ cup pineapple juice
¼ cup diced pineapple
¼ cup peeled and diced apple
1 mint sprig, chopped
1 teaspoon grated orange peel

FRENCH TOAST:

1 tablespoon ground flaxseeds
3 tablespoons apple butter
¾ cup fortified soy milk
Pinch nutmeg
Pinch cinnamon
Pinch salt
1 teaspoon canola oil
4 large slices multigrain bread (about ¾-inch thick)

In a medium skillet, bring juices to a boil. Add remaining compote ingredients except for mint and cook until fruit is soft. Add mint. Set aside.

Combine ground flaxseeds, apple butter, soy milk, nutmeg, cinnamon, and salt in a blender container and mix until smooth. Transfer to shallow pan.

Place a large skillet over medium heat and add canola oil. Dip both sides of bread into soy milk mixture and transfer to hot pan. Repeat for remaining slices. Cook until golden brown on both sides.

Reheat fruit compote and serve ¼ cup with 1 slice French toast.

MAKES 4 SERVINGS, EACH CONTAINING APPROXIMATELY:
205 calories, 37 gm carbohydrate, 5 gm fat, 0 mg cholesterol, 6 gm protein, 214 mg sodium, 4 gm fiber

Salmon Teriyaki Salad

1 pound Atlantic salmon fillet

MARINADE:

½ cup low-sodium soy sauce

2 tablespoons rice vinegar

1 tablespoon chopped fresh garlic

1 tablespoon minced ginger

1½ cups thawed apple juice concentrate

½ cup finely chopped green onions

SALAD:

1 medium green apple, julienned

½ carrot, julienned

½ red onion, thinly sliced

½ red bell pepper, chopped

½ cup diced pineapple

1 cup shredded bok choy

2 cups cooked udon noodles

Divide salmon into four 4-ounce portions.

Combine all ingredients for marinade, except green onions, in blender container and process. Stir in the onions. (Makes approximately 2 cups marinade.)

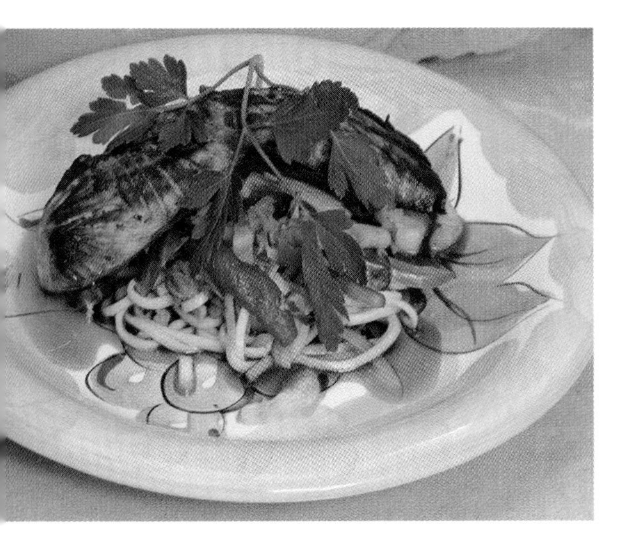

Combine salmon with ½ of marinade in a shallow bowl, reserving remainder of marinade. Marinate 1 to 2 hours in refrigerator, depending on flavor desired. Turn salmon occasionally to distribute marinade evenly.

Preheat grill or broiler. Discard marinade and cook salmon for 3 to 5 minutes on each side or until fish flakes easily.

Combine all vegetables for salad and mix well. Place ½ cup udon noodles on plate. Top with 1 cup vegetables and 1 salmon fillet. Drizzle 2 tablespoons reserve marinade over all.

MAKES 4 SERVINGS, EACH CONTAINING APPROXIMATELY:
360 calories, 45 gm carbohydrate, 8 gm fat, 60 mg cholesterol, 27 gm protein, 667 mg sodium, 4 gm fiber

3. Avoid trans-fats, also known as shortenings and margarine and as "partially hydrogenated *anything* oil."

Read food labels on baked goods, cereals, snack foods, and frozen desserts. If you find hydrogenated or partially hydrogenated oils in the list of ingredients, choose another product. Create a consumer demand for healthier products in the supermarket. Use oils that are liquid, not solid, at room temperature when cooking and baking, and keep in mind that many fast foods—especially those that are fried—are loaded with trans-fats.

Fruit Muffins

1 cup all-purpose flour
½ cup whole-wheat pastry flour
2 teaspoons baking powder
½ teaspoon salt
1 small egg
⅓ cup 2 percent milk
⅓ cup nonfat plain yogurt
2 tablespoons canola oil
⅓ cup sugar
1 cup peeled and chopped fruit or berries

TOPPING:

Pinch cinnamon
2 tablespoons sugar

Preheat oven to 350 degrees. Spray a muffin tin with nonstick vegetable coating.

In large bowl, combine flours, baking powder, and salt.

In a medium bowl combine egg, milk, yogurt, and oil. Add ⅓ cup sugar and mix well.

Pour egg mixture into dry ingredients and stir until all ingredients are moistened. Add fruit and stir until just mixed.

Fill each muffin cup with ¼ cup batter and bake for 15 to 20 minutes or until muffins are golden and toothpick inserted into center comes out clean.

To prepare topping, mix together cinnamon and sugar. Sprinkle ½ teaspoon over each warm muffin. Cool and remove from tins.

MAKES 12 MUFFINS, EACH CONTAINING APPROXIMATELY:
135 calories, 24 gm carbohydrate, 3 gm fat, 15 mg cholesterol, 3 gm protein, 87 mg sodium, 2 gm fiber

4. Minimize saturated fat.

Choose low-fat or fat-free milk, yogurt, and cheese: traditional low-fat cheeses include feta, chevre, part-skim mozzarella, and Monterey Jack. Choose skinless chicken breast and the leanest, most closely trimmed cuts of red meat. Limit your consumption of prepared foods made with butter and cream or lard, reduce your use of butter and full-fat cream cheese as spreads, and experiment with substitutes for full-fat dairy products in recipes.

Guacamole

½ cup julienned spinach
⅓ cup frozen peas
1 ounce light silken tofu
1 ½ tablespoons lemon juice
Pinch salt
Pinch cumin
Pinch cayenne
Pinch chili powder
Dash Tabasco
6 tablespoons mashed avocado
3 tablespoons peeled and minced tomato
2 tablespoons salsa
3 tablespoons minced white onions
1 tablespoon chopped cilantro
2 teaspoons chopped scallions

Steam spinach until wilted. Remove from heat and squeeze out excess water.

Briefly steam peas and rinse under cold water to retain green color.

In blender container, combine spinach, peas, tofu, lemon juice, seasonings, and avocado and process until smooth.

Fold in remaining ingredients and mix well.

MAKES 8 (2 TABLESPOON) SERVINGS, EACH CONTAINING APPROXIMATELY:
30 calories, 3 gm carbohydrate, 2 gm fat, 0 mg cholesterol, 1 gm protein, 131 mg sodium, 1 gm fiber

VII. BALANCE EACH MEAL WITH SOME PROTEIN-RICH FOOD

Including a high-protein food in each meal helps control hunger and stabilizes energy levels. Our favorite sources of protein are beans, soy foods, and fish, but there are many other plant and animal foods that will work. Don't overlook nut butters, organic low-fat or nonfat yogurt, milk, cheese, organic eggs, and antibiotic-free poultry.

HOW MUCH PROTEIN IS ENOUGH? HOW MUCH IS TOO MUCH?

Your *minimum* daily protein requirement (in grams) is
YOUR BODY WEIGHT IN POUNDS TIMES .36 (VEGANS: USE BODY WEIGHT IN POUNDS TIMES .45)

The recommended safe *upper* limit for protein (in grams) is
YOUR BODY WEIGHT IN POUNDS TIMES .9

HOW MUCH PROTEIN ARE YOU GETTING?

Animal sources

Fish, poultry, lean meat	1 oz. = 7 gm
Egg	1 = 7 gm
Egg whites	2 = 7 gm
Skim milk, nonfat yogurt	1 c. = 8 gm
Cheese	1 oz. = 7 gm
Cottage cheese	¼ c. = 7 gm

Plant sources

Beans	½ c. = 8 gm
Tofu*	2 oz. = 9 gm
Tempeh	2 oz. = 8 gm
Nut butter	2 tbs. = 6 gm
Nuts	2 tbs. = 3 gm
Pumpkin seeds	2 tbs. = 4 gm
Bread	1 oz. = 3 gm
Crackers	1 oz. = 3 gm
Quinoa	½ c. = 4 gm
Rice	½ c. = 3 gm
Pasta	½ c. = 3 gm
Cereal*	½ c. = 3 gm
Oatmeal, cooked	½ c. = 3 gm
Vegetables, raw	1 c. = 2 gm
Vegetables, cooked	½ c. = 2 gm
Potato	½ c. = 2 gm
Sweet potato	½ c. = 2 gm

*Protein content varies from one product to another. Read the Nutrition Facts label for specific information.

Raspberry Mustard–Crusted Chicken Breast

RASPBERRY MUSTARD:

4 tablespoons Dijon mustard

4 tablespoons fresh or frozen raspberries

3 teaspoons honey

FIG VINEGAR:

⅔ cup balsamic vinegar

6 tablespoons chopped figs

2 teaspoons honey

½ cup bread crumbs

2 tablespoons minced pistachio nuts

½ teaspoon salt

¼ teaspoon pepper

4 skinned chicken breasts, boned and defatted

2 teaspoons olive oil

In a blender container, combine ingredients for raspberry mustard. Refrigerate overnight.

In a small saucepan, combine ingredients for fig vinegar. Bring to a boil, reduce heat, and simmer over low heat for 1 minute. Cool and refrigerate overnight. Strain.

With a meat mallet, pound chicken breasts to ½-inch thick.

In a medium bowl, combine bread crumbs, pistachios, salt, and pepper. In a shallow pan, place chicken breasts in raspberry mustard sauce and turn to coat. Roll in bread crumbs.

Heat olive oil in a large skillet. Sauté chicken breasts over medium heat until chicken is cooked through and crust is light brown, about 3 to 5 minutes on each side. Juices will run clear when pierced with a fork.

Reheat fig vinegar in a small pan. Serve 1 chicken breast with 2 tablespoons fig vinegar.

MAKES 4 SERVINGS, EACH CONTAINING APPROXIMATELY:
295 calories, 24 gm carbohydrate, 9 gm fat, 85 mg cholesterol, 30 gm protein, 620 mg sodium, 3 gm fiber

Vegetarian Chili

1 ½ cups finely chopped onions
3 tablespoons chili powder
1 tablespoon minced fresh garlic
1 teaspoon dry oregano
2 ½ teaspoons dry basil
½ teaspoon dry thyme
1 teaspoon cumin
¾ cup diced red and yellow bell peppers
1 tablespoon chopped jalapeño pepper
5 ounces tempeh, about ¾ cup, crumbled
4 cups diced canned tomatoes
3 cups tomato sauce
⅛ teaspoon liquid smoke
2 teaspoons chopped fresh cilantro
1 tablespoon molasses
2 cups vegetable stock
⅔ cup cooked adzuki beans*
⅔ cup cooked anasazi beans*
¼ cup cooked white beans

Lightly coat a large saucepan with olive oil. Add onion and sauté with chili powder. Add garlic and sauté briefly, about 30 seconds. Add all dry herbs and peppers and sauté until peppers are soft, about 1 minute.

Add remaining ingredients except beans and bring to a boil. Reduce heat and simmer for 30 minutes. Add beans and simmer another 30 minutes.

*These pretty, flavorful beans are becoming widely available at specialty and natural-foods stores. You can successfully substitute equal amounts of any cooked beans you like or have on hand.

MAKES 8 (1 CUP) SERVINGS, EACH CONTAINING APPROXIMATELY:
175 calories, 34 gm carbohydrate, 2 gm fat, 0 mg cholesterol, 9 gm protein, 450 mg sodium, 7 gm fiber

VIII. LIMIT THE AMOUNT OF SUGAR IN YOUR DIET AND AVOID ARTIFICIAL SWEETENERS

Our American sweet tooth is getting sweeter. The average person consumes twenty teaspoons of added sugar a day. That's 156 pounds a year for every man, woman, and child!

Limiting sugar consumption is as easy as following these simple guidelines:

- Appreciate the sweetness of whole foods such as fresh fruit, vegetables, and nuts.
- Allow yourself only one small dessert per day. Canyon Ranch guidelines require that desserts contain no more than 2 to 3 teaspoons of added sugar per serving. You can easily achieve this standard at home by cutting your dessert portion in half.
- Use fresh fruit mixed with fresh juices and fruit purees as an alternative to a sweet dessert.
- Natural sweeteners such as fruit juice, honey, maple syrup, and molasses lend themselves nicely as alternatives to table sugar in marinades and sauces. "Sweeten" foods with spices such as cinnamon, vanilla, and freshly grated nutmeg.
- Be wary of fat-free foods. Many foods marketed as *fat-free* and *low-fat* are loaded with sugar. Learn to scan food labels to determine whether the fat-free choice is really a healthy choice. Remember, every 4–5 grams of sugar is equal to 1 teaspoon. Some fat-free foods have more than 25 grams (5–6 teaspoons) of sugar per serving.
- Eliminate artificial sweeteners. They may fuel cravings for ultrasweet foods and ultimately lead to an increase in sugar intake and calories.

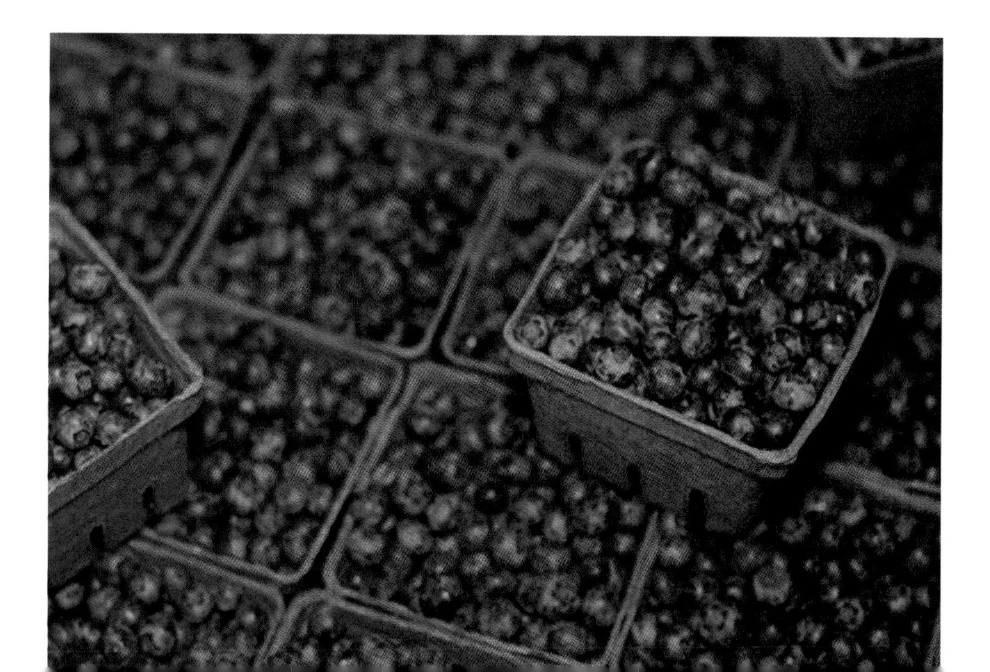

Almond Praline Cookies

3 tablespoons sugar
1 ½ tablespoons butter
2 tablespoons light corn syrup
4 tablespoons minced almonds

In a small saucepan, combine sugar, butter, and corn syrup. Simmer over very low heat until butter and sugar are melted. Remove from heat, add almonds, and mix thoroughly. Refrigerate overnight.

Preheat oven to 400 degrees.

Using a scant ½ tablespoon, spoon batter 2 inches apart onto a nonstick cookie sheet. Bake for 8 to 10 minutes. Cool before removing from pan.

MAKES 16 COOKIES, EACH CONTAINING APPROXIMATELY:
35 calories, 3 gm carbohydrate, 2 gm fat, 3 mg cholesterol, Trace protein, 16 mg sodium, Trace fiber

IX. BE SENSIBLE ABOUT SALT

Gradually cut down on the salt you add to food while pampering your palate with delectable, healing herbs and spices. These flavorful additions enhance the taste of food while gently working their restorative magic. Rosemary is a calming flavor and scent, cinnamon is warming, fresh ginger is invigorating—and a wonderful digestive and anti-inflammatory agent. Salt is a flavor enhancer, too, but if you use it moderately, you'll enhance your health, as well.

Canyon Ranch chefs know all the tricks for rapidly preparing recipes with fresh produce and herbs. Here are a few favorites.

- Peeling tomatoes: Core, throw into a deep bowl or pan, and cover with boiling water. Let them sit for a minute, then plunge into cold water. The skins will slip right off.

- Peeling garlic: Trim the hard end off, lay the cloves on the cutting board, and put the flat side of your knife down on them (sharp side *away* from you). Whack the knife with the heel of your hand. De-paper the cloves.

- Cooking onions and garlic: Start the onions first. Chopped garlic burns quickly and pressed garlic burns faster.

- Coping with fresh thyme and oregano: Wash the whole sprig. Let dry. Strip the leaves off the stem in one fell swoop, top to bottom. Any stem that comes off with them will be tender and young and can go in the dish. Chop very briefly.

- Making basil pretty: Wash and let dry. Pull off half a dozen leaves and roughly stack, then roll up into a little loose cigar-shape. Cut across the cylinder with fast, close strokes. This classic French method, chiffonade, turns basil into a lovely garnish, and it's faster and more consistent than chopping.

- Gingerroot: Fresh ginger is an incomparable ingredient but can be fibrous. If you don't want all the little strings, grate the root and then press the juice out with your hands. Discard the juiced fibers. If you have gingerroot left over, put it in a plastic bag and freeze. It grates well when frozen.

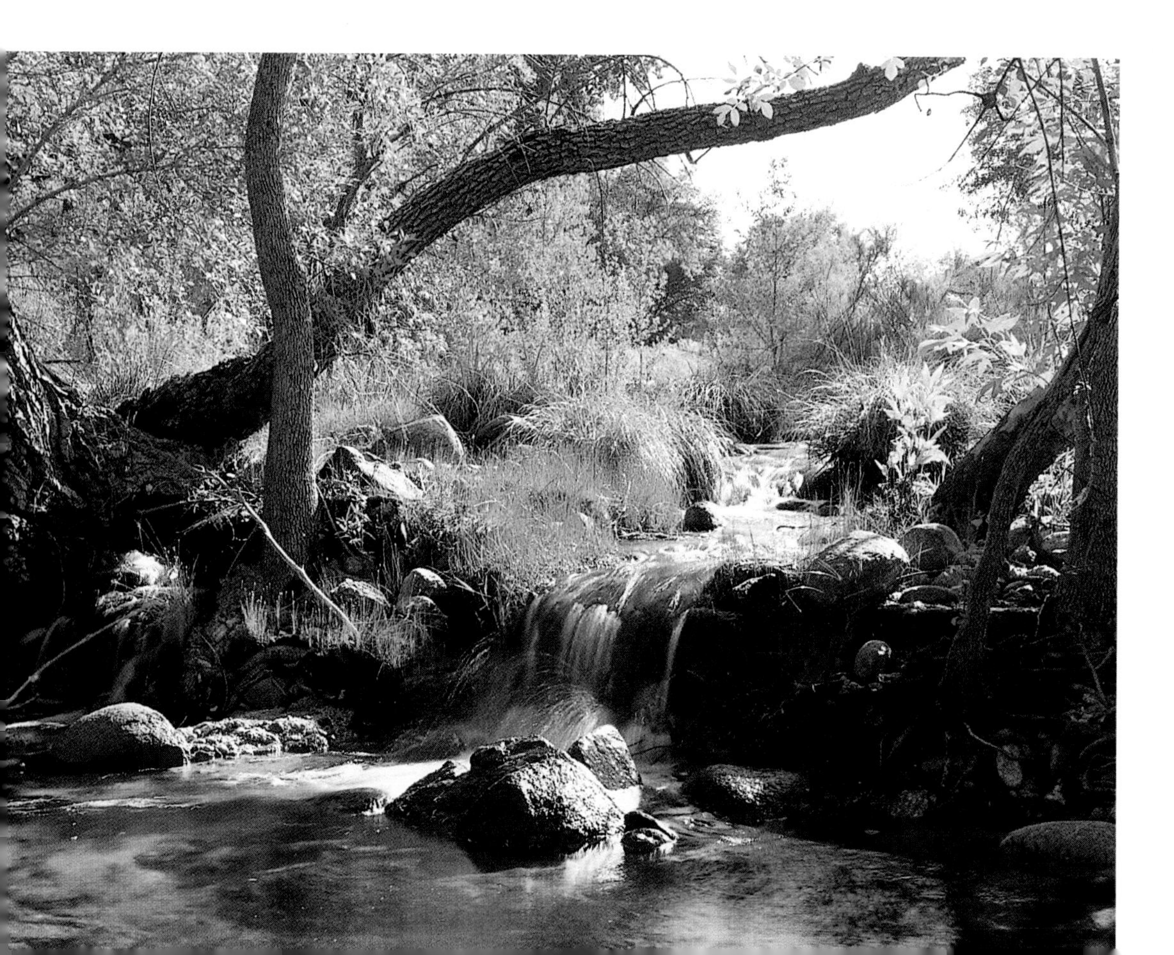

Tortilla-Crusted Sea Bass with Yellow Bell Pepper Coulis

COULIS:

2 small yellow bell peppers, seeded and quartered
½ cup diced onion
2 cloves garlic, peeled and minced
1 tablespoon chopped, fresh cilantro
½ teaspoon chili powder
⅔ cup chicken stock
2 teaspoons fresh lemon juice
2 teaspoons sugar
¼ teaspoon white pepper
Pinch salt (optional)
4 yellow corn tortillas
4 4-ounce sea bass fillets
¼ cup sweet garlic paste (see page 180)

Preheat oven to 400 degrees. Lightly coat a sheet pan with olive oil.

Lay peppers skin side up on baking sheet and roast in oven 10 to 15 minutes or until skins have blackened. Remove from oven and rinse under cold water to peel away skins.

Lightly coat a skillet with a small amount of canola oil. Sauté onions and garlic over medium-low heat until garlic begins to turn golden brown. Add peppers, cilantro, and chili powder. Sauté 1 minute and add stock. Bring to a boil. Add lemon juice and sugar. Cook, stirring occasionally, until all ingredients are soft, about 5 minutes.

Allow to cool slightly. Place in blender container and puree until smooth. Season with pepper.

Place tortillas on baking sheet. Bake in oven until very crisp, about 5 to 10 minutes. Cool. Crush tortillas between wax paper using a rolling pin.

Brush garlic paste over fish and roll in crushed tortilla mixture. Transfer fish to a baking dish that has been lightly coated with canola oil. Bake in oven for 10 to 12 minutes, or until just cooked through. Serve cooked fish with yellow bell pepper coulis.

MAKES 4 SERVINGS, EACH CONTAINING APPROXIMATELY:
255 calories, 23 gm carbohydrate, 5 gm fat, 75 mg cholesterol, 37 gm protein, 176 mg sodium, 4 gm fiber

Sweet Garlic Paste

4 ounces garlic, peeled and chopped

1 ½ cups chicken stock

In a small pot, bring chicken stock to a boil. Add garlic, reduce heat and simmer until most of the liquid is evaporated and the garlic has formed a paste.

Transfer to blender container and puree until smooth. May be stored in the refrigerator for up to 1 week.

MAKES 8 (1 OUNCE) SERVINGS, EACH CONTAINING APPROXIMATELY:
30 calories, 6 gm carbohydrate, Trace fat, 0 mg cholesterol, 1 gm protein, 5 mg sodium, Trace fiber

X. DRINK PLENTY OF CLEAN WATER EVERY DAY

The human body is about 60 percent water. Because we continuously use water in virtually every body process, it's crucial that we replenish the supply. Hydration is also an essential element in energy and hunger management. Buy a beautiful, large water tumbler for your desk at work and drink from it throughout the day. Install a water cooler in your home or office. Add a slice of lemon or lime to jazz up plain water. Carry a water bottle with you.

The Wonders of Water—Best of Beverages

Drink to your health! The standard advice to drink at least eight glasses of water a day still holds true. The key phrase is "at least"—variables such as exercise, climate, dietary fiber, sodium intake, and caffeine and alcohol consumption can all increase your fluid requirements. (At Canyon Ranch in Tucson, we know *a lot* about water needs and climate.)

Think water first, and then supplement your daily fluid intake with beverages like fruit juice mixed with sparkling water and refreshing teas—hot or iced, herbal, green, or black.

Caffeine and Alcohol Cautions

Caffeinated beverages trigger fluid loss, and alcoholic beverages cause additional fluid loss, so drink more water, at least half a cup, for every cup of these water robbers.

Canyon Ranch Bloody Mary

4 tablespoons horseradish
2 tablespoons Old Bay seasoning
3 tablespoons celery seed
⅔ cup distilled white vinegar
1 ¼ cup lemon juice
1 ¼ teaspoon black pepper
¾ cup Worcestershire sauce
1 ½ cups low-sodium tomato juice

Combine all ingredients except tomato juice in a blender container. Puree briefly. Add tomato juice and blend well. Serve over ice.

MAKES 6 (3/4 CUP) SERVINGS, EACH CONTAINING APPROXIMATELY:
35 calories, 8 gm carbohydrate, Trace fat, 0 mg cholesterol, 2 gm protein, 311 mg sodium, 1 gm fiber

Red Devil Drink

¾ cup sparkling mineral water
2 ¼ cups sliced strawberries
4 ½ cups orange juice

Place all ingredients in a blender container and puree until smooth. Serve over ice.

MAKES 10 (3/4 CUP) SERVINGS, EACH CONTAINING APPROXIMATELY:
55 calories, 13 gm carbohydrate, Trace fat, 0 mg cholesterol, Trace protein, 2 mg sodium, 1 gm fiber

JUICY TIPS

- **Look for 100 percent juices. The terms *beverage, cocktail, drink,* and *punch* indicate that a beverage is not 100 percent juice.**
- **Check the ingredients to find out what's in the juice. Avoid juices with added sugars like high fructose corn syrup sweetener, and those with additives and preservatives.**
- **Keep citrus juices in mind. They are important sources of vitamin C and, when fortified, of calcium.**

Home-Cooking Tips from the Chefs of Canyon Ranch

1. When baking or preparing recipes that use sugar, try cutting the amount called for by a third to a half. You'll usually find that the result is as good, or even better.

2. Use evaporated skim milk instead of cream.

3. Use broth instead of plain water when you cook rice and other grains.

4. Put your favorite healthy cooking oil in a high quality, hard-plastic spray bottle, and use to coat pans and grills.

5 Toast nuts and seeds called for in recipes—quickly, over medium heat—and halve the amount you use. Toasting doubles the flavor.

6. Top dishes with grated, highest quality aromatic cheeses, such as parmigiano-reggiano, pecorino romano, or extrasharp cheddar. Their intensity makes a little go a long way, and grating distributes the flavor evenly.

7. Grill over aromatic woods, such as mesquite, hickory, and applewood, for complexity and depth of flavor with no added calories.

8. Butterfly cuts of meat and poultry for quicker cooking and twice the plate coverage.

9. Look for imported Italian tomato paste at specialty markets. The flavor's incomparable, and since it comes in a resealable tube, you can use a tablespoon or two at a time and always have it on hand in the refrigerator.

10. Marinate meats and vegetables before cooking for optimal flavor.

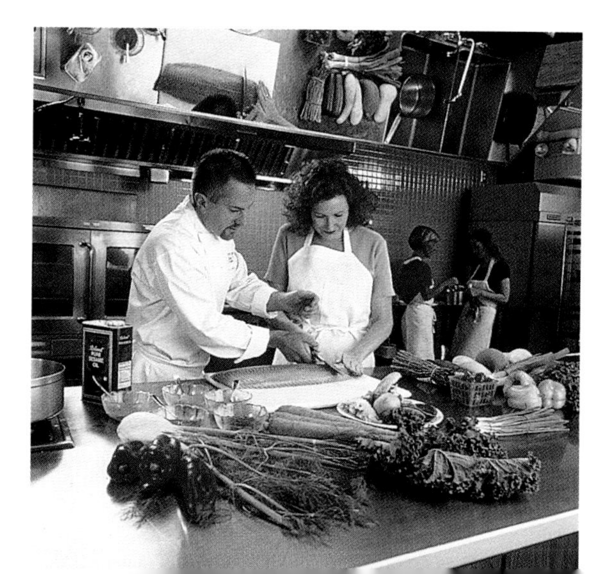

Sesame Ginger Salad Dressing/Marinade

4 cloves garlic
1 cup apple juice
1 cup rice vinegar
3 tablespoons sesame oil
2 teaspoons salt
2 teaspoons black pepper
1 tablespoon fresh ginger juice

Preheat oven to 350 degrees. Place garlic on sheet pan and roast in oven for 10 to 15 minutes or until golden brown. Cool and mince.

In a medium bowl, combine apple juice, vinegar, sesame oil, salt, black pepper, ginger juice, and roasted garlic. Mix well.

MAKES 16 (2 TABLESPOON) SERVINGS, EACH CONTAINING APPROXIMATELY:
40 calories, 4 gm carbohydrate, 2 gm fat, 0 mg cholesterol, Trace protein, 297 mg sodium, Trace fiber

A Last Word on Intelligent Eating

EATING IS ONE OF the great pleasures of living, which we should all savor to the utmost. It's sad that in our culture of abundance so many people have developed unhealthy relationships with food. It doesn't have to be this way: follow our ten rules and you can increase not only your physical health and well-being but your total enjoyment of life. *Bon appétit!*

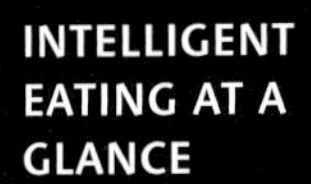

INTELLIGENT EATING AT A GLANCE

1. Begin by assessing your personal needs and goals.
2. Establish a pattern of eating regularly.
3. Be mindful of portion sizes.
4. Eat 8 to 10 servings of vegetables and fruit a day.
5. Emphasize whole grains.
6. Focus on healthy fats and oils.
7. Balance each meal with some protein-rich food.
8. Limit the amount of sugar in your diet and avoid artificial sweeteners.
9. Be sensible about salt.
10. Drink plenty of clean water every day.

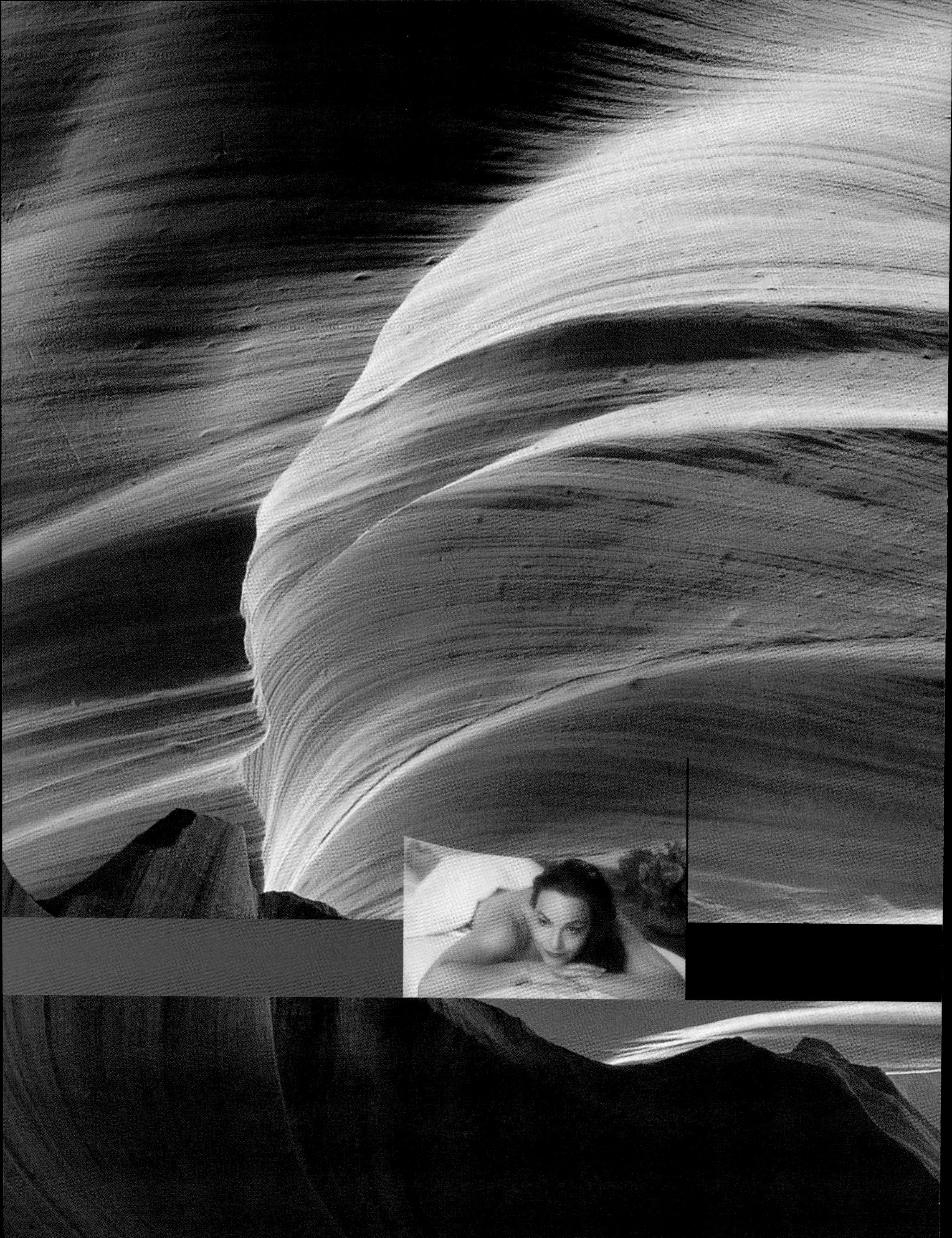

8 HANDS-ON HEALING: *Bodywork and Massage*

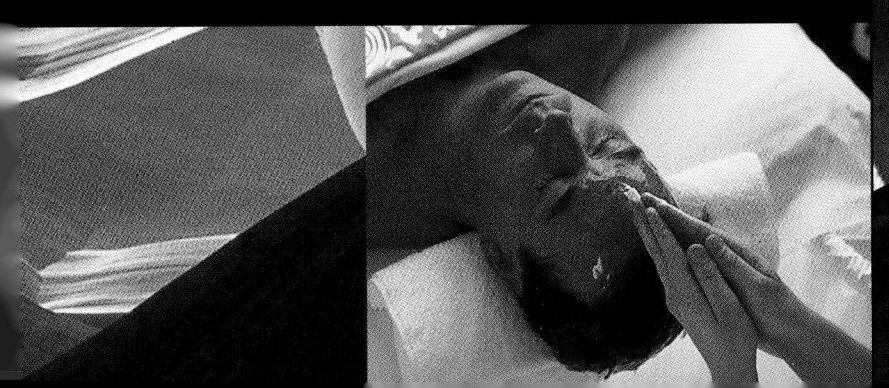

Therapeutic manipulation of the body is almost certainly the oldest of all healing traditions. The Greek physician Hippocrates, the father of Western medicine, used therapeutic touch as a key element of treatment. Touch was pushed over to the edge of mainstream Western medical practice, however, beginning in the nineteenth century. Armed with new medicines and technologies, doctors and nurses couldn't afford, and felt they didn't need, to spend as much time touching patients. They tended to relegate that side of healing to physical therapists, who, in turn, became increasingly "hands off" and technologically oriented.

No technological or chemical miracle, however, can take the place of touch, a fact that's been rediscovered in the last forty years amid an explosion of bodywork techniques and systems. As contemporary medicine swings back around to the view that the mind and all the systems of the body are inextricably connected, variations on age-old practices ranging from massage to the laying on of hands to immersion in water are rejoining the mainstream of medical treatment.

Bodywork, however, does more than alleviate specific pains, increase overall well-being, and aid in healing; it can also help us feel whole. Without our sense of touch, we are absolutely lost, and yet it's the sense least valued and stimulated in our modern, high-tech world. Every day we're exhorted not to bother with the real thing—experience we can *feel*—but to be content with simulations that come in through our eyes and ears. We should hurry up to pay eight dollars to sit motionless for two hours while we watch actors run, jump, drive fast, dance, sweat, and make love on our behalf—it's so much less trouble than actually doing it ourselves. The result is a growing disconnect between touch and the other four senses.

The Five Senses and Bodywork

VISION

The eyes use one third as much oxygen as the heart, house 70 percent of the body's sense receptors, and send two thirds of all messages received and processed in the brain.

Soothed/stimulated by: dim attractive lighting, interesting things to look at, beams of colored light, and colored bath salts.

READ ABOUT COLOR THERAPY on the Web at www.peacefulmind.com/color_therapy.htm and then try it for yourself. Select the color that most appeals to you at the moment and look at it for a few minutes.

HEARING

The ears, unlike the eyes, cannot be shut, and hearing is probably more assaulted by modern life than any other sense.

Soothed/stimulated by: recordings of pleasant music and natural sounds like waves on a beach and trickling water.

SMELL

Smell, seated in the oldest part of the brain, is the sense most closely linked to memory and to the emotions.

Soothed/stimulated by: essential oils—volatile oils derived from plants; herbs, flower petals, and fragrant leaves floated in a bath or steamed over a stove; subtle scents of muds, clays, sea vegetables, algaes, butters, and fragrant natural oils like oil of almond.

TASTE

Taste, which is almost entirely dependent on the sense of smell, also connects straight to the emotions.

Soothed/stimulated by: a concluding cup of tea, keyed to or complementing organic products used in the treatment (peppermint, rosemary, chamomile, green tea); juices and ices that reinforce the scent of treatment products based on foods (mango, papaya, citrus, coconut).

TOUCH

Touch is the first sense to develop in the womb, beginning at about the sixth week after conception, and it's the only one that involves our whole physical being—the other four senses are located in our heads.

Soothed/stimulated by: many kinds of therapeutic touch, and the application of substances with various textures (slippery, powdery, grainy) at various temperatures.

Reconnecting Mind and Body

THE RECONNECTION OF MIND to body, and of our senses to one another, is the essence of bodywork. Therapeutic treatments don't just affect the skin—the largest organ in the body—but all our senses at once. When we receive a massage in a pleasantly darkened room, as music plays quietly and we smell essential oils and taste an occasional sip of cool water, we're reintegrated as embodied, living beings. We emerge more alive, with our minds calmed and back where they belong—within the body, and in present reality.

Obtain your doctor's permission for bodywork and inform your therapist if

- You have heart problems or high blood pressure
- You are pregnant
- You have been diagnosed with cancer
- You have skin allergies
- You are allergic to iodine or shellfish (applies only to treatments involving products from the sea)

Principles of Bodywork

THE VARIED field of therapeutic bodywork rests on a number of shared understandings about body, mind, and health.

1. Improved blood circulation is beneficial for virtually all health conditions.
2. Improved lymphatic circulation—the body's filtering system—contributes to good health.
3. Release of muscular tension has important physiological and psychological benefits.
4. The structure and function of the musculoskeletal system are interdependent, and both are altered by prolonged stress, misuse, disease, and trauma.

These assumptions underlie all types of bodywork, along with the belief that therapeutic touch promotes good circulation and the release of muscular tension, and consequently promotes healing of stressed and injured tissue and better overall health.

Each of the various kinds of bodywork has its own approach, and many types—especially those derived from Asian techniques—are based on much more elaborate systems of belief than the four principles outlined above. Many have quite specific purposes. All, however, strive to improve comfort and health through touch.

Because bodywork is one-on-one, time intensive, and involves touch, it can seem very personal, and, for that reason, intimidating or self-indulgent. The field, however, encompasses therapies that do not involve actual physical contact (Healing Touch and Reiki), and many types that are received fully clothed (Reiki, Shiatsu, Thai massage, Healing Touch, Reflexology, and Jin Shin Jyutsu). Some forms are vigorous and

CONTROLLED STUDIES HAVE shown therapeutic touch to have measurable benefits for a wide variety of conditions and populations, including:

Stress

Traumatic injury to the spine

Chronic pain

Arthritis

Lymphedema (in radical mastectomy patients)

Inflammatory bowel disease

PMS

Wound healing

HIV patients

Postsurgical hospital patients

Premature infants

Depressed and adjustment-disordered children and adolescents

Post-bypass hospital patients

occasionally create minor discomfort (Rolfing, Deep Tissue Massage, and Sports Massage), while others employ only extremely gentle movements (Rosen Method, Polarity Therapy, and Trager).

Some specific styles of massage can involve minor discomfort because the tissue being worked is unhealthy, but *no* massage should cause actual pain. If something your therapist does hurts, speak up immediately. In general, communication with the therapist is essential if you want a good massage.

Bodywork professionals have a wide range of individual styles, but all are trained to be sensitive to the feelings of their clients, both physical and emotional, and to respect their clients' modesty, sensitivity to pain, and desire for communication. The bodywork practitioner is there for *you*.

Fundamentals of Touch

SWEDISH MASSAGE

This is what we tend to think of when we hear the word *massage*. Developed in Sweden in the 1830s, Swedish massage is usually brisk and vigorous and employs a combination of long strokes and kneading, generally in the direction of the heart. The emphasis is on increasing circulation in the surface muscles. Swedish massage is usually full body, and since oil is used as a lubricant, the client is unclothed and draped with sheets.

The five basic Swedish strokes:

Effleurage—A smooth, gliding stroke used to relax soft tissues. Usually applied with both hands.

Controlled studies are currently underway on the benefits of therapeutic touch for:

- Newborn children of cocaine-addicted mothers
- HIV-exposed newborns
- Infants of depressed mothers
- Infants with sleep disorders
- Infants with cancer
- Abused children
- Autistic children
- Depressed teenage mothers
- Eating disorders
- Hypertension
- Fibromyalgia syndrome
- Post-traumatic stress disorder
- Chronic fatigue syndrome
- Asthma
- Diabetes
- Juvenile rheumatoid arthritis

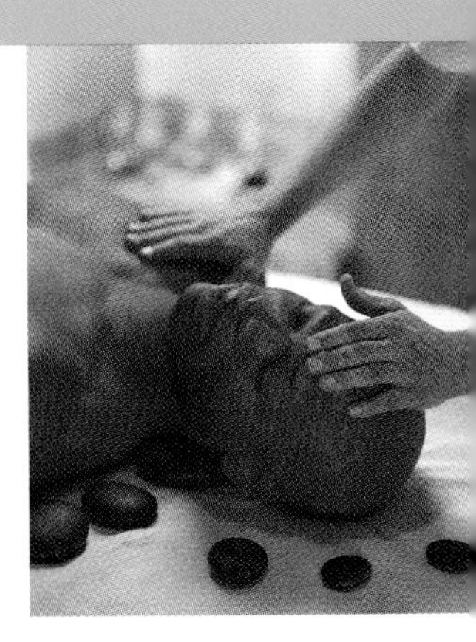

Friction—The deepest and most strongly focused stroke. This circular stroke causes underlying layers of tissue to rub against each other, increasing blood flow, breaking up adhesions, and freeing muscle fibers.

Petrissage (Kneading, or Milking)—This stroke involves squeezing, rolling, and kneading the muscles and usually follows friction to cleanse and flush an area.

Tapotement—A rapid, rhythmic tapping executed using cupped hands, fingertips, or the edge of the hand. Used to stimulate the nerves.

Compression—Rhythmic, pumplike pressure that promotes movement of blood and lymph through tissues.

COUPLES MASSAGE GUIDELINES

Couples massage is a wonderful way for two people to reconnect while helping each other relax and feel better. Fancy technique and strong pressure are not the point here: it's the quality of mutual attention and the desire to please that make couples massage something special.

DO'S

- Use old sheets and towels and a pure vegetable massage oil or lotion in a squeeze bottle. Massage can be messy.
- Breathe and relax your shoulders.
- Always use your weight, not muscle tension, to apply pressure.
- Turn down the lights and put on pleasant music: create a haven.
- Make sure both of you are comfortable. Your partner can sit or straddle a chair, cushioned with a pillow, as you stand, or your partner can lie on the floor, with pillows,

FINDING THE BODYWORK YOU WANT

TWENTY-NINE STATES currently have licensing boards for bodywork professionals, but their standards vary widely. The National Certification Board for Therapeutic Massage and Bodywork, whose members practice a wide variety of modalities, certifies practitioners and has 37,000 members. NCBTMB-certified members must take a nationally standardized test at least every four years to ensure that they meet a minimum standard of competence. The organization's Web site contains a searchable database of certified practitioners. For more information: National Certification Board for Therapeutic Massage and Bodywork
8201 Greensboro Dr.,
Suite 30
McLean, VA 22102
800-296-0664
www.ncbtmb.com

The American Massage Therapy Association, which is geared toward Swedish and other Western techniques, is a professional association with more than 40,000 members. It does not test

while you sit, leaning back against a couch. You can also work on your partner's feet in your lap or on your partner's neck and shoulders while you sit on a couch and your partner lies on it.

- Explore, feel, and pay attention to your partner's body—where it's tight, sore, relaxed, and so on.
- Encourage your partner to tell you what feels good and what doesn't.
- Alternate strokes; when you get tired of doing one thing, do something else. Relax your hands as you draw them back toward you.
- Attend to your own comfort and sensations.
- Do what you like, and ask for what you like when it's your turn to receive the massage. Be creative.
- Add a drop or two of ylang-ylang oil to your massage oil for an especially sensual effect.

AND DON'TS

- Try to give a vigorous, intense massage—you might injure your partner. Professional therapists spend hundreds of hours studying anatomy, learning technique, and practicing.
- Apply pressure to any area that's sore or sensitive. Ease off, but keep gently working the area. If your partner resists your touch there, move on, and come back to the sore area later with very light pressure. If your partner has any injuries, sprains, or bruises, leave those areas alone.
- Think your massage is a cure-all. If your partner is sore or tense afterward, don't worry. He or she may not be ready to let go of tension.

or certify members but acts as an advocacy group, a clearinghouse for information, and a provider of insurance and other benefits. The AMTA's informative Web site includes a "Find a therapist" feature that lists local professionals, along with details about their education, specialties, and hours.

For more information:
American Massage Therapy Association
820 Davis St.,
Suite 1000
Evanston, IL 60201
847-864-0123
www.amtamassage.org.
Certification by NCBTMB and membership in AMTA both cost money, and some fine therapists don't belong to either group. Other ways to find a therapist in your area, or to check out one you may be considering, are contacting your city and state licensing agencies and calling local massage schools.

Contemporary Swedish-Derived Techniques

NEUROMUSCULAR THERAPY

This form of focused, deep-muscle therapy uses strong finger pressure to relax trigger points—chronically knotted muscles and adhesions that cause spasm and pain in other muscles. Usually taken as a series of treatments, NMT is often effective in relieving neck and spinal problems and in restoring postural alignment, proper biomechanics, and flexibility. It can help rebuild strength in injured tissues and assist the flow of blood and lymph. In addition, NMT can be a valuable treatment for chronic pain.

DEEP TISSUE MASSAGE

A slow, focused style of massage that often works across the direction of the muscle fibers to flush out soft tissue, release chronic muscle tension, and break up adhesions and calcified bruises in the muscles. The recipient determines the intensity of the pressure applied.

MYOFASCIAL RELEASE MASSAGE

The fascia is connective tissue that encloses every structure in the body. In this type of massage, the therapist focuses specifically on stretching and releasing adhesions of the fascia surrounding the muscles, resulting in a release of muscular tension.

Hydrate—drink water—constantly while you receive bodywork. Virtually every form of treatment increases circulation of blood and lymph, causing thirst and often a need to urinate. Pay attention to these needs, and take care of them—that's what bodywork is all about.

SPORTS MASSAGE

A specialized form of Swedish massage developed for athletes, but useful for anyone with chronic pain or range-of-motion issues or injury; the work is usually limited to a problem area. Sports massage is also useful before and after sporting events, in which case the areas addressed will be those used in the particular activity. Sports massage emphasizes prevention and healing of injuries to the muscles and tendons.

LYMPHATIC MASSAGE

Very light, rhythmic, repetitive strokes stimulate and promote the movement of lymphatic fluids, the body's filtration and infection-control system. Especially useful for people experiencing edema (excess fluid and swelling) or general poor health.

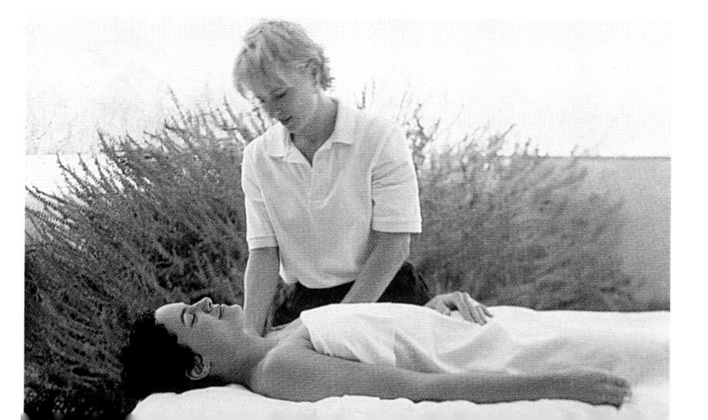

Head-Off-That-Headache Self-Massage

Most headaches start with tension held in the neck and shoulders. When you feel a headache coming on, try the following. Note: the sooner you address the tension, the better—don't wait until your head really hurts.

- Holding fingers straight and together, press firmly with the fingertips on the sides of the neck where the neck and shoulders meet.
- Press in more firmly on the right side as you bend your head to the right. Repeat on the left side.
- Go slowly, moving on an inhale and pressing on the exhale.
- Move the fingers up about one inch on both sides and repeat. Bend and press right, bend and press left, continuing to breathe in sync.
- Move up and repeat until you reach the head.
- Speed up, gently and smoothly moving the head in each direction as you work up and down the sides of the neck, paying special attention to painful or knotted-up areas.
- Now, cup the right hand around the back of the neck, working the fingers into the muscles that run along the left side of the spine.
- Bend the head to the left as your hand pulls to the right, working deeper into the muscles. Gently but firmly work any sore, knotted-up areas, continuing to breathe deeply and rhythmically. Try to release tension on the exhale.
- Using the left hand, work the right side of the spine.
- Complete by shrugging the shoulders up toward your ears and dropping them down and back several times, exhaling on the drop.

Note: for a tension headache that's already going strong, rubbing or icing the place where the thumb joins the palm often provides relief in a few minutes. Firmly rub the "thumb web" on the same side as the headache, or on both sides if the headache encompasses the head.

Functional and Movement Integration Therapies

SOME OF THESE THERAPIES, which include Rolfing, Trager, Feldenkrais, Rosen Method, Hellerwork, Astin-Patterning, and Alexander Technique, are covered briefly in Chapter 5.

The line between bodywork and movement therapy is not entirely clear-cut—touch and movement techniques have combined and proliferated into many methods, each of which offers benefits for some individuals. In general, movement therapy is sequential and focuses on the moving body, while bodywork tends to be more passively received and is concerned with underlying structure. Therapies and therapists frequently overlap.

Most forms of movement therapy involve multiple sessions to resolve long-standing problems. Some therapies, such as Rolfing, have a set and structured course of treatments, while others are open-ended and include take-home therapies and exercises. Qualified practitioners of each of these "brand-name" therapies have completed prescribed training programs for additional certifications.

Asian Techniques

THE ASIAN METHODS most common in the West use the idea of a flow of energy (*chi* or *prana*, depending on the system) that runs through the body along channels, or meridians. (This is also the theory underlying acupuncture, which is now well accepted as a therapy, not only for humans, who are clearly suggestible, but also for animals, who are not.) The goal of the therapy is to balance and regulate the energy in the body. Herbs, acupuncture, color therapy, and aromatherapy are sometimes combined with these methods.

SHIATSU

Shiatsu, which is the Japanese term for "acupressure," involves applying finger pressure (as opposed to needles) to acupuncture points for the purpose of balancing the flow of chi. It's believed that tense muscles impede the flow of energy through the body, causing pain and other symptoms. The client may also be moved through stretches to help balance the chi.

JIN SHIN JYUTSU

In this very gentle, light form of treatment, the practitioner uses pulse diagnosis to identify blockages in the flow of chi. The practitioner then holds or touches the body's twenty-six energy "locks" to release blocked energy.

THAI MASSAGE

A gentle, fluid, meditative style of massage developed 2,500 years ago in Buddhist monasteries as a healing practice. This massage is performed on a futon on the floor with the client fully clothed; the practitioner uses his whole body to produce extraordinary healing postures. While this style of bodywork can benefit anyone, it is increasingly popular with athletes, dancers, martial artists, and yoga devotees.

AYURVEDIC TREATMENTS

Ayurvedic treatments, rooted in the 5,000-year-old Indian system recently popularized in the United States by Deepak Chopra, are designed to balance and nourish body, mind, and spirit and properly begin with an identification of the individual's physical type and condition. Ayurvedic therapies emphasize the use of fragrance, color, and touch in a variety of soothing treatments. Ayurveda, however, encompasses regulation of diet, sleep, and physical activity. Cleansing treatments are just one aspect of a way of life.

Energy-Based Techniques

SOME TREATMENTS ARE based on the idea of a surrounding, universal energy that can be channeled or intensified by the practitioner.

REIKI

Reiki is Japanese for "surrounding life energy." This noninvasive, nontactile treatment stems from the idea that the practitioner is able to channel this energy (through the top of the head) and transmit it to the fully clothed client through the hands, without physical contact.

POLARITY THERAPY

Polarity Therapy is based on the observation that electricity flows from one pole to another. The therapist uses gentle touch and rocking to direct and balance the body's energies. Clients often experience deep emotional as well as physical relaxation.

Other Approaches

REFLEXOLOGY

This practice, which has much in common with shiatsu and acupressure, involves stimulation of specific points on the hands and feet that correspond to organs, glands, systems, and parts of the body. Neurological pathways to distant parts of the body link these points, and pressure or other stimulation of the reflex point has a stimulating or relaxing effect. Because the feet and hands are easy to reach and work on, reflexology is one of the few types of bodywork that you can really do for yourself. Reflexology charts are widely available; all you really need to know, however, is that patiently, attentively massaging your feet and hands, with special attention to areas that are tender, is an effective form of self-care. To begin, use no more pressure than that required to squeeze a new tennis ball.

CRANIOSACRAL THERAPY

In this therapy, the practitioner uses touch both to detect and treat problems in the craniosacral system, the closely interconnected, closed system of skull, spinal column, and sacrum. The practitioner assesses the pulse of the cerebrospinal fluid that circulates through this system and then applies gentle pressure to restore healthy circulation. The treatment is reputed to improve the functioning of the nervous system, and practitioners report success in treating many afflictions of the central nervous system.

Water Therapy

WATER THERAPIES ARE BOTH the oldest and newest thing in bodywork. The benefits of immersion in warm water have been appreciated for millennia; the Romans built baths near natural hot springs wherever they went, and the word *spa* originated as the name of a town in Belgium with a famous healing spring. (The name of the town, in turn, was an acronym for the Latin *sanitas per aqua*, "health via water.")

Still, medicine is only now quantifying the physiological effects of immersion. The enveloping pressure of water causes the entire cardiopulmonary system to work harder during aquatic exercise, making a warm pool an ideal exercise environment not only for people with musculoskeletal problems or who are undergoing rehabilitation, but for anyone who wants to improve cardiovascular capacity. The compressive effect of immersion also assists muscle blood flow, helps rid the muscles of metabolic wastes, and causes changes in the renal system (kidneys and bladder) that help lower blood pressure.

And all this in a medium "that produces an increase in relaxation and in the pain threshold." No wonder Watsu—a one-on-one therapy that combines shiatsu, movement therapy, and assisted flotation in warm water—has quickly become one of the most popular treatments at Canyon Ranch and at other spas throughout the United States.

TREAT YOURSELF

THE SOLE OF THE foot is rich in reflex points, but many people find it difficult to work on their own feet directly.

An easy way to enjoy foot massage during the day is to keep a golf ball in your desk. Several times a day, take off your shoes and roll the ball under one foot and then the other, concentrating on areas that are tense or tender. Do not push so hard that you cause real discomfort; gently work over areas that hurt, returning to them several times. After a day or two of doing this, you should notice the soreness or tension decreasing.

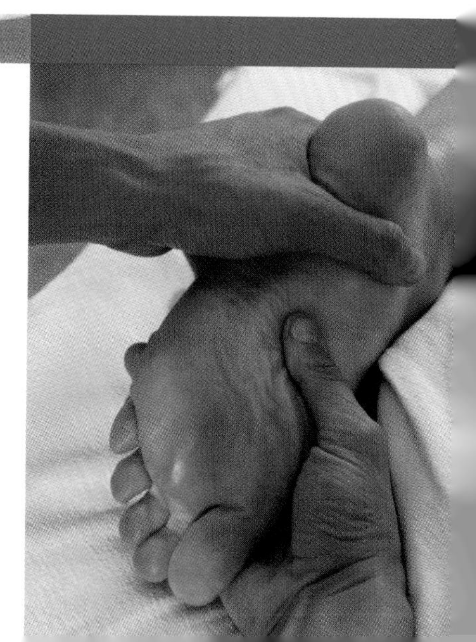

Watsu was developed in the late eighties at Harbin Hot Springs in California by the therapist Harold Dull, who combined *wat*er with shiat*su* to create a treatment that allows relaxed fluidity of movement and stretching not possible on dry land. Many people who've experienced Watsu find it physically soothing and emotionally nurturing. At the ranch, it's easy to spot folks who've just come from a Watsu session—they're the ones wearing swimsuits and blissed-out expressions.

Mud, Salts, Oils, Color Baths, and Herbal Wraps

ANYONE WHO'S EVER SOAKED a sore and tired body in a tub of warm water and Epsom salts has felt the therapeutic power of compounds absorbed by the skin. Especially when circulation is stimulated by warmth, our skin absorbs vitamins, minerals, and trace elements that our bodies need.

Therapies in which the body soaks in mineral- and algae-rich waters are standard cures in Europe; insurance plans pay for people to take the waters because the benefits are so obvious. We came out of the sea, and the blood and lymph circulating through our bodies acts as an interior ocean, supplying tissues with nutrients and carrying wastes away. Sea bathing is an ancient, ever-popular cure, even if we now call it "going to the beach on vacation." Seawater is the largest body of minerals in the world, and both evaporation and oceanic plants concentrate nutrients by hundreds or thousands of times.

The use of bath salts is probably as old as human habitation near the Dead Sea—which goes back to the dawn of civilization. Mineral-rich Dead Sea waters and muds have been credited for thousands of years with relieving pain, especially pain caused by arthritis. The ancients didn't know that it was the high concentration of potassium, calcium, and magnesium in the waters and muds that soothed sore tissue, but they knew it worked. Now, at the beginning of the new millennium, you can buy Dead Sea mud and salts in any well-stocked semialternative supermarket. The idea that the skin and mucous membranes absorb what the body needs has even come back into vogue in standard medicine, where the latest and most sophisticated drug-delivery systems are skin patches and nasal sprays.

Around the world, people use traditional treatments that depend not just on muds, algaes, and mineral salts but also on more ethereal-seeming substances like essential oils, colored light, particular sound frequencies, and poultices of herbs and spices. There's no mystery to why such treatments are effective—our senses are highways to the brain, the master gland that controls our complex biochemistry. Each of the five senses can be either stimulated or soothed to rev up or calm the whole system, or just one part of it, and Westerners are becoming more familiar with the benefits of these subtle, noninvasive approaches to wellness.

DRY BODY BRUSHING, which stimulates the nervous system and the circulation of blood and lymph and exfoliates the skin, precedes most hydrotherapy and body treatments. It's also an effective and easy self-help routine that you can do at home. We recommend it for everyone, first thing in the morning (it's too invigorating for evening), but it's particularly helpful for people suffering from

- poor circulation
- dry skin
- gooseflesh-type skin
- fatigue

Using a dry body brush—a back brush with a handle is perfect—and a gentle wrist-flicking motion so light that it doesn't redden the skin, follow the sequence and direction of the strokes in the diagram. Except where indicated otherwise, always brush towards the heart or center of the body, and start each limb at the point closest to the trunk, brushing with short strokes. Start at the shoulder when you do an arm, for example, then work your way down the arm, always flicking the brush towards the shoulder, until you reach the fingers. At that point, each light stroke of the brush should be long, running all the way up the arm to the shoulder. This technique opens the portals of the lymph first, so that it can flow freely as you move it up from the extremities. Note: brushing must be very light or the lymph, which lies just under the skin, will simply disperse.

THERMAL FOOTBATHS: A REFRESHING aerobic workout for the blood vessels of the feet. Place the feet in a bucket of cold water (45–50 degrees F) for 30 seconds. Then soak them in warm water for 2 minutes. Repeat the cycle at least twice.

ORDER OF AREAS REFRESHED (HEAD TO TOES)

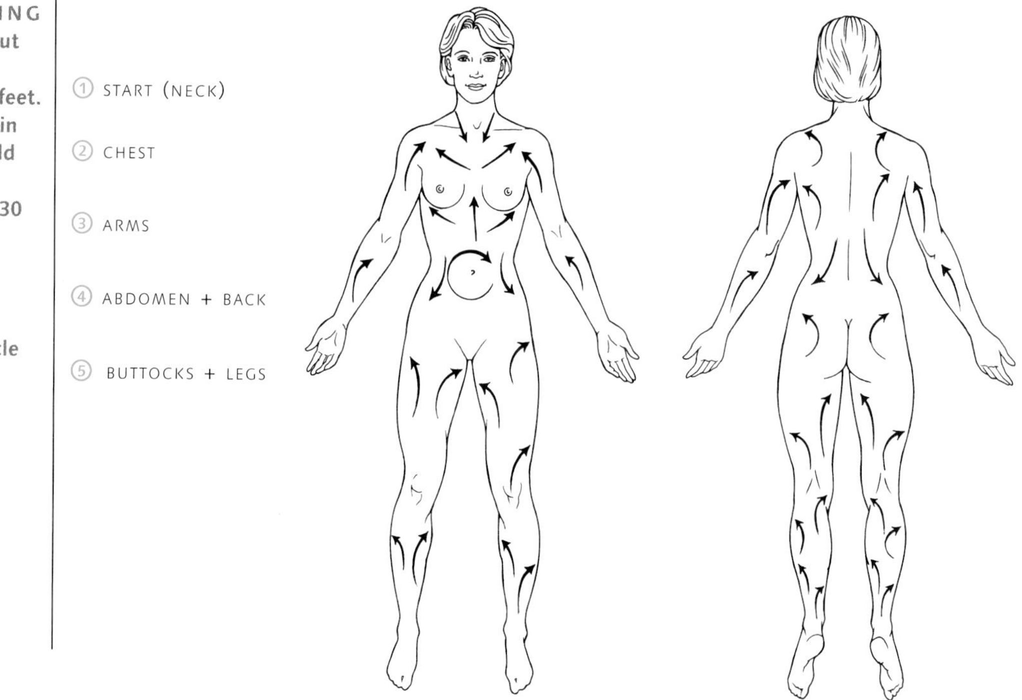

Aromatherapy

AROMATHERAPY, ANOTHER new idea as old as time, uses essential oils—volatile, highly concentrated, plant-derived extracts—to heal, alleviate pain, and regulate mood.

Essential oils have always been treasured (two of the wise men's three gifts to Jesus were fragrances) and not just because they smell nice. Essential oils, like edible phytochemicals, protect plants from environmental damage and predation and contain antioxidants. Various essential oils have antibacterial, antifungal, antiparasitic, and antiviral properties, and some contain compounds that penetrate cell walls. Molecules in some essential oils, including frankincense and sandalwood, have even been shown to cross the blood-brain barrier. Individual oils may contain 200 to 800 different constituent chemicals, only a fraction of which have been identified and researched.

Essential oils can be added to the bath, diluted with pure vegetable oil and applied to the skin in massage, dripped on the forehead or along the spine, or applied in a warm compress. They may also, of course, be diffused into the air or diluted and applied as perfume. Only buy oils that come in brown or blue glass bottles—volatile oils break down in certain wave lengths of light and interact with plastic. Store them away from heat and light.

Aromatherapy products should not be labeled "fragrance"—you want pure, concentrated, plant-derived compounds. They can be more expensive but will go a long, long way; just a drop or two will scent a bath.

For the properties of individual oils, check the publications and guides available where they are sold, or the many aromatherapy sites online; www.aromaweb.com is a good resource. Do your research: essential oils are powerful and should be treated like medicine. Always dilute them, and when in doubt, use less.

CREATING YOUR HOME SPA

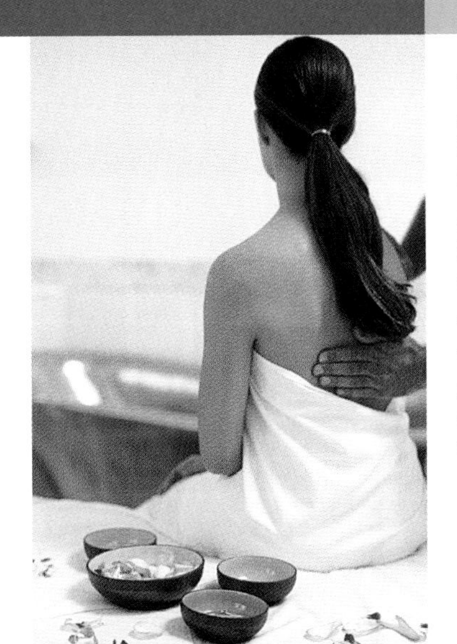

YOU'LL NEED:
a dry brush (or back brush) for morning lymphatic dry brushing

Essential oils
Bath salts
Candles
A tape or CD player

You might also like:
Muds
Seaweed or algae packs
Bath coloring

Note: when you shop for muds, salts, essential oils, seaweed packs, and other products, read the ingredient list and select products composed of naturally derived ingredients—substances you recognize, not unpronounceable mystery chemicals.

Enjoying Your Home Spa

As you learn about essential oils, create your own rituals for various moods and purposes—getting ready for a big night out, relaxing after a long day, relieving aches and pains, or treating cold symptoms.

Here's a routine to try when you need to regroup after a long day and get ready for sleep.

- Prepare a mixture of 5 drops geranium, 4 drops lemon, and 4 drops sandalwood. Combine 4 drops of the mixture with 1 tbs. pure vegetable oil and set on the side of the tub.
- Turn off the phone, light a few candles, and put on some soothing music or a nature-sound CD. Have a cup of cool drinking water within reach.
- As you run a warm bath, add a quart or two of full-fat milk and half of the essential oil mixture.
- Turn off the lights.
- Get into the tub and soak, concentrating on breathing slowly and deeply.

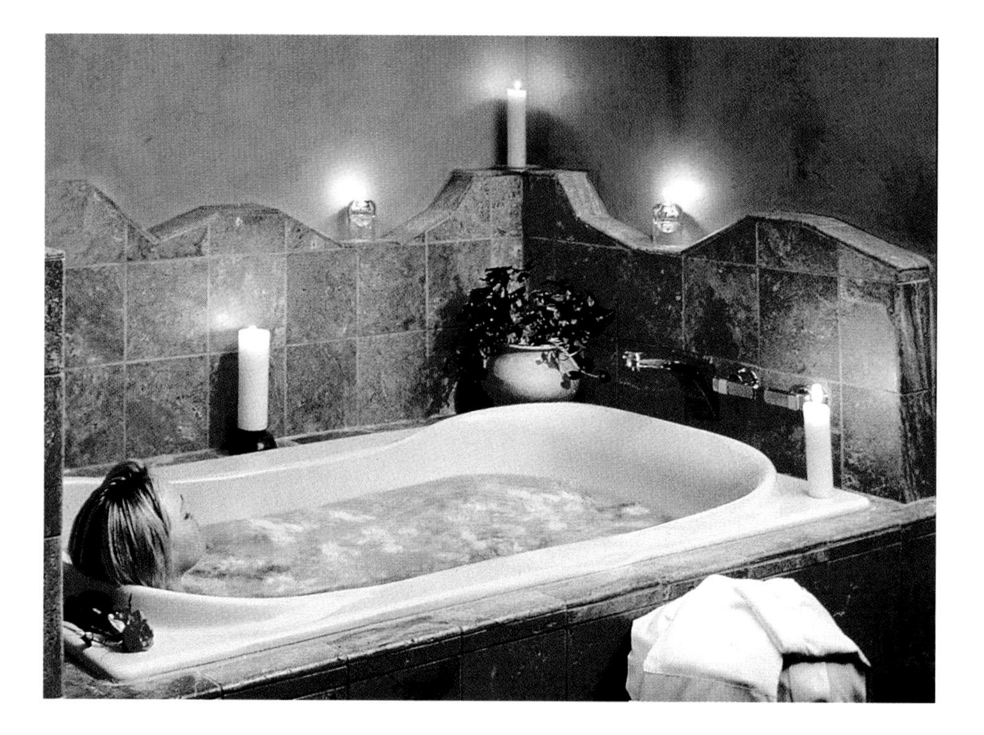

- Pour a little of the remaining massage oil mixture in one palm, and begin slowly massaging the ears, then the feet, one at a time, and, finally, both hands. Take your time and slowly, firmly massage the oil into all surfaces, paying special attention to any areas that are tender or tense.
- Keep the water comfortably warm by running more hot water as necessary.
- When you're ready to get out, step out carefully and towel off, blow out the candles, wrap yourself in a comfortable robe and sit for five or ten minutes as you sip a cup of herbal tea.
- Before you get into bed, take a few deep breaths standing up.
- When you lie down, progressively relax your muscles, beginning with your feet and moving up your body . . .
- Sweet dreams!

It's Better to Give

As bodywork and other therapeutic treatments become increasingly popular, opportunities to learn about them multiply. While professionals must have a rigorous knowledge of anatomy and physiology, and undergo hundreds of hours of training, learning to give a great neck rub or foot massage is a snap. Both the NCBTMB and AMTA Web sites offer advice to beginners, and books, videos, and community college classes are widely available.

Touching others effectively is a uniquely satisfying and practical skill, and one that strengthens our understanding of health as the positive enjoyment of our bodies, and of life.

Healing Touch

The "laying on of hands" is a very old form of healing, but it's only in the last decade that the power of compassionate human touch has become formalized as a therapeutic practice known as Healing Touch in the United States and Canada. This gentle, relaxing, and highly adaptable technique, developed by nurses, is most often performed by registered nurses with years of specialized training. At last count, there were more than 1,100 certified Canadian and U.S. practitioners, and many more nurses with some training are incorporating the practice into patient care.

In a Healing Touch session, the practitioner first interviews the patient about his or her general state of health, current treatments, and areas of concern: Healing Touch is a holistic therapy, in which the entire health picture of the individual is the starting point. The patient then lies down, fully clothed, in a comfortable position while the practitioner begins to work her way up the body—starting at the feet—balancing and releasing areas that are painful, tense, injured, or in some way problematic. The practitioner may gently touch and hold the patient, or may hold her hands just above the patient's skin, while quietly prompting the patient to relax, breathe deeply, and visualize and focus on what he or she is feeling, both physically and emotionally. Since Healing Touch is noninvasive and does not necessarily involve body contact, it is used to help relieve pain and hasten the healing of injuries, surgical wounds, and burns.

Healing Touch is an "energy" therapy, one of many techniques and practices—including acupuncture and yoga—that subscribe to the ancient Eastern concept of energy flow along pathways in and around the body. In this tradition, a flow of energy through the body that's chaotic, blocked, or out of balance is associated with pain, disease, and emotional distress; healthy energy circulation permits healing and contributes to overall health balance, relieves stress, and helps release destructive emotions. The Healing Touch practitioner seeks to balance the flow of vital energy to make healing possible. All healing is, in fact, self-healing, and Healing Touch is one more way to promote wellness of body, mind, and spirit.

It is not necessary for the patient to understand or "believe in" energy medicine to feel benefits: this is not faith healing. For many people, however, Healing Touch is a revelatory experience, producing unfamiliar and powerful sensations of warmth, flow, vibration, and release.

Patients report effects ranging from deep relaxation to sudden releases of long-held grief and anger, and from relief of physical pain to a more vivid sense of body-mind connection. Due to its power to relax and allow people to connect to their emotions, Healing Touch can be very useful to people who are undergoing life transitions; because it is nurturing and administered by practitioners with wide medical experience and knowledge, it can be highly beneficial for people who have undergone traumatic medical interventions such as chemotherapy and surgery. (Healing Touch also strongly emphasizes self-care techniques.) At the very least, it promotes a state of relaxation in which the body's healing processes can function optimally.

To learn more about Healing Touch, or to find a certified practitioner near you, contact the Colorado Center for Healing Touch, 303-989-0581, or visit the Healing Touch International Web site, www.healingtouch.net. Healing Touch International educates and certifies practitioners. You can reach them at 12477 W. Cedar Dr., Suite 202, Lakewood CO 80228; 303-989-7982.

9 EMOTIONAL AND SEXUAL INTIMACY: *The Connection Between Happiness and Health*

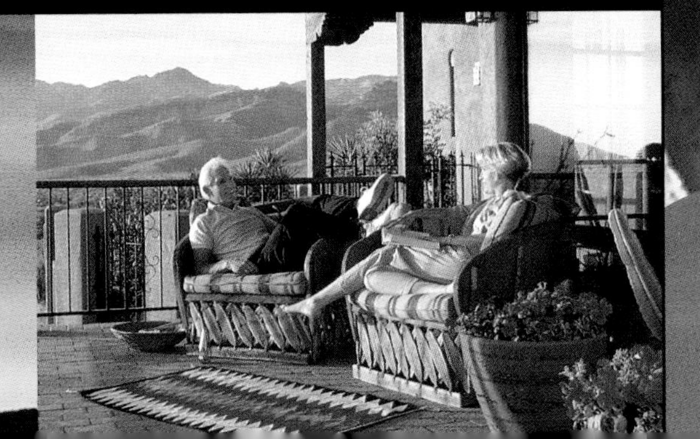

There aren't many flat-out statements we can safely make about all people, but here's one: humans beings cannot be happy or healthy without satisfying connections to others. Intimacy is good for us and disconnection is bad. If we care about our physical well-being—never mind life satisfaction and happiness—we need to acknowledge our emotions and learn how to express them in ways that help us be close to other human beings. Cultivating intimacy is as much a life-enhancing gift to ourselves as regular exercise and a good diet.

But how do we achieve intimacy? People want and need better relationships, but often have no idea how to get them. Statistics on divorce and domestic violence show that we are not a nation of experts on true love, and improving our relationships seems like a much taller order than, say, achieving physical fitness. We don't know where to begin or how to proceed.

In fact, in the last decade or so, many researchers have challenged the nearly universal belief that we should just *know* how to sustain a relationship with people we love simply because we love them. These researchers have carefully analyzed the differences between happy and unhappy relationships. Their findings are encouraging because they're more specific and concrete than the old wisdom: just "communicate," and everything will be fine.

With the high-profile research of such psychologists as John Gottman, and psychoneuroimmunologists like Joan Borysenko and Paul Pearsall, the findings of neuroscientists like Candace Pert, and the work of research biologists like Robert Sapolsky, we now have the information to successfully get around some of the old roadblocks to better intimacy. We can actually measure many of the dramatic physiological effects of trivial incidents that happen to open ancient emotional wounds. We're beginning to comprehend the process that turns a small affront into a deadly

THE NEW SCIENCE OF INTIMACY

- **John Gottman identifies four dynamics that can ruin a relationship: criticalness, defensiveness, stonewalling, and contempt.**
- **Paul Pearsall describes how heart energy—essentially, loving-kindness—affects our overall sense of well-being and contributes to connectedness with others.**
- **Joan Borysenko uses her work in psychoneuroimmunology to explain the negative effects of unresolved guilt.**

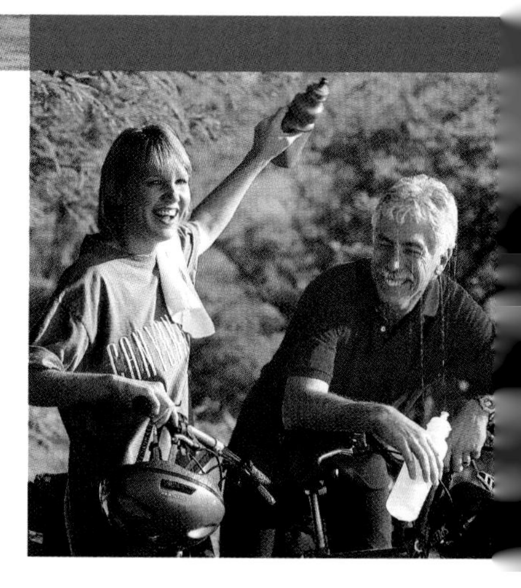

attack and a loved one into an enemy we must disable. This work on intimacy is giving us scientifically based tools for managing biologically based, relationship-shredding reactions.

The Meaning of Intimacy

LET'S DEFINE SOME TERMS. Intimacy means sharing experiences, feelings, and thoughts. In adult, reciprocal love relationships, it usually means preferring your partner's company to that of most other people. It means closeness, trust, and sometimes merging—of bodies, minds, and spirits—while maintaining a healthy sense of boundaries and self.

Intimacy cannot exist without expression. Our understanding of ourselves, of what we think and feel, and the manner in which we express our inner reality make all the difference between unhealthy self-absorption and healthy connection.

STEPS TO ENHANCING INTIMACY

I. Know yourself.

II. Accept yourself.

III. Examine and adjust your beliefs.

IV. Examine and adjust your behavior.

V. Develop your interpersonal skills.

I. Know yourself.

This ancient dictum is not a call to self-absorption. On the contrary: to truly know ourselves, as thinkers since Socrates have said, is the beginning of wisdom, and, thus, of happiness.

Knowing yourself means knowing your strengths and weaknesses, knowing what you feel and think, knowing what you need to be happy and what you simply cannot tolerate. It isn't about staring at your navel; knowing yourself is about not stumbling through life blind to your own nature, and it's a vital first step toward achieving greater intimacy with others.

Books can help. From the writings of philosophers and holy men to collections of Zen koans to the works of contemporary psychologists, there's a huge amount of information, advice, and inspiration out there. Read about emotional intelligence, the differences between men and women, the effects of stress on both body and mind, the role that the mind plays in the body's well-being: new work is emerging all the time.

"MINDFULNESS is the observance of the basic nature of each passing phenomenon. It is watching that thing arising and passing away. It is seeing how that thing makes us feel and how we react to it. It is observing how it affects others. In mindfulness, one is an unbiased observer whose sole job is to keep track of the constantly passing show of the universe within."

VENERABLE HENEPOLA GUNARATANA

Traditional approaches are also helpful. Meditation and prayer can open long-closed avenues to thought and feeling. Keeping a journal—simply sitting down and writing every day about your thoughts, fears, and hopes—helps many people get to know themselves better. And practicing mindfulness is yet another way to find clarity in the midst of the rush and distractions of everyday life.

Another important step in knowing ourselves is identifying and letting go of habits that distress the people we care about or that make us feel disgusted with ourselves. Take a good, hard look at any habits you have that trouble you. Whether your behavior is something "bad," like smoking, or something "good," like working out excessively, it can be a barrier to intimacy, and it probably originates in a desire for connection and pleasure that you are missing. Almost anything human beings do they can overdo, and many people need professional help to get control of their habits, especially those involving substance abuse. Some of the more common and destructive habits:

- Overeating and undereating
- Abusing alcohol and other drugs
- Excessive gambling
- Overspending
- Overworking

The unhappiness and limitations caused by anxiety, mood disorders, physical illnesses, and chronic pain can also stand in the way of closer and more satisfying relationships. Finding treatment for such problems is, of course, important; owning up to their emotional impact is just as crucial. It's a truism of psychology that

RECOMMENDED READING

Joan Borysenko, *Guilt Is the Teacher, Love Is the Lesson* (1990). A psychoneuroimmunologist's guide to quieting the self-blame that can interfere with relationships and health.

John Gottman and Nan Silver, *Why Marriages Succeed or Fail* (1995). Pioneers in quantified relationship studies explain their findings and their lessons.

Venerable Henepola Gunaratana, *Mindfulness in Plain English* (1991). An accessible, practical guide to an often mystified subject by a revered Sri Lankan Buddhist monk and teacher.

Jon Kabat-Zinn, *Full Catastrophe Living* (1990). A psychologist and expert in mind-body medicine offers insight into the challenges of everyday life.

Charlotte Kasl, *If the Buddha Dated* (1999). A light-hearted Buddhist approach to intimacy.

unacknowledged wounds do not heal, but medical doctors are usually too busy to address the emotional toll of serious illness, chronic pain, or loss of function. Facing and allowing yourself to express the effects of life's setbacks—*in the service of connection*—is a step toward greater intimacy.

11. Accept yourself.

Consciously try to let go of self-punishing, repetitive behavior. Christ told us to love our neighbor as we love ourselves, while the Buddha taught that compassion for all living things is the highest virtue. Compassion for ourselves can be a difficult lesson, but it's a necessary one. We can't love anyone very well if we don't love ourselves first.

Cultivate a nonjudgmental, observing mind; work on observing yourself with tolerance.

Meditation practice can help us in learning to love and accept ourselves because it nurtures the detached, calm part of our consciousness and gives the emotions a safe place to come to the surface. It also helps us notice when we start to brood, worry, or obsess and encourages us to let thoughts that torment us go on by.

Meditation requires a quiet place, a focus for your attention, a few moments, and your breath—that's all.

As you observe the breath flowing in and out of your body, observe the thoughts that flick in and out of your mind. Gently remind yourself that you are not responsible for the occurrence of thoughts and emotions and sensations—only for your actions. Thoughts and emotions just are.

When a thought comes to the surface, practice thinking, "That's only a thought, and it's okay that I have it." Do the same with physical sensations, images and sounds—anything that enters your awareness. To the observing mind, even painful

"A person who has consciously worked through the whole tragedy of her own fate will recognize another's suffering more clearly. . . . She surely will not keep the vicious circle of contempt turning."

ALICE MILLER, THE DRAMA OF THE GIFTED CHILD

Harriet G. Lerner, *The Dance of Intimacy* (1989). The psychologist author of *The Dance of Anger* offers a guide to healthy intimacy for women.

Robert Ornstein and David Sobel, *Healthy Pleasures* (1989). A brain researcher and preventive medicine specialist discuss the proven medical benefits of pleasure, including "the virtues of sensuality."

Paul Pearsall, *The Heart's Code* (1998). A psychoneuroimmunologist presents recent findings on cellular memories and their role in the mind-body-spirit connection.

Candace Pert, *Molecules of Emotion* (1997). A neuroscientist reports revolutionary findings—emotions are in every cell of the body.

Robert M. Sapolsky, *Why Zebras Don't Get Ulcers* (1994). A research biologist explores the correlation between chronic stress and illness, including depression and sexual dysfunction.

thoughts become as light, insubstantial, and flowing as breath. The more fully you are able to notice and accept the quality and content of all your thinking, the closer you can come to living in the present moment as a whole person.

III. Examine and adjust your beliefs.

The only intimacy training most of us ever have is in our family of origin; we learned how to be close to others from our parents, who learned from their parents, and so on. What we learn from family is so much a part of us that it's often difficult to even identify the deeply embedded mistaken beliefs that keep us from achieving satisfying relationships as adults. But as long as we remain unconscious of our early training and experiences, we automatically reenact scenarios from the past rather than acting like constructive, loving, and lovable adults.

If the scared, angry two- or three-year-old inside us keeps popping out, we can do enormous damage to the relationships we care most about. When a loved one does or says something that touches an old, unresolved hurt, the panicky, primitive responses of the irrational child within are wildly out of proportion. Researchers have documented the physiological changes that occur when the person we love best suddenly becomes for us "not just the schmuck who has hurt and betrayed me today, but my mother, whom I could never please." Emotional storm surges like this kill intimacy before it ever has a chance to grow, and they're very, very common.

Before we can adjust the beliefs that clutter our lives, we must become as fully aware of the ones that remain unconscious as we can be, and examine those that we do acknowledge, however vaguely. Since it's difficult to be objective about the most subjective aspects of ourselves, professional help is often necessary if we don't want to remain asleep at the wheel of life. Once exposed to the light of day, many mistaken beliefs simply disappear. We wake up.

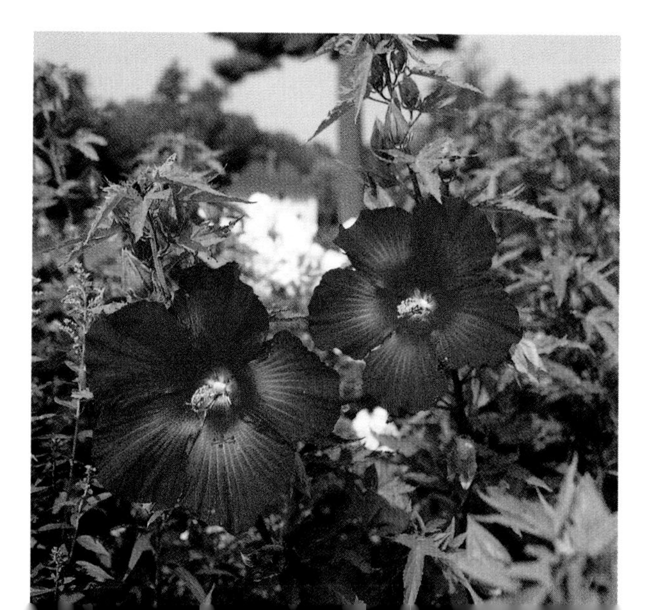

TEN COMMON MISTAKEN BELIEFS ABOUT RELATIONSHIPS—AND THE REALITY.

1. Mind reading is the essence of true love. People who love each other can anticipate and satisfy each other's every need.

   Only little children can confidently expect some mind reading from their parents. Adults need to identify their thoughts and feelings and express them in healthy ways. Dependence on mind reading can lead to chronic feelings of disappointment, anger, and sadness.

2. No one will love you as you are. To get love, you must hide certain parts of yourself.

   Feeling unworthy stems from unconscious or unresolved childhood hurts. Healthy adults are confident that they are ultimately lovable. Gaining approval is not the same thing as creating intimacy, and our intimate relationships cannot be our sole source of self-worth.

3. Relationships must be fifty-fifty. If you carefully keep score, you can whip up righteous indignation at a moment's notice and always have a good reason for feeling bad.

   The female partner is likely to be the "natural" keeper of the intimacy in a heterosexual relationship, for both biological and cultural reasons. The health benefits of learning to love are just as real for men, however. Scorekeeping by either partner deadens intimacy.

4. Romance should naturally last forever. Something is wrong with the relationship if the chemistry isn't always there.

   The falling-in-love feeling typically lasts between eighteen and thirty-six months. In healthy intimacy, the feelings of the adrenaline-pumped early stages are gradually replaced to a large extent by the sensations created by oxytocin, a hormone responsible for feelings of well-being and calm. Romance can be created over and over in a healthy intimate relationship.

5. Your parents did everything right in raising you, so don't pay attention to your thoughts and feelings—just act as you were taught. Conversely, your parents did everything wrong; you must never do anything they did.

   No one grows up in a perfect family; we all experienced hurts and disappointments. To love someone, we have to see that person clearly, not through a haze of automatic responses and moldy resentments. We need to co-create our relationship, moment to moment, like a work of art.

6. Stress comes from negative events. If nothing bad is happening, you can forget about practicing stress-management techniques.

   Stress is a fact of life. If you do nothing to manage it, you will be more irritable than you need to be and less likely to think before speaking and acting.

7. You should be honest all the time, about everything, with those you love.

   Constant criticism destroys feelings of closeness and safety. Don't confuse openness and truthfulness with a compulsive need to criticize.

8. Conflict is damaging to intimacy. Avoid it at all costs.

   Conflict happens, so conflict-resolution skills are crucial. Couples feel closer when they discover that they can disagree without wrecking the relationship.

9. Sex should happen spontaneously in healthy love relationships. You shouldn't ever have to plan it.

   Intimate sexual connection is a by-product of relaxation and play. When both partners have busy, rushed lives, they need to set time aside to be together.

10. If you have a good relationship, you should feel happy all the time.

    Balance—states of both sadness and happiness—creates a "healing hardiness" that's basic to our overall sense of well-being.

Lying deep in our minds, unexamined and fully amped with emotional energy, mistaken beliefs are massive roadblocks to achieving greater intimacy. The truth is that we can achieve fulfilling adult relationships only if we think and behave as adults, as people who can distinguish between reality and thoughts. If we are to love the people we care about as they deserve to be loved, we must examine and reframe our mistaken beliefs and cultivate optimistic trust.

PAULA AND DAN'S STORY

"If he finds out, I don't know what he'll do."

Her skin was a ghostly gray, she was sickly, and the look in her eyes varied from dull to terrified. At thirty-four, Paula appeared to be years older. In a lifestyle consultation with a Canyon Ranch behavioral therapist, she told her story.

Married eight years, with a one-year-old and a three-year-old, Paula was an attorney who'd become a stay-at-home mom, and she'd lived nearly a decade with a secret that was devastating her. She was a smoker, but no one knew.

When they'd gotten engaged, Paula had promised Dan that she would quit—he was not going to marry a smoker. Paula, however, only pretended to quit. She never smoked in the house, or in the company of her friends—even with friends who smoked—or in front of adult family members. She smoked in her car, even if her kids were with her, as they often were. She was increasingly worried that soon her children would be old enough to understand that smoking was "bad" and that they would tell their father. And then the marriage would be over.

> "Optimists know intuitively that there are always choices that can be made. . . . They also tend to be able to laugh at themselves, to have a positive sense of humor. . . and a spirit of engagement in life. . . . Their social traits include valuing relationships, honoring them, and feeling a sense of goodness and basic trust in people."
>
> JON KABAT-ZINN

Paula felt hopeless and scared. She hadn't been able to quit, because she'd been using smoking for stress reduction since she was fifteen and didn't know any other way to cope. For her, smoking was a break from her routine, from the kids, from her husband. She smoked to stay thin, and she smoked when she was lonely, disappointed, or angry. In her isolated life at home, cigarettes, which had always been her friend, had become her best friend.

But now she was in a horrible bind. She was terrified that if she didn't quit, Dan would find out and would see her as a liar and a lousy mother. She was sure he'd divorce her. She also believed that quitting was impossible.

The therapist agreed with Paula that the challenge of quitting would be big, but, unlike Paula, the therapist knew of approaches that might work. Paula had to agree to do several things. First she would need to accept the idea that quitting is a process, not an event: she would have some short-term tasks and some that would take longer. She would need to accept help. And, most important of all, she needed to reveal her secret so that she could begin to heal.

Since Dan and Paula were at the ranch together, the therapist suggested that the first step would be for Paula to bring Dan to her next counseling session. The session would require Paula to prepare for three things. She would have to:

1. Tell Dan her secret and reveal that she'd been keeping it from him the entire time they'd been married.
2. Describe for him, as she had for the therapist, how frightened and ashamed she felt, every day.
3. Ask for his support.

At the next session, the therapist set guidelines at the outset, asking Dan to hold his response until Paula had said all she needed to say.

At this point, Dan looked almost as frightened as Paula, and said, "I have no idea why I'm here." The therapist asked him to *listen with his heart,* and when Paula had finished what she had to say, to make his best effort to *speak from his heart.*

Shaking and crying a little, Paula told Dan her whole truth and then said, "I need your help if I'm going to do this." Without missing a beat, Dan replied, "I'll do anything it takes." Then they cried and hugged.

With further treatment, Paula came to realize that her habit was a true addiction. She understood that, for her, cigarettes functioned not only as a stress reducer but also as an antidepressant. She decided to have a consultation with a psychopharmacologist, who gave her a prescription for medication to replace the cigarettes.

When she returned to Canyon Ranch a year later, she'd been a nonsmoker for more than ten months, and she practiced relaxation techniques, including conscious deep breathing and visualization, instead of smoking. Her skin was rosy and her eyes bright. She'd begun to exercise regularly and had added ten very necessary pounds to her formerly emaciated frame.

At her two- and three-year ranch anniversaries, Paula came back. She was still a nonsmoker, and she'd been able to discontinue all medication. But the most wonderful effect of her healing journey was the change in her relationship with her husband. She told the therapist on her fourth anniversary visit, "My marriage is better than it's ever been!"

Paula had let go of a dreadfully mistaken belief about her marriage—that Dan would leave her if she told the truth—and overcome her fear that she'd fall apart without cigarettes.

IV. Examine and adjust your behavior.

1. MANAGE STRESS

Uncontrolled, chronic stress is harmful to mind and body, and to relationships. When we're in the throes of a full-fledged stress response, or stretched to the limit by chronic stress, we *cannot* behave lovingly, kindly, or appreciatively to those we love. Either we learn to manage our stress or we suffer, becoming "human doings" instead of what we long to be—human beings.

Deep breathing is one of the best and easiest ways to control stress. Slow, even, deep, unhurried breath is to your body and mind what a lullaby is to a baby. Breathing slowly and consciously for a moment or two signals both body and mind that in spite of everything—the traffic jam, the baby-sitter waiting, the flood of stress hormones that just poured into your bloodstream when you looked at your watch—things will be okay. "Look," you're saying to yourself, "my breathing is relaxed, so *I* must be relaxed." Amazingly, this actually works. The body ceases to read thoughts as "Danger!" and begins to believe that it's safe to rest for a moment.

2. LEARN TO COPE WITH MOODS

Moods, like stress, are a fact of life. And, like stress, they're manageable if we acknowledge and attend to them.

At the very least, we need to pay attention to the subtle and sometimes not-so-subtle fluctuations in our moods, and learn to control the moody behavior that alienates or hurts our loved ones. Learn to recognize your difficult moods, and avoid discussing anything charged until you feel better. As adults in reciprocal relationships, we can consciously choose to behave in such a way as to attract those we love—or at least not to push them away. Sometimes it's enough just to say, "I'm in a rotten mood; it has nothing to do with you. Let's talk later."

If a bad mood persists beyond a couple of weeks, though, and if you're not mourning a loss—grief is "normal depression"—you may be clinically depressed. Sometimes depression lifts spontaneously, and sometimes regular walking or jogging helps (avoid excessive exercise, however). And sometimes talking things over is enough.

If you find that your bad mood is so strong and persistent that you have no power to act, or if it begins to affect your eating or sleeping patterns, or if you feel a pervasive lack of joy in anything, then you need to seek help. You should also consider help if someone close to you thinks you're depressed. One of the most insidious things about depression is that it seems rational to the victim: "The world is absolutely dreadful, so of course I feel sad, frightened, and irritable."

Depression is hazardous to your health, and it can be lethal to intimate relationships, "infecting" entire families and ruining marriages. It is treatable, however: a combination of cognitive-behavioral therapy and medication helps in at least 70 percent of cases.

GARY AND PAT'S STORY

"Just too many social events . . ."

On the couple's eighth visit to Canyon Ranch in as many years, Gary, age sixty-three, showed up with slightly elevated blood pressure and about twelve extra pounds. He'd retired a few months before after thirty-five years as CEO of a company founded by his father. Pat had been a schoolteacher before the couple had their four children. At sixty-two, she loved spending time with their children and grandchildren, traveling, doing philanthropic work, and seeing friends. With Gary at last free to join her, life should have been good.

But Pat had just given Gary an ultimatum: quit drinking or leave. Gary wasn't sure Pat was being fair; his view was that he was just a little moody and sometimes drank too much. He knew that he ought to be enjoying his new freedom, but instead he felt "flat" and had a hard time resisting alcohol at the many social functions the couple attended. He came to the ranch willing to take a look at the way he was handling retirement. So he decided to book a stay designed specifically for stress management, to see if he could reduce his blood pressure, lose weight, get control of his drinking, and, most important, save his marriage.

Very quickly, Gary learned that he had a form of depression. It had never occurred to him that he could be depressed because he'd always been busy and successful. But as he talked, he realized that lately nothing gave him joy. He was also burdened by his thinking, which was frequently negative and obsessive. He lacked energy and was often cranky or withdrawn, and he admitted that he'd been drinking more than he ever had in the past and that he drank to excess at every social occasion. He and Pat hadn't slept together in more than a year.

Gary consulted a doctor who prescribed a course of antidepressant medication. With the nutritionist, he created an eating plan to help increase his energy and reduce his caloric intake. A consultation with an exercise physiologist got him back into a schedule of walking and playing tennis. In a series of movement therapy sessions, he and Pat reconnected without words, through play.

In his sessions with the behavioral therapist, Gary came to realize that his expectations for retirement had been unrealistic. He needed to find ways to feel a sense

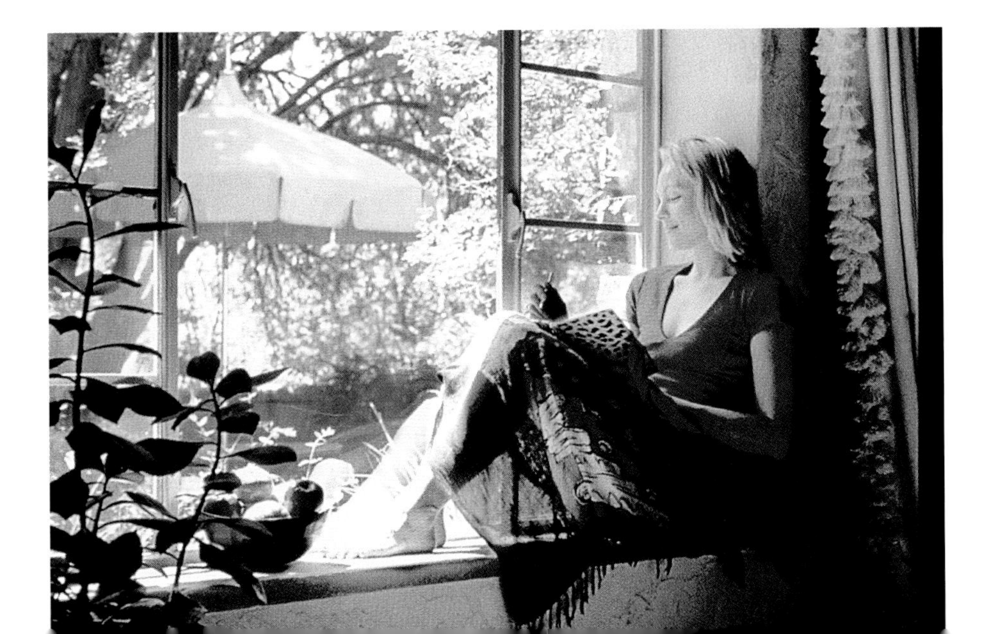

of purpose every day; his life had to be about more than showing up at various social events, sitting on boards, and giving away money. He also learned to identify and acknowledge his thoughts and feelings.

He and Pat saw the therapist together about their desire to reconnect sexually. During the session they tried a partner breathing technique and discussed their hopes and dreams for the next stage of their relationship. They learned about the ancient approach to sexuality called tantra and agreed to read more about it and practice tantric techniques at home.

Gary had "homework" of his own. He agreed to attend Alcoholics Anonymous at home, after being introduced to it at a meeting at the ranch. And, in accordance with his plan, he interviewed four psychotherapists, selected one, and began regular weekly cognitive-behavioral therapy.

About seven months later, we received a call from a more animated and much happier Gary. Not only had he lost some weight and experienced a drop in his blood pressure, he'd attended several social events where he'd been able to abstain from alcohol. He was also pleased to report that since returning home, he and Pat practiced tantra every morning, on waking, "from fifteen minutes to a full hour! Sometimes we make love and sometimes we don't," he said, "but we both enjoy the time together. It's made us fall in love all over again."

Nice retirement, don't you agree? What appeared to be a simple case of too little to do and a bit too much drinking turned out to be a complex set of factors that created tension in both partners, a subsequent distance between them, and a growing sense of despair in two previously happy, stable people. With some self-disclosure leading to understanding and acceptance, and with determined work, Gary and Pat became closer than ever before.

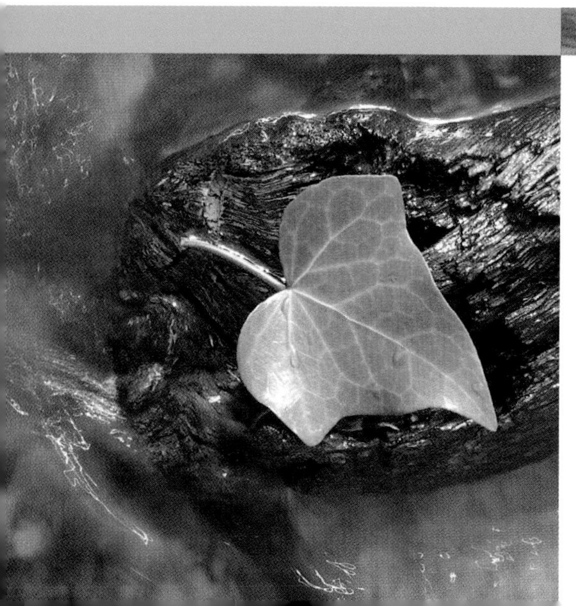

"SOME OF US HAVE been conditioned not to recognize fear. Here's a brief list of behavior that often overlays fear:

1. Blaming, attacking, being defensive
2. Chattering, staying busy, being restless
3. Boredom, anxiety, sleepiness
4. Picking at people, being critical
5. Making excuses
6. Engaging in addictive or compulsive behavior
7. Wearing a mask of any sort."

CHARLOTTE KASL

3. FACE YOUR FEAR

Many of our actions in intimate relationships are motivated by unacknowledged fear. It might be fear of our essential aloneness in the world, fear of uncovering childhood pain or secrets, fear of rejection or abandonment. It might be the fear of living with relentless physical pain. Fear can be very confusing: sometimes it looks like anger, sometimes like indifference. It can take the form of substance abuse, isolation, or even physical pain or disease.

Fear disorders, like depression, often respond quickly to treatment, but fear tends to immobilize us and perpetuates itself by keeping us from looking inside. But unless we do precisely that, we stay stuck.

It's easier to accept an unsatisfying or even disastrous relationship and a wasted, dreary life than to do the conscious, determined, and often difficult work that change requires. It's easier to numb ourselves with food or alcohol or overwork than to feel our hurts and heal them. It's easier to be a sketch of a person than to be a whole human being—but it's only when we take the trouble and make the effort that we are able to love with all our hearts.

LIZ AND MIKE

"Jumping out of my skin . . ."

At only twenty-nine, Liz had suffered for years from multiple chemical sensitivities, irritable bowel syndrome, chronic aches and pains, and a constant, overwhelming sense of dread. She'd been in a bad car accident ten years before that had terrified her, but after seeing a counselor had found some relief. Therapy had helped enough so that she was able to finish college and establish a relationship with Mike. They had been married for four years when Liz developed the nearly paralyzing fear that brought her to the ranch, seeking help.

Her goals were to learn to be less anxious and to find ways to reduce the physical pain that was her daily companion. She recalled that while she'd felt somewhat better early in her relationship with Mike, lately she was growing increasingly fearful and found herself avoiding people, including Mike. Her pain, both physical and emotional, worsened whenever the couple discussed what Liz wanted more than anything in the world—a baby. She found herself pulling away from the husband whom she dearly loved, and whom she later described as "the only person who really knows me and loves me for who I am."

Just after she arrived at the ranch, Liz became so anxious that she started to pack and leave. Luckily, a nurse noticed her, teary-eyed and tense, and suggested that they speak for a few minutes. This brief, informal meeting led to a series of events that ultimately transformed Liz's life.

The program set up for her included a comprehensive nutritional-medical approach, movement therapy, dance classes, yoga, and behavioral sessions. Within days of beginning her new ways of eating, moving, breathing, and thinking, Liz looked more relaxed, and, by the end of her first eight-day stay, even happy. She accepted a referral to a psychiatrist near her home who was willing to support her efforts to help herself using this approach—she was firmly opposed to taking medication for her anxiety. She stayed in monthly phone contact with the staff members at the ranch who'd helped her.

Six months later, Liz returned to the ranch looking better and reporting, "For the first time since I was two years old, I've been able to eat without pain." She said that she loved her husband more than ever and that she'd taken training to work in the hospice movement and was now doing work she believed in.

A year later, Liz sent a card to her "team" at the ranch announcing the birth of a healthy, seven-pound baby girl.

V. Develop your interpersonal skills.

Even a perfectly balanced, totally rational, and loving person—assuming such an individual exists—would have trouble maintaining a personal relationship without a working set of interpersonal skills. We all need not just love but the toolbox of human intimacy that helps us express love and attract the love of others.

"Small pleasures, whether they're sensual or mental . . . can absorb some of the shocks and difficulties of life and contribute to ongoing happiness. Make sure you have enough of the small, daily things of life, and attend to pleasures of smells, tastes, and sounds, rewarding relationships, and meaningful work."

ROBERT ORNSTEIN AND DAVID SOBEL

1. Learn and practice conflict resolution. Think about this as respectful disagreement. Avoid hurting the other person just to make a point, just to be right. Remember: the only subject about which two people can talk without any possibility of disagreement is arithmetic. (Maybe.) Literally everything else two people might discuss can be complicated by stress level, mood, opinion, perception, and the recapitulation ("triggering") of buried hurts. Recognize that you can disagree without going to war, and without losing mutual respect.

2. Ask for time when you want to discuss something, and be brief. Plan simply to begin a discussion: resolution doesn't have to happen the first time you bring a subject up. By being succinct you demonstrate respect for the other person's priorities, which are probably different from yours.

3. Play together. Some research shows that to maintain a healthy balance in a love relationship, we need to have five positive experiences for every negative one.

4. Apologize whenever you have been unkind. This does not mean that you have to change your opinion or betray your real feelings. It does mean that you recognize and take responsibility for your failures to be considerate in your choice of words, tone of voice, and body language. Avoid shaming people you love, especially in front of others. Apologizing out of the blue can help reconnect you with your beloved: surprise apologize.

5. Stretch yourself emotionally. Love must be demonstrated, spoken, and acted if you want to connect with another person. If, for example, you partner wants to hear, "I love you," and you have a hard time saying it, try, even if it feels awkward at first. All skills must be practiced before we're good at them. Over time, your loving efforts will feel more familiar and natural, and you'll see those efforts returned.

6. Take disappointment like a grown-up. You will not have all your wants and needs met by another person—and you're guaranteed disappointment if that's what you expect from love. On the other hand, if a relationship is constantly disappointing and you never feel gratified, you may want to consider a healthy separation.

7. Express appreciation. Don't just think nice things about the people you love, say them. Don't just plan to do sweet things for them, do them. Offer compliments and encouragement often, freely, and without ulterior motive. Behave as if you see the best in the people you love, all the time. Act as if your relationship, even in the most difficult moments, is a mirror that helps you stay conscious and loving—because it is. Behave as if you are capable of giving the deepest love possible, and as if you are capable of receiving it as well.

You just might get it.

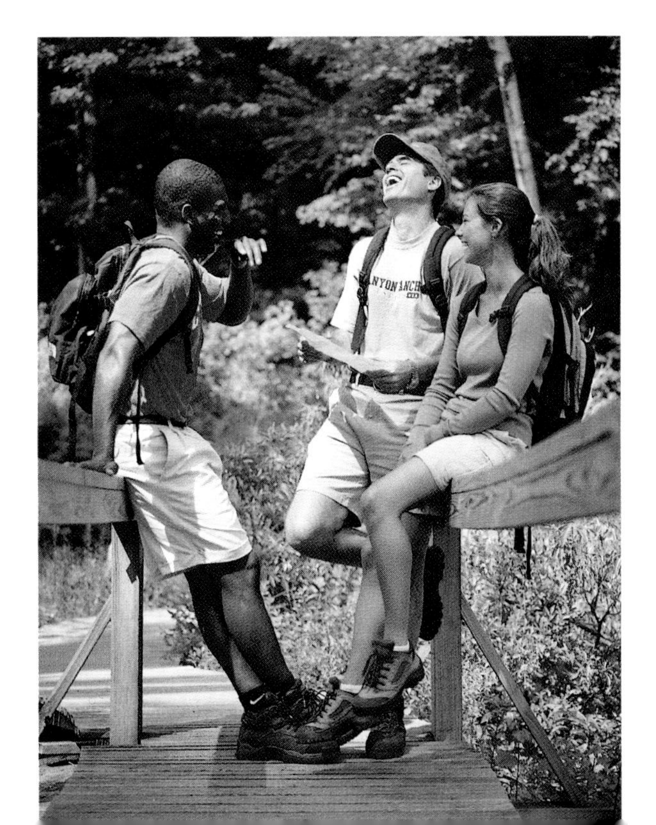

Sexual Intimacy

THE BASICS OF ACHIEVING and maintaining satisfying sexual intimacy are the same as those for achieving emotional intimacy—except more so.

Mechanical problems in sexual relationships are certainly real, but they're the easier ones to solve; there's a cure for just about every purely physical difficulty people have with sex. Some medications, including antidepressants, beta-blockers, and drugs that control high blood pressure, can cause sexual dysfunction in both men and women, but prescriptions can be adjusted, and other medications for the same conditions may have fewer side effects for some individuals. Lubricants, hormone replacement therapies, Viagra, and implants can help, and usually do. If you have any questions about your health with regard to sex—effects of medication, medical issues, possible hormonal changes—check with your doctor. Many people struggle needlessly with solvable performance problems just because they don't bring them up at the doctor's office.

There are also specific, effective, time-tested therapies for most types of dysfunction, not to mention an ancient spiritual system, tantra, that can help transform okay sex into great sex.

There's no implant or medication or exercise that will help with most of our sexual dissatisfactions, though, because they originate not in our genitals but in our heads and hearts. More and more couples are coming to sex therapists and counselors not because they can't have sex, but because they don't. Professionals are seeing more unhappily celibate couples today than ever before. These problems of desire often boil down to intimacy.

Sex is an incalculably powerful force. We think about it constantly, our culture tantalizes us with it incessantly, and yet we hardly ever discuss it. It's an absolutely vital part of who we are, but it only comes out at night. Sex is the secret everybody knows.

A DO-ANYWHERE SEX EXERCISE

TENSE THE MUSCLES that run from your pubic bone back toward your tailbone. If you have trouble locating them, pretend that you are urinating and suddenly have to stop the flow—those are the muscles you want. Tense, hold, and release ten or twenty times, as often as you think about it during the day. The exercise is invisible—if you keep a straight face—and improves both vaginal and urinary control for women and ejaculatory control for men. And it can also make a boring meeting a little more amusing.

More exercise for better sex: overall physical conditioning that includes toning and flexibility around the hips, knees, and pelvis. Yoga and dance classes are perfect.

Is it surprising, then, that we have trouble getting the sex we want? If we're embarassed to say, "I love you," how on earth are we going to get up the nerve to say, "What I'd really like for you to do is . . . ?"

The Golden Rule, do unto others, does *not* work with sex. If the woman in a heterosexual relationship, say, gently and softly strokes her partner, thinking that this will show him how *she* likes to be touched, he's unlikely to get the message and will start wondering when the heck he's going to get to feel something. Conversely, if he starts stimulating her in a way that would feel great to him, she's likely to jump shrieking out the window.

Bottom line: you've got to talk.

Sex with a near stranger is perfectly possible—the excitement of the unknown is an amazing turn-on. But unless you happen to be one of the few individuals who's genuinely contented with a lifetime of brief encounters, you have to find a way to sustain and nurture sexual attraction and excitement in a long-term relationship. To do that, you need to watch for and clear away the life debris that short-circuits desire.

CLEARING THE WAY FOR BETTER SEX

1. Manage stress.

Chronic stress not only distracts us from sex, it derails desire on a biochemical level, before it ever has a chance to develop. The last thing a zebra galloping full tilt from a lion thinks about is mating: he's too busy staying alive.

Stress in humans is the same mammalian fight-or-flight response, but intensified and soured by lack of appropriate physical outlet. When we live in such a way that stress hormones keep circulating through our bodies, *we* aren't able to think much about mating, either.

The pace of contemporary life makes it hard to slow down and relax enough to feel desire. Many of us, in our genuine need to unwind at the end of the day, turn down the noise in our heads and in our blood with numbing, self-calming habits, including excessive use of alcohol and other drugs, mindless TV viewing, computer use, and talking on the phone. None of these ways of calming ourselves is likely to bring us closer to the people we love, and some, such as excessive drinking, actively impair sexual performance and enjoyment.

DAILY DE-STRESSING FOR BETTER SEX

Remember all the great sex you've had on vacation? Sadly, we don't get to spend our whole lives at the beach, but we can try to make the end of every day a conscious escape from the workaday world. Set up a buffer between your personal life and the world outside.

- If you work at home, limit the space it takes up in your house. Shut the door to your home office, or put it all away when work time is over.

- Make a physical space for sex. We make room for every other important activity—cooking, eating, sleeping, hanging out—why should sex be the only big part of life that doesn't have its own dedicated space?

- Whether or not one of you stays home with the kids, establish a routine that allows time both for the family and for you as a couple most evenings. Remember that while your children need your attention, they need your relationship to be strong even more: their parents' bond is the rock on which their world rests. Restructure your lives if you have to—one extracurricular activity per kid, maximum, is a good rule for both parents and children. Overscheduling is one of the big pitfalls of modern life.

- If one or both of you needs time alone, take it. Go for a walk, read for a while, meditate. When you've attended to your need for solitude, you'll be better company. Be sure that your partner knows that this isn't rejection or withdrawal, but a mental-health time-out—and that you'll be back. Conversely, accept your partner's need for downtime as nothing personal.

- Talk over your day. Sharing the big and little things, the sad and funny details, the frustrations and triumphs of your separate lives keeps you close. Tell your loved one about your thoughts and feelings when you were apart. Besides making you feel more in the loop, it also helps both of you not take each other's moods to heart.

A WOMAN, MARRIED for many years, joined a better-sex workshop and in the course of conversation revealed that her husband had had an affair. When asked how she found out, she explained that she had intercepted a letter from her husband to the other woman. When she'd confronted him with the evidence, he'd ended the affair.

Then she pulled the letter out of her purse and showed it to everyone. When asked why she'd brought it with her, she explained that she took it with her wherever she went, so that if he ever tried to look for it and destroy it, he wouldn't be able to find it, and she'd have the upper hand if she decided to divorce him.

By coming to a workshop on sex, this woman was trying to put a Band-Aid on a marriage that was bleeding to death.

If there's been an affair, you and your partner almost certainly need help from an objective third

2. Get some sleep

A tired bedfellow is not a lively bedfellow. If your schedule is such that you typically do not have enough time for sleep, see if you can make changes. Researchers are increasingly convinced that most of us need eight hours a night for health and longevity. If you have insomnia or often wake at night, see Chapter 1 for help.

This is important. Not only are passion and sleepiness incompatible, you risk your overall well-being when you habitually don't get enough rest.

3. Resolve your anger

Unresolved anger is the highest, widest, and most substantial roadblock to sexual joy in most long-term relationships. When an experienced therapist hears someone—usually a wife—say, "I honestly don't care if we never do it again," the therapist's first question is, "What exactly are you angry about?"

The answer, as you might guess, is almost invariably a furious, "Angry? I'm not angry!"

The grudges you hold stand solidly between you and your loved one: it's hard to make a soft bed on rocky ground. It's also impossible to make love with someone you hate, whether you *know* you hate that person or not.

Anger feels like a dangerous emotion; deep inside all of us dwells the toddler who believes his rage can destroy the world. Since global annihilation would be the obvious outcome of expressing our rage, we suppress it. The worst thing about this strategy is that when you put a lid on one emotion, you put a lid on all of them.

And when you take the lid off, in therapy or in an honest conversation, it's the anger that inevitably pours out first. The sudden release of pent-up rage can be very

party. The German word for adultery is *Ehebruch*, "marriage-break," which neatly sums up the destruction adultery can wreak, even for couples who vigorously pretend it doesn't matter. Getting past that kind of hurt is very hard, and nearly always requires professional help.

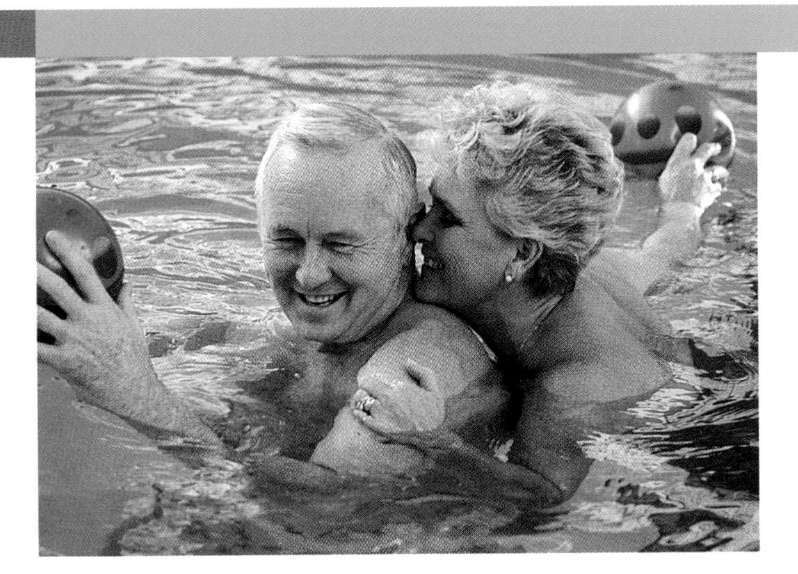

upsetting to both parties concerned. After it's come out, though, all the other feelings that have been bottled up can begin to flow: tenderness, affection, love, sexual passion.

Holding on to our wrongs like treasures, taking them out every so often and polishing them, is bitterly satisfying and certainly makes us feel superior to those we love. Enjoy those feelings, because if that's the situation you're in, you're not going to feel much else.

FOUR STEPS TO LAYING ANGER TO REST

For garden-variety marital grudges, anger resolution can work—if you, as the self-declared injured party, undertake it in good faith. Say there's an issue, an old hurt, that comes up every time you argue, or that you often find yourself stewing about. Give that gruesome, zombielike grudge a decent burial:

1. Bring the issue up once more, with the understanding that this is the very last time you'll hash it through. Promise your partner that if he says he's sorry one more time, you'll never bring it up again.
2. Listen to the apology.
3. Confirm that it's officially over and done with. Ideally, at this point you go to bed together to celebrate and reconnect.
4. Now you must do your part. When you find your thoughts running in their old pattern, rehearsing the eternal wrong done you, deliberately turn your mind away and think about something else. Remember: you're letting it go not because you're a saint, but because you're done brooding, and that's good for your marriage, good for you—and great for your sex life.

A SPECIAL NOTE FOR WOMEN

THE EMOTIONAL part of intimacy tends, in general, to be harder for men; the lust part tends to be harder for women. There are good reasons for women's inhibitions.

Girls are just as interested in sex as boys, but the message that their sexuality is a bad, dangerous, embarrassing thing starts very early, loud and strong. Mommy jokes in front of her four-year-old daughter that she's not going to be allowed to date until she's thirty-five; Daddy gets upset when she runs around the house without clothes on but just laughs when her brother does the same thing.

At puberty, the warnings become more anxious and come from all directions: if you have sex you'll get pregnant, you'll get a disease, you'll disgrace your family, you'll get a reputation, your life will be ruined, you'll be dirty. And you cannot trust boys or men: they're all just after one thing.

And then—poof!—all that conditioning is supposed to drop away when a woman walks down

EXPLORING SEX

Managing stress and exhaustion and releasing anger are the groundwork for exceptional sex. The next lesson is for both partners to learn to more easily unlock the cupboard in which they keep their sexuality locked all day.

If you want exceptional sex, you'll have to make an effort: no big change in life comes without conscious action. If your partner is reluctant or doubtful, forge ahead on your own—the warmth and eroticism in the air will be hard to resist. Here are just a few of the things you can do.

- Get new ideas about what is possible and what sounds worth trying from outside sources like books and videos.
- Become aware of the time you spend "in your head," and begin to decrease it in favor of time spent just noticing the sensations you are having at a given moment.
- Play Sense of the Day. Put the name of a sense—touch, smell, hearing—on your refrigerator door or bathroom mirror to remind you to attend to the world using that sense throughout the day.
- Make a conscious decision to give up your anger about one thing.
- Practice building sexual charge between you and your partner outside the bedroom—for example, kissing while you watch a movie.
- Imagine that you can open and close your heart at will, and decide to spend the next two hours with an open heart. The habit of withholding warm feelings and generous impulses is often just that, a bad habit. Work on breaking it.

the aisle. Suddenly, sex is a wonderful expression of love. Oh, right.

At the same time, the word girls get from the media is that their sexual attractiveness is the most valuable thing about them, their big bargaining chip in the game of life. Few males in this culture fully understand how thoroughly this stream of urgent mixed messages complicates and confuses women's feelings about sex. All this stuff can get in the way, even in the most loving and passionate relationships.

Most women need time to let go of the dreck, to let down their mental barbed-wire fence, relax with the person they love and trust, and revel in the pleasures of the body. For most couples, most of the time, sex is better when both partners take time to slow down and consciously jettison the debris. Together, they can make a safe place to set aside the inhibitions acquired over a lifetime.

- Notice your tendency to need to be right, and practice consciously letting this go in favor of being close.
- Make love with the lights on and your eyes open. Take small steps at first if this is hard.
- Become aware of the curse of perfectionism and the habit of criticism, and do what you can to let go of them.
- Notice one beautiful thing each morning, noon, or night for a week, and share it with your partner.
- Create a beautiful space in which to make love.

BETTER SEX THROUGH TANTRA

Fine. But say you've been married for twenty years and sex has become just a pleasant part of daily life. The passion that was once there seems to have leaked away. How do you change the comfortable, if slightly boring, patterns the two of you have settled into?

Tantra, a branch of the classical practice of yoga, offers a step-by-step guide for doing just that. Practicing certain aspects of tantra—in its entirety, a sophisticated, detailed instruction manual for achieving transcendently great sex and spiritual enlightenment—can be a way for Western couples to create something big and grand and powerful between them.

Tantra, according to the sutras, is one path to enlightenment, the path to bliss that runs through sensuality and ritual. It's a highly stylized practice, beginning in closeness and mutual appreciation, in which the man and woman take on the roles of gods, eternal masculine and feminine entities. More properly, the lovers fully perceive and honor the sacred in each other as the male partner awakens the sacred sexual energy, *shakti*, that belongs to the female. The goal of tantra is to fully unite male and female, heaven and earth, mind, body, and spirit in a great flow of energy.

Tantra emphasizes control and slow, focused, disciplined stimulation, building to prolonged and transcendent climax. Tantra's insistence on the holiness of sex—the opposite of the deep-lying Western suspicion of everything sexual as dirty and furtive—can be both liberating and refreshing, and its disciplined ritual introduces a new dimension of anticipation and arousal to the bedroom, one that reminds some people of the intensity of their first sensual experiences and the almost unbearable, delirious eroticism of "making out."

The idea of sex as a spiritual duty strikes many people as odd, but there's deep wisdom to it, as the ancient yogis perceived. If busy, long-married people wait to have sex until they both happen to be overwhelmed by passion, well—we're back to the failure of desire and the proliferation of celibate marriages. The sacred energies lie dormant.

Loving, intimate sexual connection is an inexhaustible source of personal energy and happiness, and there's much to be said for approaching it, at least sometimes, like exercise: maybe you don't really feel like it right now, but you know it's good for you, and you know you'll feel wonderful afterward. Tantra offers a framework and instructions for developing that discipline about sexual connection.

You can begin by Soul Gazing, with a comfortable setting, a few quiet minutes, and your partner.

- Sit across from one another, clothed or unclothed, holding hands.
- Look into the eyes of your beloved.
- Maintain eye contact and breathe together.
- Let time pass. There is no hurry. There is nothing else to do but this. There is no goal.
- Visualize energy flowing between you with each breath.
- Keep your attention focused on the eyes of your lover. See and know your beloved.
- Attend to your heart, and let feelings and sensations rise from within your chest as you continue to look into your lover's eyes.
- If you wish, say what is in your heart.
- Finish with a kiss.

For more information, we recommend *How to Have Magnificent Sex: The 7 Dimensions of a Vital Sexual Connection* by Lana Holstein, M.D. (2001).

INTIMACY FOR LIFE

Like the old song says, you won't get the love you want by just wishin' and hopin'—you have to talk, and act. The self-revelation necessary for intimacy can be terrifying, but the rewards are immeasurably larger than the risk.

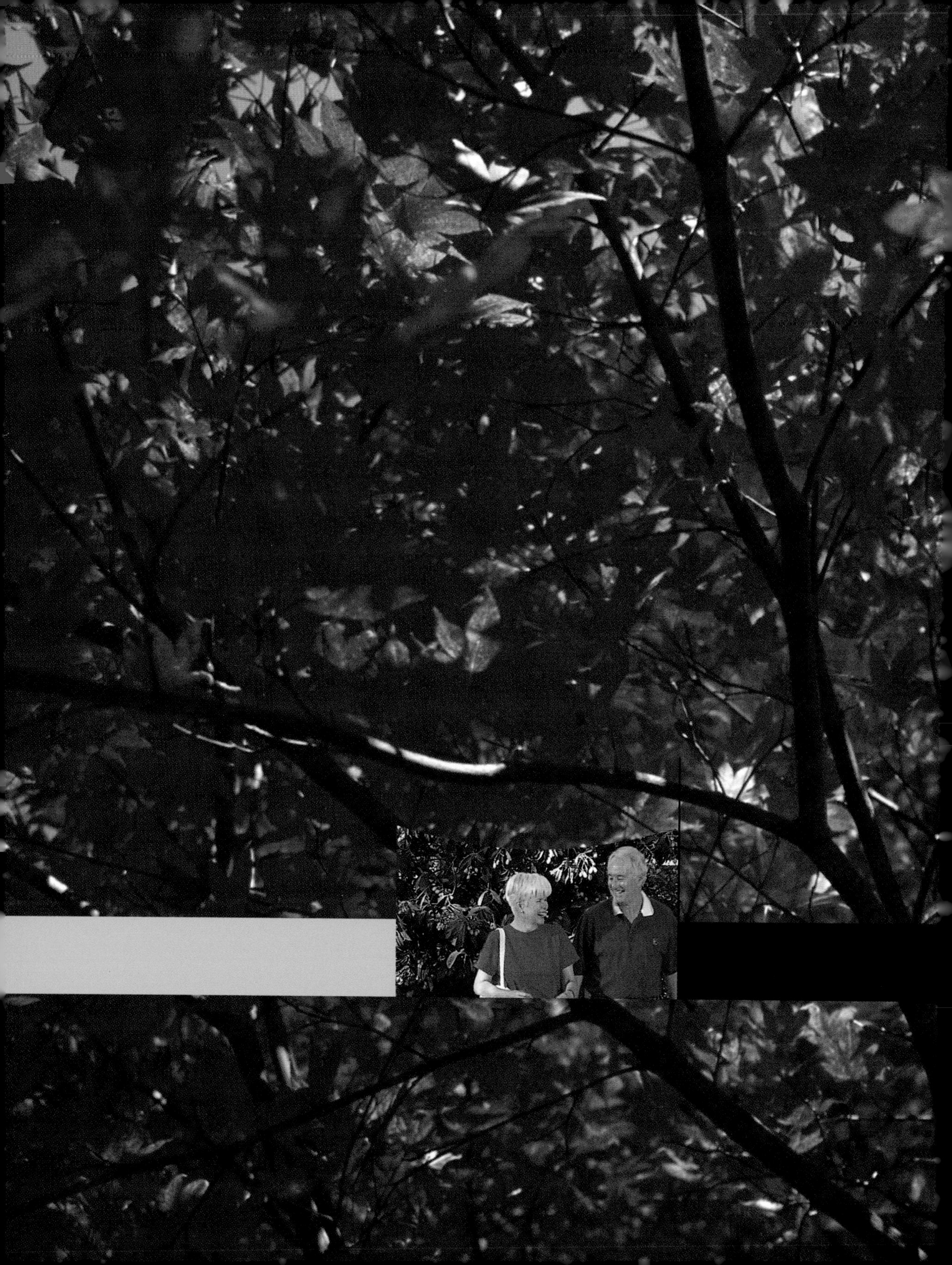

10 LIVING YOUNGER LONGER: *Optimal Aging and You*

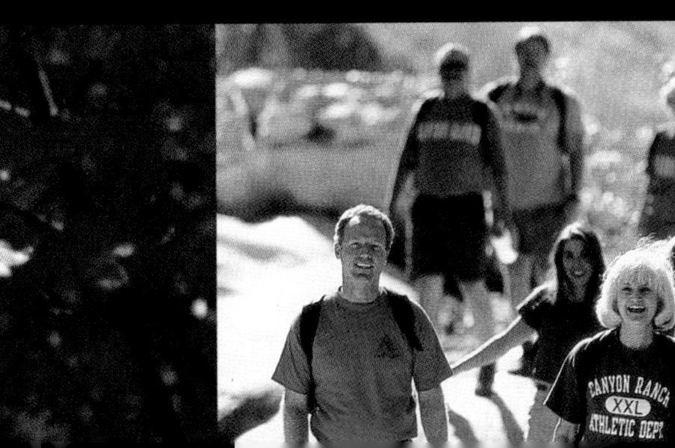

Optimal aging sums up everything Canyon Ranch is about. Optimal aging means more than living to a great age; it's about increasing our potential for living every day we're given, at every stage of life, with vigor, purpose, and joy. The goal is not necessarily to increase the absolute number of our days; the real promise of optimal aging is to increase the number and pleasure of our best days—the sum of days we spend feeling good and doing what we enjoy.

Turn that around, and what we're talking about is minimizing the percentage of our lives we spend ill or disabled—in medical terms, "compressing the period of morbidity." Most of us don't fear age itself; what frightens us about getting older is the pain, debility, and loss of independence that all too often come with advancing years. If you could feel as good at ninety as you did at forty, think how little the number of candles on your cake would mean. You, and only you, can order your life so that the years take the minimum possible toll.

"And may you stay forever young."

BOB DYLAN

There are no guarantees, of course, and physical immortality remains a dream. Very few human beings achieve 120 years, the theoretical upper limit for our species. The boundary of life is still fixed, and many factors that shorten lives remain beyond our control: accidents, environment, and genetic inheritance are facts, and some people with great lifestyles get sick for reasons no one understands. Nobody stays forever young.

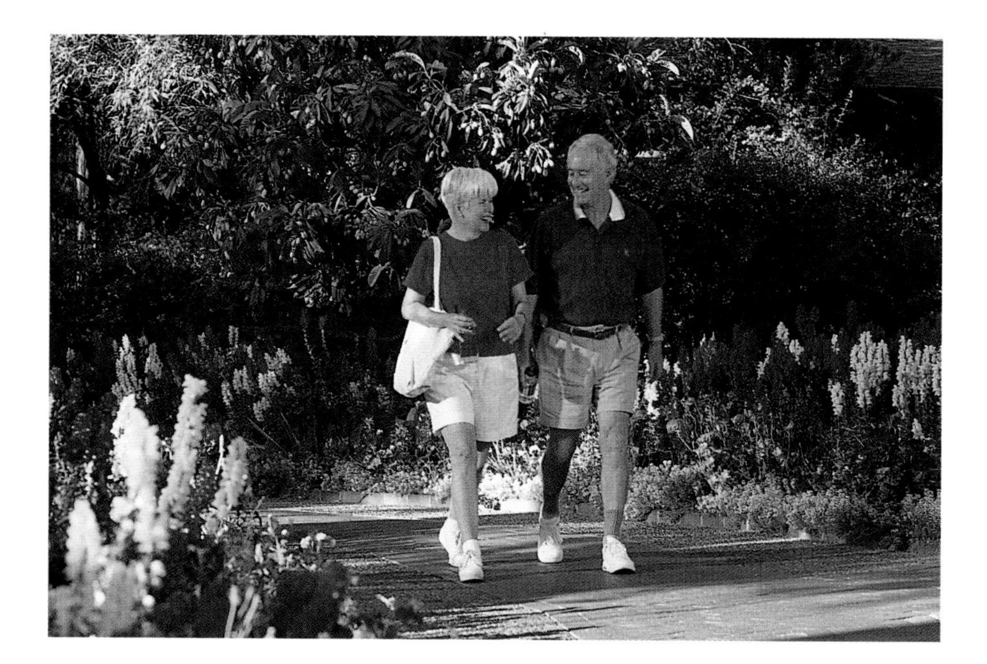

There's startling variation in the rate at which individuals age, however. Some people remain biologically young for decades longer than others, and the difference between a robust ninety-year-old and the person who begins shutting down before he's even eligible for senior discounts has obvious relevance for each of us.

Research on human aging has unleashed a flood of information about the impact of lifestyle on the rate of aging. More and more people are living, and living well, to one hundred and beyond. And as we have come to understand more about the healthy elderly, and about the microprocesses of aging itself, researchers have begun to view biological aging as a process of damage that erodes resilience and function—in short, as the loss of health.

We know that the way we live, day in and day out, influences our health profiles, and we have every reason to think that lifestyle is just as important in determining how healthy we'll be in years to come. This chapter is about choosing health, strength, and life, for your own sake. Bottom line: your best bet for living well and long is developing and maintaining healthy habits, starting now.

As the new science of aging keeps producing fascinating results, depressing "truths" about aging—the frail elderly cannot build muscle, for example—have turned out to be false. At the same time, some of the most unlikely sounding old wives' tales—eating fish is good for your brain, for instance—have proved to be right on the money. And the most extraordinary thing about the new microbiology is that scientists can tell us exactly *how* a diet rich in cold-water fish helps us stay healthy and smart.

Stay tuned for further developments in this fast-moving field of research: each new discovery has the potential to help every one of us extend our prime of life. In the meantime, read on to learn what you can start doing today to improve your chances of living to be very old chronologically, and as young as possible biologically.

Living Longer 101

RESEARCH INDICATES THAT OUR individual cells have a life expectancy of about 120 years. It's the rare individual who'll come close to that mark, although a handful of people have exceeded it. But while few of us will come close to the upper limit, we all maximize our chances for a good, long life when we follow the basic rules of health.

It's becoming clearer all the time that most of us are born with a good shot at a long life: only 20 to 30 percent of age-associated disease now appears to be genetically determined. In other words, the old joke about picking your parents carefully if you want to live to one hundred contains a grain of truth. If you have one or more close relatives who've lived past ninety, you do start off with an edge over someone whose family is not particularly long-lived. Nonetheless—except for people with certain untreatable inherited conditions—environment, lifestyle, personality, and individual health history are much stronger predictors of individual life span than genes.

Aging is inevitable, but it's a malleable process. Once we reach our physiological peak at around age thirty, nearly all functions slowly begin to deteriorate. Variation in the rate of change among individuals, however, is dramatic, and is largely a function of the way we live. The oxygen-carrying capacity of a couch potato's unfortunate heart and lungs, for example, declines by about 2 percent a year after age thirty, while the person who burns off 3,000 calories a week in aerobic exercise can expect to lose only one half of 1 percent a year of his heart-and-lung capacity—at least until age eighty or ninety. This single difference in lifestyle works out to a potential *fifty-year difference* in functional life expectancy. In fact, a completely sedentary lifestyle is such bad news for your health that it's now considered to be risk-taking behavior. Lying around doing nothing is twenty times more risky than commuting on a motorcycle.

Most of what you can do to improve your chances of living long and well is simple common sense:

- Practice safe sex.
- Don't use dangerous drugs.
- Fasten your safety belt.
- Be physically active on a daily basis.
- Eat sensibly, and drink lots of water.

THE BIGGEST HEALTH RISKS

NATURALLY, ANYONE who'd like to live to a ripe old age must first avoid falling victim to the most common causes of pain, disability, and death. Roughly speaking, about half of Americans die of heart disease or stroke, while the other half die of some form of cancer. (Of course there are many other causes of death, but those are the big two.)

Cancer is a world unto itself, a complex of many different diseases. You can substantially lower your risk for many of them by following the basic health rules—see below—but beyond that, it's complicated. (Harvard's School of Public Health has a Web site that can assess your personal risk for the most common cancers and guide you to lifestyle changes that can lower your risk for each: www.yourcancerrisk.com.)

Your cardiovascular system, on the other hand, is simple. Your heart is a pump and your blood vessels are hoses. If your heart stops beating, you die. Anything that adversely affects your heart is something you need to attend to.

- Take a multivitamin with minerals.
- Drink alcohol only in moderation.
- Don't smoke. Please don't smoke. If you do smoke, see your doctor about quitting. Effective help is available.
- Get plenty of sleep and fresh air.
- Floss your teeth.
- Avoid noxious chemicals.
- Keep your weight, blood sugar, and blood pressure under control.
- Have regular checkups and follow medical advice.
- Consult your doctor when anything seems to be amiss.
- Take time to relax and do things that make you happy.
- Care about others.
- Wear sunscreen.

Earlier chapters offered detailed help on the larger topics, like diet and exercise, but overall, this list is hardly rocket science. (That's coming up shortly.) You should take this unglamorous advice very seriously, however; every single "action point" above can prolong and improve your life.

But, please, don't go to bed early, eat your broccoli, or take up weight training because you're "supposed to," or because Canyon Ranch "says so"—that won't keep

- **Don't let stress wear the pump and hoses out any sooner than necessary. Learn stress-reduction techniques, use stress-avoidance strategies, and work on smoothing out your responses with meditation and, if necessary, counseling.**
- **Don't let the hoses get rough and inflamed. Eat a diet high in anti-inflammatory, heart-protective agents (omega-3 fatty acids), and take one aspirin a day if your doctor advises it.**
- **Keep all the parts in good working order with regular maintenance: cardiovascular exercise.**
- **Don't plaster cholesterol on roughened spots by consuming a diet high in saturated fats and trans-fats.**
- **Don't indulge in a high-carbohydrate diet full of simple sugars that will turn to hard fat around your waistline and raise your insulin levels.**
- **Do not smoke.**

you going for long. Instead, approach changes you make for good health as daily, conscious gifts to yourself and to the people who love you. Of course you want to live long and well—we all do. If you embrace healthy living with the clear intention of increasing the length and beauty of your life, it can be an easy and even joyful path.

Aging Under the Microscope

SO. HOW OLD COULD A FIT, well-nourished, well-rested, and exceptionally lucky person live to be? Based on both observation and the way our cells function and reproduce themselves, about 120 years. The question of the absolute upper limit on life leads down into the microscopic realm of the cell for a look at the very nuts and bolts of life. Significantly, what cellular biologists are learning about aging at the micro level doesn't so much change the old rules for health as it helps explain why they work. The new research is also adding a constantly more refined set of weapons to the antiaging arsenal. (For an overview of the latest on modifiable risk factors for premature aging, see Appendix A.)

Age tends to thicken, slow, and stiffen our bodies in ways we can see all too well. The ultimate cause of the changes we see and feel is, basically, a simultaneous thickening, slowing, and stiffening at the microscopic level. In the course of a lifetime, the fluid that fills cells gets thick, changing from clear broth into cloudy glue as waste from cellular processes and other molecular junk accumulates. Chemical signals vital for life travel sluggishly through this increasingly dense fluid. At the same time, the originally flexible, permeable walls of cells become rigid, creating a further hindrance to intercell communication. When the individual cells that make up

> "Flexibility is the discipline of life; rigidity is the discipline of death."
>
> LAO-TZU

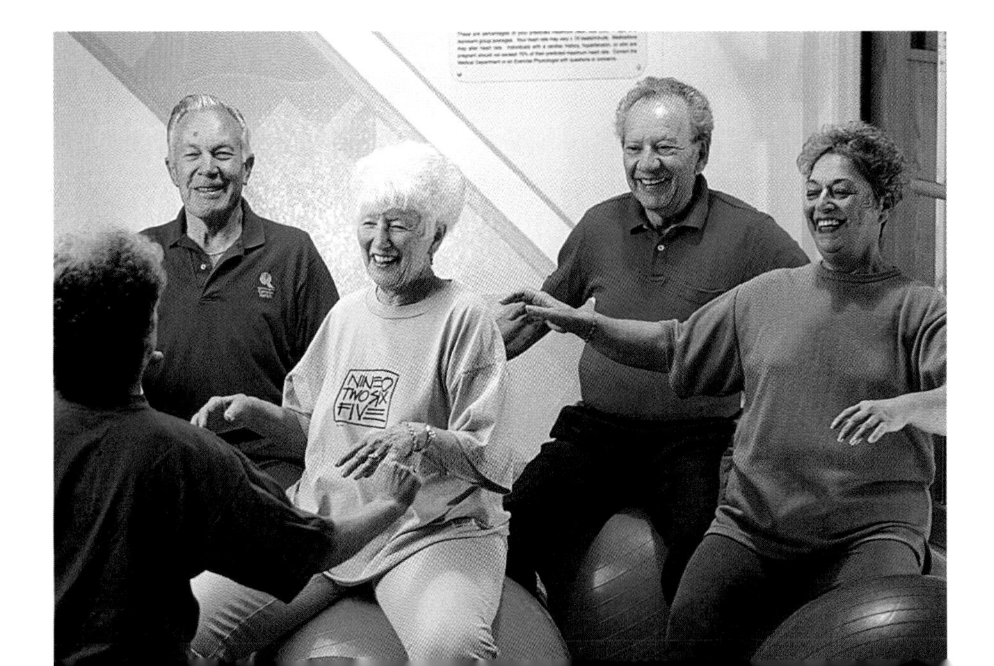

a system—such as the heart, liver, or brain—communicate badly with one another, the system as a whole doesn't work very well. The result of declining cell membrane permeability is gradual degeneration of all function and physiological processes—in short, aging.

The good news is that it appears the processes of aging can be slowed. Like the thickening of our waists and stiffening of our joints, loss of cell membrane permeability is caused by a combination of destructive factors over which we have con siderable control.

No matter how subtle the details, the basics remain the same: eat right. Exercise. Learn to relax and take time to enjoy living. Find out if you'd benefit from a modified diet and special supplementation. And don't let the polysyllables keep you from getting a good night's sleep.

Nutrition for Optimal Aging—The Latest Word

THERE IS SOME EVIDENCE from animal studies that a very low calorie, nutrient-rich diet can prolong the lives of individuals beyond the normal life span of the species. The animals studied have enjoyed good health, their only significant change, other than leanness, being a greatly reduced fertility rate. There's no evidence yet that calorie restriction—a reduction by one third to one half of normal calorie intake—prolongs life in human beings, although hundreds of people are reportedly trying it, hoping to live to be 150 or more. (Many report reduced libido and persistent chilliness, and all are very thin, but they report feeling healthy.) Unless calorie restriction is shown to prolong human life, the severity of the life change involved will probably not attract large numbers of people. It's an interesting theory, however, and the only age-reversal intervention proven effective in other mammals.

A more conservative approach to diet and longevity is to consider including these supplements and foods in a healthy diet:

- Vitamin C (250—500 mg) twice a day
- Vitamin E (400—800 IU of natural, mixed tocopherols) daily
- Folic acid (400 mcg), B_6 (100 mg), and B_{12} (100 IU) daily
- Natural selenium (from yeast, 200 mcg) daily
- Calcium (up to 1,500 mg daily, including dietary intake) with vitamin D (400 mg) and magnesium (400 mg)
- Dark chocolate (phytophenol antioxidants, 1.5 ounces) daily

- Red wine or grape juice (1 small glass) daily
- 3 servings of fish weekly. Coldwater fish such as salmon, tuna, and mackerel have the highest amount of omega-3 essential fatty acids. If you don't care for fish, take omega-3-rich fish oil capsules or flaxseed (1,000 mg) daily
- 10 servings of tomato paste or sauce weekly, preferably accompanied by monounsaturated fats such as olive oil to improve absorption of lycopene

Free Radicals vs. Antioxidants—and Why You Care Who Wins

YOU'VE UNDOUBTEDLY HEARD about free radicals, frightening-sounding entities running wild in your body. They're simply molecules that are highly reactive because they're short one electron. These compounds are constantly created throughout the body by metabolic reactions, particularly by reactions involving oxygen. To chemists, such reactions are "oxidizing reactions," thus the term *antioxidant*. The oxidizing reaction we know best is rusting, and a vivid mental picture of interior rust may help you resolve to pass up that burger for the fruit plate.

Because free radicals are so unstable, they tear other molecules apart, many of which become new, hungry free radicals scavenging for electrons in previously well-organized cells. Uncontrolled free-radical chain reactions muck up cell fluid, damage cell walls, and are implicated in degenerative diseases including arteriosclerosis, diabetes, and osteoarthritis. They may also exacerbate neurodegenerative diseases such as Parkinson's, dementia, and multiple sclerosis.

Healthy cells produce enzymes that, under normal conditions, neutralize free radicals before they do serious damage. However, the body's native antioxidant enzymes require certain trace minerals to work optimally. If you don't get enough zinc, iron, copper, manganese, or selenium, your body's native antioxidants can't perform their mission.

We also get antioxidant protection from foods; vitamins C and E, for example, are antioxidants. In the last few years, a score of other effective antioxidant compounds have been identified in fruits, vegetables, and nuts. These chemicals protect the plants in which they're found from damage from various causes, and they seem to perform similar functions in our bodies. A diet rich in the "new" antioxidants—phytochemicals including coenzyme Q10, beta-carotene, carnitine, lycopene, lipoic acid, and phenols—is healthy for everyone but is especially good for people with a heavy load of free radicals. Immune reactions, infections, injury, and detoxification processes in the liver and gut create floods of these bandit molecules. Other causes of oxidative stress include overeating, obesity, and excessive exercise.

You don't need to know which antioxidant is which, or where each one occurs. The vital point about phytochemicals is that they fight internal rust, and fruits, vegetables, nuts, and plant-based beverages are loaded with them. And they're so easy to locate: a rather delightful fact about antioxidants is that they're typically the very compounds that give fruits and vegetables their vivid colors. The chemicals that make grapes purple, blueberries blue, carrots orange, and tomatoes and peppers red brighten up the world, *and* keep us healthy.

In a late-breaking development, some plant-based products long assumed to be mostly bad for us, or at least not particularly good, have partially redeemed themselves in nutritionists' eyes by packing quantities of powerful phytochemicals. Coffee, tea, red wine, chocolate, and wholesomely brewed ales and stouts all contain useful plant compounds. For more specifics, see the section on phytochemical-rich foods and beverages in Chapter 7.

Antioxidants are great allies in the battle against disease and premature aging. That's why every time you turn around, the number of recommended daily servings of fruits and vegetables seems to go up. No study—*not a single one*—has ever indicated that eating lots of fruits and vegetables is anything but very good for human beings. Everything we learn about cell function underlines the importance of eating your vegetables—and your fruits, nuts, and chocolates, too.

Exercise for Optimal Aging

WHILE THE BENEFITS OF exercise are well known, few physicians make specific exercise recommendations, especially for older adults. This is unfortunate: exercise can be an effective complement or even alternative to purely "medical" treatment for many common conditions associated with advancing age, including osteoarthritis, osteoporosis, heart disease, and diabetes.

The human frame of bones, muscles, and connective tissue is a miracle of organic engineering, beautifully adapted to the needs of active, hungry hunter-gatherers. Unless you're one of the few people currently leading a fully Neolithic lifestyle, however, you'll need to make an effort to keep your bones, joints, and muscles healthy. Why? Because our way of life may have changed radically in the last 150 years, but our bodies' needs are the same as they were during the last ice age. We must have regular exercise, lots of sleep, and a moderate diet to be healthy in the long run, or even reasonably comfortable.

Without a strong frame, no house can stand, and without a strong, well-maintained musculoskeletal framework, the body collapses, everything hurts, and we have no health. This, sadly, is the inevitable result of a completely sedentary lifestyle, and it's the all-too-common experience of older people in our culture. The life of sitting, driving, and more sitting that modern technology makes so easy causes troubles that modern medicine cannot cure. Most exercise physiologists agree that sedentary people, as they approach medicare age, can expect to live with chronic aches and pains—simply from lack of exercise.

"Regular exercise" is probably not the miracle antidote to aging you were hoping for—there's no denying that swallowing pills is easier—but we cannot lie to you. Physical activity is so vital to your health and well-being that (as you may have noticed) we have returned to it throughout the book.

Level of physical activity and length of sleep are the strongest predictors of optimal aging. Other aspects of life, such as diet, emotional resilience, spiritual well-being, connections to others, and genetics, can all have a significant impact on longevity and life satisfaction. The scientific evidence is clearer every day, though, that getting regular exercise is the most important positive step you can take to slow and even reverse the effects of time, and to make the time you have worthwhile. In the uncompromising words of the MacArthur Foundation report on fitness and aging, "Exercise can literally mean the difference between life and premature death; between living at home or in a nursing home; between enjoying life or merely enduring it."

Every one of the top ten biomarkers of age, as identified by William Evans and Irwin Rosenberg in *Biomarkers: The 10 Keys to Prolonging Vitality,* is related to an individual's proportion of lean to total body mass. Lean muscle mass, in turn, is largely determined by how much you move your body. If you want to burn calories more efficiently, sleep more soundly, regulate blood sugar more effectively, tolerate extremes in temperature more easily—be physically active. If you want to look younger, be physically active. If you want to *feel* younger, be physically active. If you want to increase your chances of spending your last years in your own home rather than in a nursing home or hospital, *be physically active.*

(See "Exercise and Age" in Chapter 3 for guidelines for older people on starting to exercise.)

What's the best physical activity for longevity? That, at least, is uncomplicated: the best exercise is the one you like, because that's the one you'll stick with until you're doing it for at least thirty minutes every other day and then keep doing forever. (Or until you're bored with it, at which point, if you're committed, you'll find something else.)

It's true that various types of exercise have different advantages: weight-bearing activities like walking promote more bone-mineral deposition than, say, swimming. On the other hand, a person with joint problems may be more comfortable in a pool than on a treadmill, but not if she really hates water. The point is that the benefits of one form of exercise versus another are minor compared with the good things that flow from moving your body regularly, in any way you choose. Exercise alone or with a friend or in a group, indoors or out, morning or afternoon, mindfully or while listening to books on tape—it's your call.

And if you don't know what you like, try various things to see what suits you. Cross-training—doing one exercise for ten minutes, something else for five minutes, a third exercise for ten minutes, and so forth—has particular advantages for older people because it minimizes both overuse injuries and boredom. If you have access to a gym with cardio machines, try going from the stairclimber to the treadmill to the cross-country skiing machine—just as you please. Try a few of the Cybex or Nautilus machines. Balance on a big ball. Stretch. You'll get a good workout and, just as important, you'll be practicing neotony (medicalese for "acting like a kid") at the same time. Behaving as if we were young helps keep us young.

And that leads us to the last factor for optimal aging: how you think, feel, and respond to others—your mental, emotional, and spiritual health.

Only as Old as You Think You Are

CELL MEMBRANE PERMEABILITY, level of physical activity, and length of sleep per night are powerful predictors of longevity. Personality traits like optimism, sense of humor and purpose, curiosity, belief in a higher being, close emotional ties, childlike playfulness, serene acceptance of the fact of death, and a large web of social contacts are equally powerful determinants of happy and successful aging.

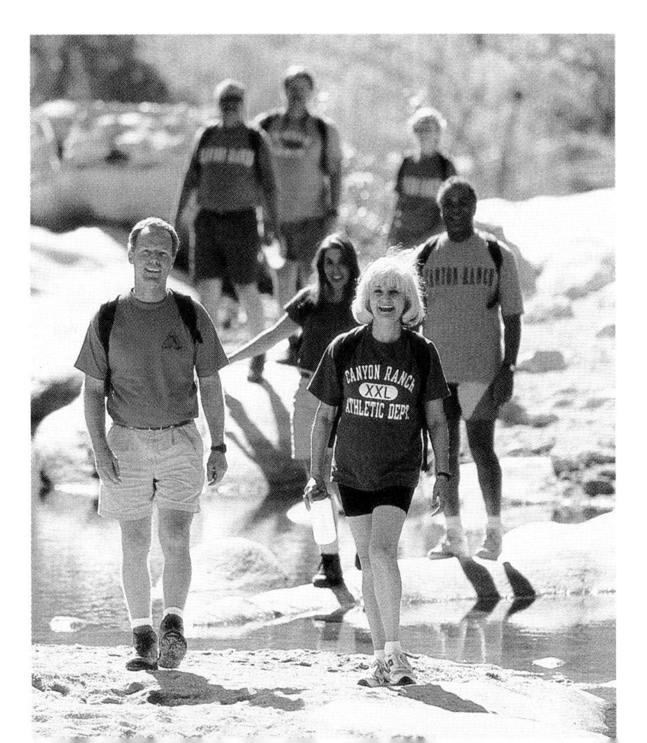

Consider these findings from various studies of personality and physical health:

- In a study of the Type A personality, people who persistently used "me" words had twice the incidence of heart disease of more altruistic participants.
- Five times as many depressed heart attack survivors died within a year as did survivors who were in good spirits.
- Two to three times as many socially isolated heart attack survivors died within a year as did survivors who had many contacts with family and friends.
- Smokers who regularly attended church (or temple or mosque) had lower mortality than smokers who didn't, and churchgoers in general had lower levels of stress hormones than people who never went.
- Of 118 law school students tested, 20 percent of those with the highest levels of hostility were dead twenty-five years later; only 4 percent of those judged to be "least angry" had died during the same period.

"A healthy mind in a healthy body" isn't just something they chisel over gym doors at fancy schools; it's a practical rule. People who live to be very old share a number of characteristics, all which can be summed up in one seemingly banal word: *resilience*. The way they live offers a window not only into longevity but into the nature of human happiness itself.

Centenarians are the fastest increasing segment of the population in the developed world, and they're rapidly becoming the most studied. Characteristically, these adventurers in time rarely smoke and tend to be lean, although few follow a low-fat diet. More than half drink alcohol moderately. They have low blood pressure and

TOP SECRETS

THE TOP "SECRETS" of people who live to be one hundred or more:

- Work hard throughout your life, and never functionally retire
- Exercise for fun and pleasure—keep "playing"
- Make and maintain social connections
- Be a contributing member of one or more close-knit social systems
- Stay curious, explore, learn—and keep laughing
- Follow a disciplined, regular daily schedule; live efficiently
- Cherish and preserve your independence
- Eat and drink in moderation
- Lighten your emotional load
- Accept what can't be changed
- Find meaning and purpose in living
- Believe in something bigger and better than yourself
- Stay in contact with the young and share your wisdom

excellent posture and are much healthier, on average, than most seventy-five-year-olds. Centenarians are mostly female, and nearly all of them worked hard long past age sixty-five.

In general, centenarians are also:

- Interested in everything, obsessed with nothing
- Inquisitive and willing to try new things
- Cheerful, calm, and unselfconscious
- Realistic, and unafraid of death
- Busy, creative, and autonomous
- Ready to make new friends

All the research into the genes, traits, and habits of centenarians suggests that liveliness of mind and generosity of spirit are as important as any physical factor for living long and well.

Live Well, Live Long

VOLTAIRE, THE FRENCH writer and philosopher, observed that if we lived every day as if it were our last, we'd behave exactly as if we knew we'd live forever. In either case, we'd live with care, cherishing the people we love and consciously choosing the things that give us the most joy and satisfaction. Voltaire, by the way, lived to a vigorous eighty-three in a time of appalling medical practice, deplorable sanitation, and raging epidemics, and he kept on planting young fruit trees at his country house until he died. Our best chance of living long is living well today. Choose life—you'll never be sorry you did.

Epilogue

IN THIS BOOK, we've tried to reproduce, as far as possible, what it's like to be at Canyon Ranch. Of course we can't give you the beautiful settings, the actual taste of the delicious meals, the feel of a massage, the cheering sight of endless heaps of white towels in the locker rooms, or the expert, one-on-one attention of our staff.

What we have given you is access to the deep wellness resources of one of the world's foremost centers for the promotion of health. Canyon Ranch is, among other things, a vast and growing library of health knowledge. There's help and information here for everyone, from the thirty-year-old amateur athlete to the eighty-year-old postbypass patient with crunchy knees. The danger in this all-inclusiveness for you, as for our guests, is overload: the stacks in this library are just about endless, and it's possible to get lost in them.

We always worry about the wildly ambitious guest who leaves the ranch with five different forty-minute exercise routines—one for stretching, one for weights, one for cardiovascular conditioning, and so on—and recommendations to do them all every day. There's nothing more discouraging than the idea that you have to give up everything else in life to be healthier.

You don't, honestly. You shouldn't even try. Put the thought of "the perfect lifestyle" right out of your mind. The picture of healthy living as grim, boring self-denial—a gruesome round of unfamiliar vegetables, high-impact aerobics, and no fun ever—has probably done as much harm to the health of the American population as the french fry and the internal combustion engine.

All you have to do to improve your health and well-being is . . . something. Not everything. The direction in which you move is more important than the size of the step, and small improvements result, over time, in large benefits. Very moderate regular exercise, very moderate improvements in your diet, and very simple life-management rules and stress-reduction techniques can and will make you measurably stronger, healthier, and happier.

You can count on positive results if you begin to make small changes that you can comfortably live with, and keep at it.

We emphasize "small, gradual, doable, step-by-step" change because we know all too well that it's nearly impossible to maintain big, radical transformations: need we say more than "liquid protein diet"? Moderation and small steps work, because just continuing to move in a healthier direction, at your own pace and in your own way, is the best strategy known for long-term lifestyle improvement. (Occasional lapses are inevitable and meaningless; don't let them get you off track.) An apple a day, a brisk walk a day, and a good laugh a day will propel you toward a healthier, happier life. That's a promise.

We've poured all this information and advice into one book not because you should do it all this minute, but so you can readily find the information and inspiration for making that first small improvement in your way of life. And then, when you're ready, it will all be here waiting when you decide to take another small step, and all the steps after that.

Just in case we haven't given you enough ideas for healthy change, here are a few more, contrasted with the sort of dramatic, doomed actions belonging to the awful, drastic process unfortunately known as "getting healthy":

Healthy step	Self-punishing, unsustainable action
Buy 1 percent instead of 2 percent milk	Switch from whole to fat-free milk.
Walk ten minutes before breakfast and twenty minutes after dinner.	Start getting up at 4 a.m. to go jogging. Start with several miles. Ignore the pain.
Try an introductory yoga class at a nearby center. Go with a friend.	Having never done yoga, spend $300 on videotapes, outfits, and equipment.
Add a big green salad to lunch every day.	Go on the cabbage-soup diet for a month.
Practice balancing on one foot, then the other, whenever you stand in line.	Join a health club and lift weights for 90 minutes the first day.

Actions like those in the left column, while they may seem too small to count, are in fact effective over time—just because they *are* small, and very reasonable. Most people can stick with incremental changes, and build on them as time goes by.

Feel good about the small improvements you make; when you take any positive action for health, give yourself credit. Rejoice in every sign of progress. Don't concern yourself with what others do, or measure yourself against people thirty years younger with different body types, or beat yourself up when you slip a bit. Try various things. Don't worry. And have all the fun you can.

Lifestyle change is a project for the rest of your life, and, let us repeat, moving in the right direction is more important than the speed with which you travel. Changing your life in small, healthy ways pays off every day in substantial, pleasurable benefits like sound sleep, the ability to try new things, and the energy to keep up with a changing world.

Wonderful things can come of slightly better habits in the long run—and a good, long run is our fondest hope for ourselves, and for you.

Appendix A: An Overview of Biomarkers

HERE'S A QUICK SUMMARY of recently identified risk factors for less-than-optimal-aging, and the current thought on how best to minimize them. Much of what follows is quite new science, so don't be surprised if you find new things to worry about. The point, of course, is not to make you anxious—stress ages us faster than almost anything else—but to give you the knowledge you need about how you can help yourself.

DYSGLYCEMIA

What it is: A condition also called pre-diabetes or glucose intolerance, it often leads to insulin resistance. Associated with diets high in food that converts into simple sugar (high glycemic-index foods).

What it does: Accelerates various aging processes—connective tissue damage, autoimmune disease, and degeneration of tissues and organs. Accelerates diabetic complications. Strong correlation with increased risk of heart disease and high levels of inflammation-promoting compounds.

Diagnosis: Blood test, torso-centered obesity ("apple-shaped" obesity).

Treatment: A diet rich in foods with a lower glycemic index (see Chapter 6); small, frequent meals; regular physical activity; weight and stress reduction; chromium picolinate (200 mg twice a day); glucose-balancing herbs, including rosemary, fenugreek, and bitter melon.

CHRONIC INFLAMMATION

What it is: Widespread, low-level inflammation that increases the rigidity of cell walls, impairing communication between cells. Caused by individual susceptibility, and by a diet high in omega-6 essential fatty acids (polyunsaturated vegetable oil), low in omega-3 fatty acids (abundant in coldwater fish such as salmon and in flaxseed), and deficient in certain other nutrients, including vitamins B3, B6, and C, biotin, zinc, and magnesium.

What it does: Increases risk for a large number of chronic conditions, including cardiovascular disease, autoimmune diseases, arthritis, asthma, and inflammatory bowel disease. Inflammation can also affect coronary arteries, the brain, and the digestive system, leading to such degenerative conditions as heart disease, stroke, dementia, and ulcers.

Diagnosis: Personal and family health history.

Treatment: Improved diet high in omega-3 fatty acids (from coldwater fish, fish oil supplements, and flaxseed) and other crucial nutrients. Anti-inflammatory herbs include curcumin (turmeric and its relatives), ginger, and boswellia. Bioflavanoids plentiful in fruits and vegetables also help reduce inflammation.

ELEVATED HOMOCYSTEINE

While cardiovascular disease remains the number one cause of death among people over sixty-five, traditional risk factors—high blood pressure, high cholesterol, and smoking—account for only 50 to 60 percent of all such disease. This long-standing medical mystery may have been solved by recent findings that connect elevated levels of certain compounds in the blood with increased risk of heart disease. The most significant new risk factor is a high level of an amino acid called homocysteine.

What it is: The process by which molecules are transferred in chemical reactions within cells tends to become flawed with age, resulting in rising levels of harmful compounds such as lipoprotein and fibrinogen—risk factors for heart disease and other circulatory disorders. The compound most strongly predictive of cardiovascular and other serious disease is homocysteine.

What it does: Elevated homocysteine is a strong indicator of risk for many of the classic afflictions of advancing age, including heart attack, stroke, blood clots, peripheral artery disease, rheumatoid arthritis, and osteoporosis.

Diagnosis: Blood test.

Treatment: Vitamin B complex supplement containing folic acid, B6, and B12, which clear homocysteine from the blood. Note: excess homocysteine is such a striking risk factor, and prevention is so easy, that many doctors now recommend that everyone take a vitamin B complex supplement containing folic acid.

IMPAIRED DETOXIFICATION CAPACITY

What it is: Reduction in the efficiency of the liver, kidneys, and bowel—the organs responsible for clearing the body of toxins. Often caused by overexposure to toxins, including alcohol and trans-fatty acids (major sources of trans-fats include margarine, shortening, and the "partially hydrogenated" oils in fried foods and baked goods). Exposure to bacterial, fungal, and parasitic infections; chemical toxins in the environment; and compounds resulting from injury and inflammation can also result in impaired detoxification. Overexposure damages the liver and leads to gastrointestinal imbalances, "leaky gut" syndrome, and functional bowel disease.

What it does: Allows toxins to circulate through the body, causing widespread damage.

Diagnosis: Personal and family health history.

Treatment: Regenerative supplements such as l-glutamine, insulin, fiber, essential fatty acids, ginkgo biloba, glycerrhiza, folic acid, and phosphatidyl choline; reinoculation of the gut with beneficial bacteria (lactobacilli and bifidibacteria); elimination of ongoing infections and avoidance of toxic exposure; reduction of animal protein in the diet; replacement of digestive enzymes.

POOR IMMUNE FUNCTION

What it is: A decline in the efficiency of the immune system that may be due to one or more of the following: genetic predisposition, environmental influences, poor nutrition, physical inactivity, leaky gut syndrome, low levels of hydrochloric acid in the stomach, and/or maldigestion. Food allergies also weaken the immune system.

What it does: Increases risk of cancer and infections.

Diagnosis: Observation of low resistance to disease and infection.

Treatment: Elimination diet to identify and control food allergies; astralagus and spirulina supplements.

CHRONIC STRESS RESPONSE

What it is: Overactive fight-or-flight response resulting in sustained high levels of cortisol, glucose, and insulin.

What it does: Prolonged exposure to high cortisol levels is a risk factor for developing many serious conditions, including heart disease, depression, and Alzheimer's disease.

Diagnosis: Blood test.

Treatment: Meditation, yoga, and other stress-reduction strategies.

LOW HEART-RATE VARIABILITY

What it is: Lack of healthy variation in the heart rate, beat to beat. More common with advancing age and closely associated with chronic stress response.

What it does: The mechanism is not well understood, but flattening of the sine-wave pattern of healthy heart-rate variability is a strong predictor of sudden death after a first heart attack, of in-hospital mortality, and of sudden death in the general population.

Diagnosis: Computerized analysis of electrocardiogram strip and Holter monitor studies available at about a dozen sites in the United States (Canyon Ranch is one).

Treatment: Stress reduction, including meditation, yoga, and life change. Note: diagnosis is hard to come by, but exercise and stress reduction improve heart-rate variability for everyone, so you might as well get moving and get control of your stress as a preventive measure.

WHAT TESTS DO YOU NEED?
Tests recommended for all: fasting lipid profile and homocysteine. For people near, during, or after middle age who are symptomatic: estradiol and testosterone. Otherwise, customized testing based on personal and family medical history.

HORMONAL IMBALANCE

What it is: Changes in hormonal balance that come with menopause in women and andropause in men.

What it does: Decreased estrogen levels among men are associated with greater risk of osteoporosis and fractures. Men experience Type II osteoporosis, usually after age seventy, when their natural estrogen levels tend to decline markedly. The onset of andropausal symptoms in men begins as early as age thirty, however, and include fatigue, depression, irritability and anger, reduced libido, and impaired erectile function. Low testosterone has been associated with increased risk of coronary artery disease, low muscle mass, and weight gain. Deficiencies or imbalances of female hormones cause or contribute to decreased libido, depression, osteoporosis, fatigue, poor memory, loss of motivation, and appearance of fine wrinkles in the skin.

Diagnosis: Blood levels of hormones; DEXA bone density studies.

Treatment: Hormone replacement therapy, exercise, a diet rich in soy products and DHEA supplementation all have beneficial effects on hormone levels and help reduce secondary problems like osteoporosis.

Appendix B: An Introduction to Healing Herbs

As you look for ways to take the best possible care of yourself and those you love, you'll want to explore the world of botanical remedies. People have been using herbs for thousands of years, and their discoveries about how the body responds to various botanicals are easily accessible.

Humans use herbal remedies because they work. When modern chemists began to synthesize drugs, they often used herbs as a base: digitalis, aspirin, and quinine are just the most famous of the many medicines derived from or based on plant remedies.

In recent years, research has verified the effectiveness of many herbs. Chemical studies show, for instance, that feverfew does relieve migraines, garlic lowers blood pressure and cholesterol, and aloe helps skin heal.

Classic herbal remedies are inexpensive, easily obtainable, and safe when used correctly. This is not to say that herbal remedies are harmless if misused: nothing could be further from the truth. Remember: one of the elements of the periodic table itself is arsenic, a deadly poison. "Natural" does not mean "safe."

HERBAL GUIDELINES

- **It is of the utmost importance that you use herbs or extracts prepared by a reliable company**. The herb industry is essentially unregulated. While many reputable suppliers exist, others are sloppy or downright unscrupulous. A limited but valuable and rapidly expanding source of help is www.ConsumerLab.com, an independent laboratory that tests herbal products for potency and truth in labeling.
- Before you use an herb, do your homework. Consult a reputable guide for proper dosage and method of use.
- Don't take herbs casually or for no good reason. Pregnant women and children under two should use herbs only under medical supervision.
- Stop taking any herb that causes adverse side effects. Different people have different responses: it's up to you to monitor yours.
- Fresh, organic herbs are best if you use the whole plant. Concentrated extracts of medicinal plants prepared by reputable companies are also fine. Some common herbs, such as chamomile, are widely available from many good sources, but most dried, loose herbs are useless.

- Some useful herbs are toxic when taken internally. Before you swallow anything, know what you're taking and the correct dosage and use. Among the most common herbs that should never be taken internally are arnica, pennyroyal oil, comfrey, coltsfoot, foxglove, jimsonweed, ergot, belladonna (deadly nightshade), henbane, bittersweet, and poison hemlock.
- It's a big botanical world out there. Start learning about and using herbs on a small scale, with a basic herbal medicine chest.

COMMON HERBS AND THEIR USES

Aloe

Long recognized for its healing properties, the hardy, prolific aloe vera plant will grow on any sunny windowsill, ready to provide relief for injuries to the skin. Cut a large "leaf," trim off the spiny edges, then split it. The clear, nearly odorless gel inside soothes and speeds healing of cuts, scrapes, burns, sunburns, fungal infections, and other skin irritations. Bottled gel is available if you don't want to grow the plant: buy pure, unscented gel and keep it refrigerated.

Arnica

Rub tincture of arnica on bruises, sprains, and sore muscles and joints to reduce pain and swelling and encourage healing. Do not use on broken skin or take internally.

Chamomile

The applelike, mildly sedative aroma of chamomile tea has soothed many an upset stomach and relieves heartburn, indigestion, and colic. Chamomile is safe for small children: its airborne essential oil has even been used to calm fretful newborns. It can relax tense muscles and is often useful for menstrual cramps, jumpy nerves, and sleeplessness. Note: chamomile is a ragweed, and people who are allergic to ragweed may react to it.

Comfrey

This herb, which is used only externally, has a remarkable ability to heal even the ugliest wounds. Apply a poultice of dried comfrey root—prepared by grinding the root to a powder, mixing with water to make a paste, and packing directly onto the wound—once a day to bedsores, diabetic ulcers, staph infections, spider bites, and other wounds that refuse to heal.

Don (or dong) quai

This Chinese herb is the female counterpart to ginseng. It acts as a tonic for women and the female reproductive system, helping other "women's" herbs work better. Try using it in combination with specific remedies for PMS, menstrual cramps, menopausal symptoms, and weakness after childbirth.

Echinacea

The Plains Indians relied on this natural antibiotic and immunity enhancer. It's helpful as a first line of defense against colds, flu, sore throat, and episodes of lowered resistance. Try a dropperful of tincture or two capsules of freeze-dried extract four times a day for up to two weeks. Don't use echinacea habitually or it will lose its effectiveness.

Eleutherococcus (Siberian ginseng)

Unlike true ginseng, eleutherococcus is not a stimulant or sexual enhancer; it's a tonic that tones the whole system and helps the body cope with stress. Both men and women who suffer from chronic illness or fatigue, or who are generally run down, may find it helpful. Follow dosage instructions on the label—product strength varies.

Garlic

The old superstitions about garlic's efficacy against vampires and other evils certainly derive from its real power as a shield against infection. Garlic is a potent antiviral, antibacterial, and antifungal remedy, in addition to being a wonderful flavoring. Take several raw cloves daily to enhance the immune system. (If you can't swallow fresh, uncooked garlic, you can take the less potent dried form in capsules.) Eat several cloves of garlic at the onset of a cold, or take regularly as a preventive measure, especially if you are prone to infection. (Obviously, garlic is nontoxic.) A few drops of warm garlic oil in the ear canal during the early stages of an ear infection can clear it up. Garlic has recently been discovered to have even more virtues: research shows that it can lower blood pressure and blood cholesterol in some individuals and may block the action of certain chemical carcinogens.

Gentian

Europeans have long used "bitters" to aid digestion, poor appetite, and flatulence. Try a few drops of Angostura bitters—a tincture of gentian—before or after meals if you have poor digestion.

Ginkgo biloba

This most studied of all traditional remedies comes from the oldest living species of tree on earth and is usually taken in extract form for many of the ills of aging. Ginkgo has been shown to increase memory performance and learning capacity in older people and to reduce swelling in the brain and retinas. It acts as an antioxidant and blood thinner and improves circulation at the microscopic level. A standardized extract should be taken in two or three doses a day for both treatment and prevention of circulation problems. Higher doses may be useful for early-stage dementia, depression, and head trauma. Note: since ginkgo is a blood thinner, it can interfere with other anticoagulants and can cause headaches and gastrointestinal upset.

Ginseng

Ginseng has been a staple of Asian medicine for thousands of years. According to the Chinese view, it's a vitalizing and harmonizing agent that repairs the yang or male energy. It's not regarded as a cure, per se, but as a tonic that strengthens organs, glands and systems so they can better ward off disease. In traditional Chinese medicine, ginseng is used to relieve fatigue, impotence, and the general effects of aging. The Western perspective is that ginseng is a balanced stimulant: it stimulates both the adrenergic (adrenal) and cholinergic (calming) systems. Ginseng may be most directly helpful in reducing release of the "bad" stress hormone, cortisol. Regular use of ginseng may tone the adrenal glands, making them more efficient in turning adrenaline production on and off. Some studies have shown that ginseng also heightens cognitive function. People with high blood pressure or who are taking hypertensive medication should use caution and monitor their blood pressure closely when taking ginseng.

Goldenseal

Widely used by Native Americans, goldenseal is a good disinfectant that promotes scab formation and wound healing. One-half teaspoon powder made from goldenseal root and one-quarter teaspoon salt dissolved in a cup of warm water makes a useful gargle for sore throats, canker sores, tonsillitis, and infected gums. Omit the salt and use this mixture as an eyewash for eye infections or as a douche for vaginal irritations.

Milk thistle

This nontoxic extract of the seeds of the milk thistle plant is sometimes labeled "silybum" or "silymarin" and is widely available in health food stores. European research has shown that milk thistle extract helps liver cells regenerate and may protect the liver from damage by toxins.

Peppermint

Long familiar in the form of after-dinner mints, peppermint is a powerful aid to digestion. Drink peppermint tea for indigestion, nausea, and heartburn, or take enteric-coated capsules to soothe irritable bowel syndrome, diverticulitis, and other chronic intestinal ailments. Note: peppermint can cause gastric reflux and should not be given to infants or small children.

St. John's wort

This weedy flowering herb, often harvested in late June—near the date of the feast of St. John the Baptist—was introduced to North America by early European settlers, and it's now a common roadside and field weed in the eastern United States. A classic and highly valued remedy, this herb (or "wort") was once believed to have great power in driving out evil spirits that afflicted the mind. Over the centuries, our way of thinking about mental illness has changed, but the efficacy of St. John's wort has not. In recent years, it's once again become popular, as a less toxic alternative to drugs like Prozac for the treatment of mild to moderate depression. (It is not recommended for severe depression.) People with mood disorders should take the herb regularly for at least two months before deciding whether it's helpful. Note: animals who graze on St. John's wort sometimes develop photosensitivity. While this side effect has not been documented in humans, it's wise for people taking St. John's wort to protect themselves from the sun.

Saw palmetto

The scruffy, low-growing palm that produces saw palmetto berries used to be viewed as a pest plant throughout its native Florida; now stands of saw palmetto are valuable, and the berries are regularly poached by freelance harvesters. Research shows that extract of saw palmetto berries protects and shrinks the prostate gland, a trouble spot for most men as they grow older. Dried, ground berries and alcohol-based preparations are useless; look for standardized oil-based extract. Saw palmetto is nontoxic and can be taken indefinitely.

Slippery elm

You can usually find slippery elm lozenges on the shelves of your grocery or health food store. Their soothing quality, which can relieve both sore throats and irritated gastrointestinal tracts, stems from the herb's ability to restore the normal mucous coating on irritated tissue. Slippery elm poultices, made from the powdered bark mixed with water, can also be used on simple wounds, burns, boils, and inflamed tissue.

Tea tree oil

This Australian import with powerful disinfectant properties is a clear liquid that has a clean, antiseptic smell similiar to eucalyptus. Paint the oil on fungal infections of toenails and fingernails and on skin infected with athlete's foot, ringworm, or jock itch. Apply full strength to boils and other localized infections. Use a 10 percent solution to rinse infected wounds or to use as a douche for yeast and trichomonal infections.

Uva ursi

Called kinnikinnik by Native Americans, this herb is helpful with inflammations of the urinary tract, such as cystitis, and may reduce painful and heavy menstrual bleeding. It may also help dissolve kidney and bladder stones.

Valerian

This mildly sedative herb was widely used before the discovery of barbiturates. If you have trouble falling asleep, try a dropperful of valerian tincture at bedtime.

Contributors

CHAPTER 1

Philip S. Eichling, M.Th., M.D., M.P.H., developed the department of medical services at Canyon Ranch in Tucson and has been its director since 1991. His practice is centered on "lifestyle medicine," which encompasses all medical conditions that can be affected by lifestyle and behavior change; his particular interests are cardiovascular risk and sleep medicine. He holds a degree in theology from the University of Chicago, a medical degree from NYU, and a master of public health degree from Harvard. He is board-certified in both internal medicine and family practice. He is clinical associate professor of medicine at the University of Arizona College of Medicine, where he teaches preventive medicine to residents and medical students. Hundreds of CEOs and executives from around the world use him as their medical touchstone and come to Canyon Ranch for their annual exams.

Mark A. Hyman, M.D., is the codirector of medical services at Canyon Ranch in the Berkshires, where his practice combines the best of conventional and alternative medicine. He has practiced in rural Idaho as a family doctor, in Beijing, and in an inner-city emergency room. He lectures on natural approaches to common health problems, health promotion, optimal aging, and biochemical and nutritional approaches to disease prevention. He has been interviewed many times on radio and television. He participated in the White House commission on Complementary and Alternative Medicine, formed to make policy recommendations to the president and Congress. His book, *The Myths of Modern Medicine: Stop Falling for the Lies That Are Making You Sick and Start the Program That Will Make You Healthy*, will be published next year.

Mark Liponis, M.D., codirector of medical services at Canyon Ranch in the Berkshires, is certified in both internal and critical-care medicine and has been at Canyon Ranch since 1994. There he has pursued his interest in treating individuals rather than diseases through prevention, lifestyle change, and cutting-edge interventions. He is a regular contributor to *Men's Health* and *Prevention* magazines and appears on radio and TV. With Mark Hyman, M.D., he developed and maintains a health and wellness Web site, www.ultraprevention.com.

Robert Rhode, Ph.D., has been teaching and practicing clinical psychology since 1980. He is an award-winning faculty member of the departments of family and community medicine and psychiatry at the University of Arizona Health Sciences Center. For fifteen years he was part of a team that developed and delivered a substance-abuse prevention program for the U.S. Navy, and he has trained more than 1,000 medical professionals in habit change. An ardent biker and swimmer, he specializes in helping people do what they know they should but don't do regularly.

CHAPTER 2

Dan Baker, Ph.D., medical psychologist, has been the director of the Life Enhancement Center at Canyon Ranch in Tucson since its inception. The Life Enhancement Center offers an experiential, goal-oriented program that assists people in achieving healthy lifestyle changes. He also directs the Family Business Program. In his thirty-year career, he has assisted numerous people in finding fulfillment by teaching them to lead life from their strengths and to envision possibilities. He has held full-time appointments in psychiatry and pediatrics at the University of Arizona department of community and family medicine.

Jeffrey Rossman, Ph.D., has been director of behavioral health at Canyon Ranch in the Berkshires since 1993 and is also associate director of the ranch's Healthy Families in Business Program. His work with individuals, couples, families, and corporate groups focuses on helping them realize their potential for creativity and healthy functioning. He has been a facilitator in the Family Business Program at Harvard Business School and is an adjunct faculty member in psychology at the Union Institute, Antioch College, and Tufts University.

CHAPTER 3

Jane Roberts, M.S., is fitness director at Canyon Ranch in Tucson. She is certified through Cooper's Institute for Aerobics Research as a health promotion director, physical fitness specialist, and group exercise leader. She is also certified as a health and fitness instructor with the American College of Sports Medicine and as a personal trainer with the National Academy of Sports Medicine. She has seventeen years of experience in the fitness industry, including programming for corporate facilities, community health clubs, and spas.

CHAPTER 4

Robert Hughes, M.S., is an exercise physiologist at Canyon Ranch in Tucson. He holds a bachelor's degree in movement science and a master's degree in exercise physiology. He has worked in the health and fitness industry since 1978, studying many different exercise modalities, and lecturing internationally for organizations such as the American College of Sports Medicine and the Physical Education Association of Great Britain. He has published more than twenty articles.

CHAPTER 5

Rebecca Gorrell is a movement therapist at Canyon Ranch in Tucson, where she served as director of movement therapy from 1997 to 2000. Previously, she was fitness director at Canyon Ranch in the Berkshires from 1989 to 1995. A former modern dancer, she is certified by the American College of Sports Medicine. She is also a certified Pilates and N.I.A. instructor, and is pursuing a graduate degree at the University of Arizona, researching the role of movement therapy as a healing modality for cancer patients. She is also a contributing editor of *Shape* magazine and is the host of the *Spa Workout* video series. She has made many national and local television appearances and has been featured in national magazines. She contributed a body-shaping chapter to *The Female Body Owner's Manual*, published by Rodale Press.

Carol Marks graduated college with a degree in education. Several years later she began the study and practice of yoga, and in time took her skills as a teacher from the classroom to the yoga studio. She has been actively teaching for the past twenty years. She has studied and continues to study with some of country's most respected teachers, including Judith Lassiter, John Friend, John Schumacher, and Sandra Summerfield-Kozak. She has been spiritual coordinator at Canyon Ranch in Tucson since 1998. She teaches yoga to ranch guests as well as training her staff.

CHAPTER 6

Michael J. Hewitt, Ph.D., is director of health and healing at Canyon Ranch in Tucson; he was previously director of exercise physiology for eight years. He has worked with many hundreds of guests, in addition to conducting research and writing about metabolic and physiologic measurement techniques. He established body-composition test procedures for skinfold and DEXA methodologies for the ranch and introduced the cardiometabolic stress test there. Before coming to Canyon Ranch, he had diverse experience in education, health, and industry. He lectures, gives interviews, and educates the public about fitness and body composition topics and was a partner in developing Canyon Ranch Healthy Weight Philosophy. A devoted sailor, he is a division staff officer in the U.S. Coast Guard Auxiliary.

Kathleen Johnson, M.S., R.D., has been involved with Canyon Ranch since 1989 and served as program director of the nutrition department and as nutrition development coordinator. As such, she was instrumental in developing the Healthy Weight Philosophy and training staff ranch-wide about nutrition. She is also involved in educating physicians about nutrition at the University of Arizona.

MINDFUL EATING

Kathleen Johnson (see above) wrote this section.

CHAPTER 7

Jennifer Flora, M.S., is food development coordinator at Canyon Ranch in Tucson. For five years she has worked closely with the executive chef and kitchen staff to develop recipes that meet ranch nutritional guidelines. She has also worked as a nutrition and food-service educator in the Tucson area. She holds a master's degree in clinical nutrition and dietetics.

Kathleen Johnson (see above) contributed to this chapter.

Marilyn Majchrzak, M.S., R.D., corporate food development manager for Canyon Ranch, coordinates menu development for all Canyon Ranch properties. She has worked in the commercial food industry, served as a nutrition consultant and educator, and worked with food service employees and community agencies.

Lisa Powell, M.S., R.D., director of nutrition at Canyon Ranch in Tucson, has worked for the ranch for fourteen years. During that time, she also served as director of nutrition at Canyon Ranch in the Berkshires and opened the nutrition department at Canyon Ranch SpaClub in Las Vegas. She is Canyon Ranch's media spokesperson for nutrition. Formerly a research nutritionist for the University of Arizona, she has also worked as a nutrition consultant to private businesses and the food industry.

Kathie Swift, M.S., R.D., has been nutrition director at Canyon Ranch in the Berkshires since 1991. She has been recognized as one of the top ten nutritionists in the country and is credited with developing the cutting-edge Functional (Nutritional) Medicine Program for Canyon Ranch. She is a frequent presenter at symposiums for the spa and dietetic industries, has been featured on many television, radio, and web programs and in magazine articles.

CHAPTER 8

Diane Trieste, corporate spa treatment director of Canyon Ranch Health Resorts, has a business degree and has been involved in therapeutic bodywork and spa treatments for a decade. A licensed massage therapist certified in sports massage, she has worked on many professional athletes, including members of the 1992 U.S. Olympic Track and Field team and the 1996 U.S. Gymnastics team. She has consulted widely, designing facilities, developing treatments and products, training staff, and creating spa programs for massage schools. She also guest-teaches and lectures, and serves as chair of the Standards Review Committee of the Commission on Massage Therapy Accreditation.

HEALING TOUCH

Sue Kagel, R.N., B.S.N., has been a registered nurse since 1979, and was fully certified in holistic nursing in 1995 and in Healing Touch in 1997. She practices and teaches Healing Touch at Canyon Ranch in Tucson and trains and mentors Healing Touch students. She is active in raising public awareness about Healing Touch and often lectures and gives interviews about her specialty. Like many other nurses, she came to Healing Touch through her observation of the power of compassionate touch in traditional hospital settings.

CHAPTER 9

Marcia Bernstein, M.S.W., B.C.D., has been a member of the behavioral health staff at Canyon Ranch in the Berkshires for eight years. Since earning her master's degree in 1974, she has also worked in residential treatment centers for disturbed children, with homeless families and battered women, with chemically dependent people in both inpatient and outpatient settings, and in Manhattan Family Court. She has served as manager of a national employee assistance program, directed a partial hospital program for dually diagnosed adults, and was an adjunct assistant professor at Fordham University School of Social Service. She is also a certified hypnotherapist. She has a particular interest in working with people to counteract the psychological and emotional effects of living in a high-speed, low-touch, nonstop society.

Lana Holstein, M.D., a Yale-educated physician and well-known, widely quoted sex expert, is director of women's health at Canyon Ranch, where she has established innovative programs on menopause, osteoporosis, and midlife balance. She also developed and conducts workshops at Canyon Ranch for individuals and couples—

often with her physician husband, David—on sexuality, intimacy, and romance. Her work appears in magazines, syndicated newspaper columns, and scholarly publications, and she has been a guest on the *Today* show. She is the author of *How to Have Magnificent Sex*, published in January 2001.

CHAPTER 10

Evan W. Kligman, M.D., a board-certified family physician and geriatrician, practices longevity medicine in various settings; he has been practicing at Canyon Ranch in Tucson since 1998. He is clinical professor of public health and family and community medicine at the University of Arizona's Colleges of Public Health and Medicine, codirector of the Arizona Center on Aging, and medical director of the Center of Physical Activity and Nutrition. He designed and served as medical director of a longitudinal research study in healthy aging, Project Age Well, in the late 1980s. His private practice integrates primary care with nutritional counseling, Chinese medicine, psychotherapy, and spiritual direction. His Web site to assist people to live younger longer, www.liveyoungeronline.com, began in 1999.

APPENDIX A

Evan W. Kligman (see above) wrote this section.

APPENDIX B

Janelle White, M.D., who is board certified in internal medicine and geriatrics, began integrating complementary therapies with conventional treatment some years ago when she noticed her patients using herbs and other alternative treatments with benefit. She took a year off to study the use of herbs and has since expanded her practice at Canyon Ranch in Tucson to include functional medicine—combining nutrition, lifestyle change, and biochemical evaluation for patients. Her other interests include preventive medicine, memory fitness, and women's health, and she is active in advancing the use of complementary medicine in hospitals and hospices.

Index

A

B

F

I

M

N

O

S

T

Y

Z